Ertan Sarıdoğan, Gokhan Sami Kilic, Kubilay Ertan (Ed.)
Minimally Invasive Surgery in Gynecological Practice

Minimally Invasive Surgery in Gynecological Practice

Practical Examples in Gynecology

Ertan Sarıdoğan, Gokhan Sami Kilic,
Kubilay Ertan (Ed.)

DE GRUYTER

Editors

Assoc. Prof. Dr. Ertan Sarıdoğan
University College London Hospital
Elizabeth Garrett Anderson Wing
25 Grafton Way
London WC1E 6DB
UK

Prof. Dr. Gokhan Sami Kilic
University of Texas Medical Branch
Dept. of Obstetrics & Gynecology
301 University Boulevard
Galveston
TX 77555-0587
USA

Prof. Dr. Kubilay Ertan
Dep. of Obstetrics & Gynecology
Hospital of Leverkusen
51375 Leverkusen
Germany

ISBN 978-3-11-053073-5
e-ISBN (PDF) 978-3-11-053520-4
e-ISBN (EPUB) 978-3-11-053362-0

Library of Congress Control Number: 2019950551

Bibliographic information published by the Deutsche Nationalbibliothek
The Deutsche Nationalbibliothek lists this publication in the Deutsche Nationalbibliografie; detailed bibliographic data are available in the Internet at http://dnb.dnb.de.

© 2020 Walter de Gruyter GmbH, Berlin/Boston
Cover image: Courtesy of Alexander di Liberto
Typesetting: Compuscript Ltd., Shannon, Ireland
Printing and binding: CPI books GmbH, Leck

www.degruyter.com

Foreword

Change alone is eternal, perpetual, immortal.

Schopenhauer

I am pleased to have this opportunity to pen some words at the beginning of this interesting book "Minimally Invasive Surgery in Gynecological Practice." The book is comprehensive, well written and illustrated by internationally recognized authors in their field.

The book covers the field within 26 chapters starting from the basics- retroperitoneal anatomy, preoperative imaging, anesthesia, principles of electrosurgery, laparoscopic entry techniques, suturing, and adhesions- followed by chapters on procedures including hysterectomy, myomectomy, endometriosis, benign adnexal masses, tubal microsurgery, cesarean section scars, Müllerian anomalies, followed by three chapters on urogynecology; three chapters on cancer-cervical, endometrial and ovarian, one on Neuropelveology, a new expanding field, three chapters on hysteroscopy, two chapters on complications – laparoscopic and hysteroscopic-, and one on endometrial ablation.

Medicine is a permanently developing field that experienced a significant acceleration in the last five decades. In medicine, progress frequently follows scientific innovations and improvements in technology. That laparoscopy provided a surgical access became evident in the early seventies. The advantages of laparoscopic access as opposed to conventional laparotomy in performing a gynecologic procedure were already evident more than 30 years ago. Operating within a closed peritoneal cavity eliminates the need to use surgical pads and decreases the potential for bacterial and foreign body contamination. The surgeon can achieve excellent illumination, visibility, and magnification by bringing the distal end of the laparoscope close to the area of interest. The pressure effect of the pneumoperitoneum diminishes venous oozing and permits spontaneous coagulation of minor vessels. In addition, there are the well-known advantages for the patient associated with the avoidance of a large abdominal incision.

In the 70's hysteroscopy was described as "a technique looking for an indication." The impact of hysteroscopy in our specialty has been radical. This came about when hysteroscopy started to be used as a new mode of surgical access into the uterus. This revolutionized and greatly simplified many procedures that previously required a laparotomy and a hysterotomy to access the uterine cavity: lysis of severe uterine synechiae, metroplasty for septate uterus, excision of symptomatic intra-uterine fibroids. These, after all, are common conditions; hysteroscopy has simplified these procedures and significantly reduced their morbidity. Direct access to the uterus led to the introduction of interventions such as endometrial excision and endometrial ablation that offer a less invasive, yet effective alternative to hysterectomy in the

https://doi.org/10.1515/9783110535204-202

treatment of abnormal (dysfunctional) uterine bleeding refractory to medical treatment.

Both laparoscopic and hysteroscopic surgery are "minimal access surgery", but what is minimal is only the access; not the procedure, the level of skill required, nor the potential of the rate and the degree of complications. Hence, proper training, use of proper surgical technique and vigilance are of foremost importance.

Schopenhauer said it so well: "change alone is eternal, perpetual, immortal."

Professor Victor Gomel
Vancouver
January 2020

Preface

"One must examine what concerns it, not only on the basis of the conclusion and the premises on which the argument rests, but also on the basis of things said about it." Aristotle says in *Nicomachean Ethics*. Our common aim as the Editors is to improve the quality of women's health globally. Surgical practice continues to evolve fast and it brings new advantages by improving efficacy and reducing risks. As the technology advances rapidly and new evidence on safety and effectiveness is gathered, we feel obligated to cover all aspects of minimally invasive gynecologic surgery in a fair, balanced way to include laparoscopic, robotic-assisted, and hysteroscopic approaches. That is what we set out to achieve in this book.

Our target audience are those who wish to further extend their knowledge in minimally invasive gynecology. Our priority is to provide practical guidance to the reader. The Editors are from Great Britain, United States and Germany and the chapter authors represent a broad international experience. They are well respected leaders who are shaping current practice and have been invited to contribute to this book due to their expertise in their respective fields. Our previous positive experience with De Gruyter press led us to work with them again as we expand our portfolio from robotic surgery to all aspects of minimally invasive gynecology.

We have spent countless hours writing and editing this comprehensive text. We would like to extend our appreciation to our families for encouraging us. We could not have done it without their support.

https://doi.org/10.1515/9783110535204-203

Contents

Rufus Cartwright and Natalia Price

Rainer Kimmig

Kirsten Huebner, Alexander di Liberto, Catharina Luck and Kubilay Ertan

Principal contributing authors

Dr. Alexis McQuitty
Jennie Sealy Hospital
Department of Anesthesiology
301 University Blvd
Galveston, TX 77555
USA

Prof. Arnaud Wattiez
IRCAD France–Hôpitaux Universitaires
1 place de l'Hôpital
67091 Strasbourg Cedex
France

Prof. Arnold P. Advincula
Department of Obstetrics and Gynecology
Columbia University Medical Center
Sloane Hospital for Women at
New York-Presbyterian/Columbia
622 West 168th Street
New York, NY 10032
USA

Prof. Attilio Di Spiezio Sardo
Department of Public Health
University of Naples "Federico II"
80131 Naples
Italy

Dr. Davor Jurkovic
University College London Hospitals
Women's Health Division
250 Euston Road
London NW1 2PG
United Kingdom

Assoc. Prof. Dr. Ertan Sarıdoğan
University College London Hospital
Elizabeth Garrett Anderson Wing
25 Grafton Way
London WC1E 6DB
UK

Prof. Dr. Gokhan Sami Kilic
Urogynecology and Minimally Invasive Gynecology
University of Texas Medical Branch
301 University Boulevard
335 Clinical Science Building
Galveston, TX 77555-0587
USA

Dr. Ibrahim Alkatout
Department of Obstetrics and Gynecology
University Hospitals Schleswig-Holstein
Campus Kiel
Arnold-Heller-Str. 3
Haus 24
24105 Kiel
Germany

Prof. Javier Magrina
Department of Gynecology
Division of Gynecologic Oncology
Mayo Clinic Arizona
5779 East Mayo Boulevard
Phoenix, AZ 85054
USA

Dr. Jon I. Einarsson
Division of Minimally Invasive Gynecology
Brigham and Women's Hospital
75 Francis Street
ASB 1-3
Boston, MA 02115
USA

Prof. Justin Clark
Birmingham Women's Hospital
Birmingham Women's NHS Foundation Trust and
University of Birmingham
Birmingham, B15 2TG
United Kingdom

Prof. Dr. Kubilay Ertan
Dep. of OB&GYN
Klinikum Leverkusen
Am Gesundheitspark 11
51375 Leverkusen
Germany

Prof. Dr. Liselotte Mettler
Department of Obstetrics and Gynecology
University Hospitals Schleswig-Holstein
Campus Kiel
Arnold-Heller-Str. 3
24105 Kiel
Germany

Prof. Marc Possover
International School of Neuropelveology
Witellikerstrasse 40
8032 Zürich
Switzerland

Dr. Mark Hans Emanuel
University Medical Center
Heidelberglaan 100
3584 CX Utrecht
The Netherlands

Dr. Mary Connor
Sheffield Teaching Hospitals
Jessop Wing
Sheffield S10 2SF
UK

Dr. Mohamed Mabrouk
S. Orsola- Malpighi Academic Hospital
Bologna University
Via Massarenti 13
40138 Bologna
Italy

Dr. Mohsen El-Sayed
Darent Valley Hospital
Darenth Wood Road Dartford
Kent DA2 8DA
UK

Dr. Mostafa A. Borahay
Department of Gynecology and Obstetrics
Johns Hopkins University School of Medicine
Johns Hopkins Bayview Medical Center
4940 Eastern Ave
Baltimore, MD 21224-2780
USA

Dr. Natalia Price
John Radcliffe Hospital
Headley Way
Headington
Oxford OX3 9DU
United Kingdom

Prof. Olivier Donnez
Institut du sein et de Chirurgie gynécologique
d'Avignon (ICA)
Polyclinique Urbain V (ELSAN Group)
Chemin du Pont des Deux Eaux 95
84000 Avignon
France

Prof. Dr. Peter O'Donovan
Bradford Teaching Hospitals
M.E.R.I.T. Centre
Bradford Royal Infirmary
Bradford BD9 6RJ
UK

Prof. Dr. Rainer Kimmig
Universitätsklinikum Essen (AöR)Klinik für
Frauenheilkunde und Geburtshilfe
Hufelandstraße 55
45147 Essen
Germany

Prof. Rudy Leon De Wilde
Clinic of Gynecology
Obstetrics and Gynecological Oncology
University Hospital for Gynecology
Pius-Hospital Oldenburg
Medical Campus University of Oldenburg
Georgstreet 12
26121 Oldenburg
Germany

Prof. Dr. Sara Y. Brucker
Forschungsinstitut für Frauengesundheit
Universitäts-Frauenklinik Tübingen
Calwerstraße 7
72076 Tübingen
Germany

Prof. Sven Becker
Klinik für Gynäkologie und Geburtshilfe
Klinikum der Johann Wolfgang
Goethe-Universität Frankfurt am Main
Theodor-Stern-Kai 7
60590 Frankfurt
Germany

Mohamed Mabrouk, Diego Raimondo, Manuela Mastronardi and
Renato Seracchioli

1 Practical fundamentals of retroperitoneal spaces for safe pelvic surgery: possible answers to difficult questions

1.1 Does a general gynecologist need to know about retroperitoneal pelvic anatomy?

Separate works report a strong association between knowledge of pelvic anatomy and surgical competency [1]. The ability to manage several surgical procedures is considerably influenced by the level of training in anatomy and the ability to identify key anatomical structures [2]. The importance of applied anatomy is suggested also by a 7-fold increase in claims made to the UK Medical Defence Organizations between 1995 and 2000 [3].

The most easily identifiable anatomical structures are pelvic organs and blood vessels. In contrast, retroperitoneum, nerves, and lymphatics are the least identifiable. Furthermore, whilst laparoscopy has become the standard of gynecological surgical care, the ability to identify pelvic structures at laparoscopy is found to be less than laparotomy [4].

Preliminary data of ongoing multicentric study conducted by Bologna University, assessing the necessity and level of training of retroperitoneal anatomy among gynecologists, have provided an overview of the poor knowledge and confidence of surgeons with this topic. Most of gynecologists sustain retroperitoneal anatomy as an essential topic in their work, but they perceive limitations in their anatomical knowledge and training.

Recognizing retroperitoneal structures is essential for the management of complex surgery (i.e., deep endometriosis, oncology) but can also be crucial for the so-called "everyday" surgery [5–7].

In this chapter, we aim to provide practical and basic knowledge of the retroperitoneal pelvic anatomy, referring to other chapters for the remaining anatomical topics.

1.2 What are the superficial anatomical landmarks of retroperitoneum?

Most pelvic organs are covered by the peritoneum, a serous membrane with openings at the lateral end of both uterine tubes. The peritoneum can be described in two parts: *parietal peritoneum* and *visceral peritoneum*. The parietal peritoneum is attached to the osteomuscular wall by extraperitoneal connective tissue; the visceral peritoneum,

https://doi.org/10.1515/9783110535204-001

instead, is firmly adherent to the underlying viscera and often blends with connective tissue in the wall of the organs. The potential space between the two layers is called the *peritoneal cavity*.

The peritoneum is reflected from the anterior and posterior uterine surfaces to the lateral pelvic wall forming the *broad ligament* of the uterus, which divides the pelvic cavity in the anterior and posterior compartments. Dorsally, the peritoneum covers the anterolateral surface of the upper rectum, a part of sacrum concavity and pelvic lateral walls, forming *a retro-rectal peritoneal reflection*. The presence of the uterus and the vagina produces two median pouches: the *recto-uterine pouch (of Douglas)* and the *vesico-uterine (VU) pouch*. It is important to note that the depth of the two pouches is variable and the peritoneal reflection of recto-uterine pouch of Douglas is more caudal than the VU one. Ventrally, the peritoneum that covers the dome of the bladder is reflected on the posterior surface of the lower anterior pelvic wall forming a *prevesical reflection*, when the bladder is empty (Fig. 1.1).

In patients with average weight, some retroperitoneal structures can be recognized through the peritoneum:

–   The peritoneum on the lower anterior abdominal wall is raised into five folds (reported as "ligaments"), which diverge as they descend from the umbilicus. They are the median, right and left medial, and right and left lateral umbilical folds.

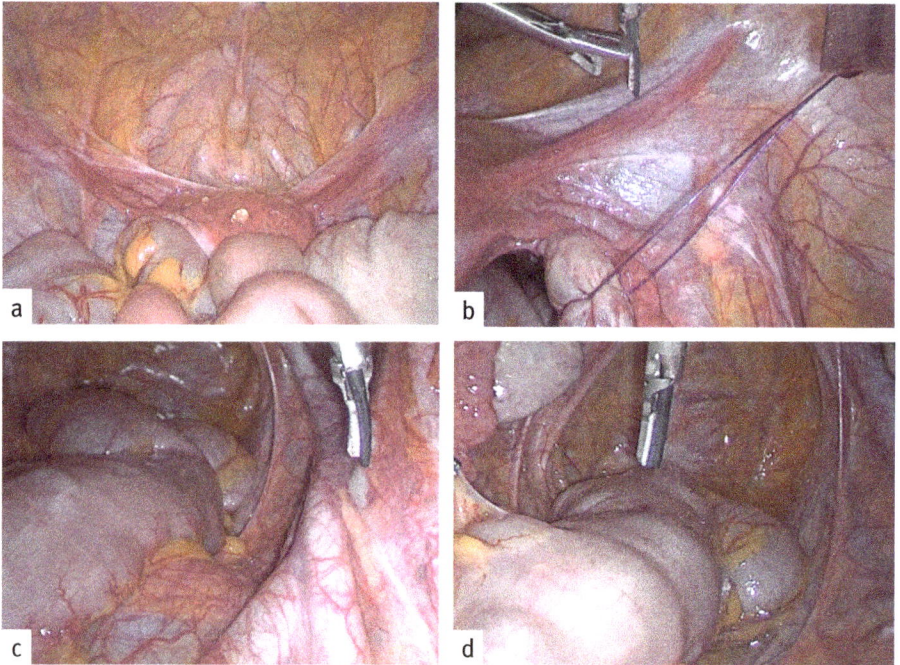

Fig. 1.1: Overview of the pelvis: (a) prevesical peritoneal reflection; (b) round ligament; (c) ureter at the pelvic brim and sacral promontory; (d) pouch of Douglas.

The median umbilical fold extends from the apex of the bladder to the umbili-cus and contains the *urachus*. The medial umbilical fold covers the *obliterated umbilical artery*. Under the lateral umbilical fold, the *deep inferior epigastric vessels* can be found, below their entry into the rectus sheath.

– *Superior vesical arteries*, on both sides, form the *transverse vesical folds* on the bladders dome.
– *Uterine artery*, on both sides, passes between the two peritoneal layers of the broad ligament, within the cardinal ligament (of Mackenrodt or lateral parame-trium), and crossing over the ureter.
– *Pelvic ureter* enters the lesser pelvis at the level of the sacral promontory, anterior to the end of the common iliac vessels (more frequent on the left side) or at the origin of the external iliac vessels (more frequent on the right side).
– *Uterosacral ligaments* form the *recto-uterine folds*, containing some pelvic auto-nomic nerve fibers in its postero-lateral part. In some patients, it is also visible a more medial and caudal folder, enveloping the *hypogastric nerves (HNs)* and the inferior hypogastric plexus (or pelvic plexus) [8].
– *Bifurcation of aorta* (at the level of the fourth lumbar vertebra or the L4/5 interver-tebral disc, to the left of the midline) and the *left common iliac vein. Middle sacral vessels* and *the superior hypogastric plexus* are located in the interiliac triangle (or Cotte triangle) at the level of *sacral promontory*, the starting point of pelvic cavity.
– Laterally, three somatic nerves from lumbar plexus: *genitofemoral nerve* lying on the psoas major muscle, and the *iliohypogastric* and the *ilioinguinal nerves* [9–11].

1.3 Is there a general scheme for the retroperitoneal space?

In the pelvis, three major layers can be identified: *peritoneum; retroperitoneum*, containing anatomical structures enveloped by connective tissue; and *pelvic walls* (muscles and bones covered by connective tissue). In a transversal section of the pelvis, it is possible to identify on the midline three main organs: bladder, cervix, and rectum (Fig. 1.2).

The *functional organization* of retroperitoneum (known as *endopelvic fascia*) is provided by dense connective structures—visceral "ligaments" and fasciae—leaving areas of looser connective tissue in contact with viscera and abdominal walls, forming spaces or septa (coalescence of fasciae). The method of dealing with these spaces rep-resents the basis of retroperitoneal surgical dissection [12–15].

The endopelvic fascia has different characteristics according to its components, and it is divided into:

Membranous: parietal and visceral pelvic fasciae
The *parietal pelvic fascia* (PPF), which covers bones and muscles limiting the pelvic cavity and adjacent structures (vessels, nerves, and nerve roots), is reflected on the pelvic organs (except ovaries and tubes), forming the *visceral pelvic fascia* (VPF).

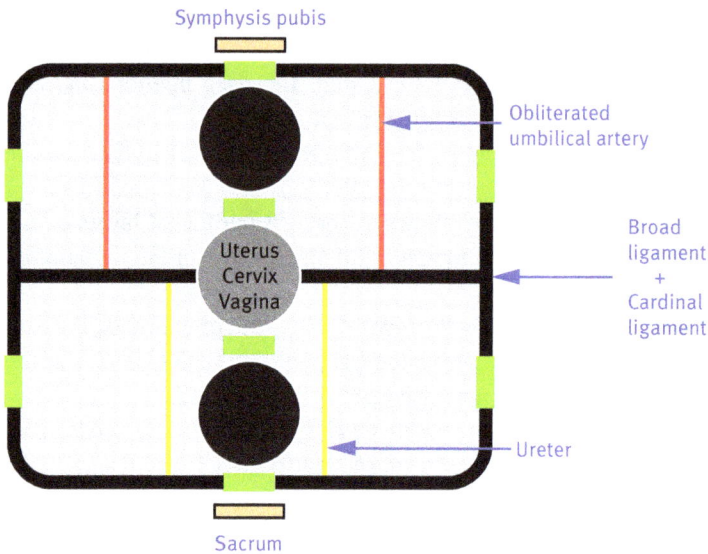

Fig. 1.2: General scheme of the retroperitoneum (the "exit doors" are represented by green boxes).

Fibro-areolar: visceral "ligaments"

The *extraserous pelvic fascia* (EPF) is defined as the connective tissue between the VPF and the PPF and acts as a mesentery, containing vessels and nerve branches. In some anatomical locations, the connective tissues of EPF is denser and referred to as visceral "ligaments."

Visceral "ligaments" can be divided into:
- *sagittal ligaments*: pubo-vesical ligaments, VU ligaments and uterosacral ligaments; and
- *lateral ligaments*: parametrium, paracervix, lateral ligaments of the bladder and lateral ligaments of the rectum.

Areolar: septa or spaces

According to the Toldt's law of fascial coalescence, the areas bordered by at least 2 independent fasciae and filled with areolar connective tissue are considered "avascular spaces" that can be safely developed.

It is possible to identify *lateral* and *median spaces*:
- *lateral spaces* can be split into *anterior* and *posterior compartments* by the internal genitalia, broad ligament and Mackenrodt's cardinal ligaments (or lateral parametrium), called, respectively, *paravesical (PV)* and *pararectal (PR) spaces*.
    - *PV space* can be further divided by obliterated umbilical artery into medial and lateral PV spaces.
    - *PR space* can be further divided by pelvic ureter in *medial (of Okabayashi)* and *lateral (of Latzko) PR spaces*.

It is important to consider that these spaces are not perfectly matched, because the ureter and obliterated umbilical artery have different course.
- *median spaces* correspond to peritoneal reflections:
    - prevesical space,
    - VU and vesico-vaginal spaces,
    - rectovaginal (RV) space, and
    - retrorectal and presacral spaces.

1.4 How to develop retroperitoneal spaces easily

The core skills of a competent surgeon are *knowledge and exposure of the anatomy*. It is always true that we cannot expect good surgical outcomes without a good surgical dissection. The principal aim of surgical practice is not the exposure of the retroperitoneal structures, but the preservation of their anatomical and functional integrity.

In order to perform an efficient surgery in a reasonable time, we need to learn and apply adequate surgical dissection techniques.

General rules of retroperitoneal dissections are as follows:
- Have a *strategy* (start point, end point, and a roadmap).
- Identify *anatomical landmarks* and find the avascular spaces.
- Apply *traction-counter traction*, push, and spread.
- Use all ways of dissection, including CO_2 dissection, surfing into the *spider-web* structures of retroperitoneal area.
- Keep the surgical field *clean and dry*.
- Going slower makes your surgery faster: gradual and controlled thinning out of connective tissues to reveal structures within and maintain correct orientation of dissection.
- Separate several anatomic layers progressively ("onion-like concept").

Concerning the site-specific rules, we have to consider the entry way and the flow of dissection. We could access the retroperitoneum everywhere in the pelvis, lifting the peritoneal fold and cutting it. However, functional organization, embryological origin, and the need for relevant structures preservation impose us to find specific *entry points* and appropriate pathways between fasciae into virtual and avascular anatomical spaces, same like emergency *exit doors* in a closed room or an airplane.

Exit doors: Some doors can be used to access to the retroperitoneum. They are very useful in case of complex surgery (deep endometriosis, broad ligament fibroids, coagulation of uterine artery at the origin in case of hysterectomy for a large uterus, isthmic myomas) or complications (hematoma, ureteral damage).

In the midline, from ventral to dorsal, there are:
- prevesical door,
- VU door,

– recto-vaginal door, and
– retro-rectal door.

Laterally, from ventral to dorsal, there are:
– division of the round ligament and
– lateral or medial to infundibulo-pelvic (IP) ligament at the level of pelvic brim.

Flow of dissection: laparoscopic surgeons must adapt to the altered appearance of anatomy due to the effects of pneumoperitoneum and Trendelenburg positioning, two-dimensional images on monitor, fixed visual axis and magnification. Therefore, progression and flow of dissection between the fascial structures are essential to avoid the loss of the pathway.

1.4.1 Surgical tips and tricks

1.4.1.1 Round ligament exit

The *PV spaces* are two bilateral spaces located laterally to the bladder and VU ligaments and medially to external iliac vessels. To reach this space, we can divide the round ligament and, if needed, apply the incision parallel to the external iliac vessels.

It is divided by the obliterated umbilical artery and umbilico-vesical fascia into *medial* and *lateral* sections. The limits of these spaces are the posterior face of the superior ischio-pubic ramus, ventrally; the cardinal ligaments of the uterus, dorsally; and the internal obturator and the iliac-coccygeal muscles, separated by the tendinous arch of the levator ani muscle, caudally.

Deeply into the lateral PV space, it is possible to identify the *obturator nerve and vessels*, going into the obturator canal, and the obturator lymph nodes. In 83% cases, an anastomosis between the obturator and the external iliac arteries or veins (called "corona mortis") can be found [16].

Medially to the obliterated umbilical artery, we can recognize the superior vesical artery (*superior vesical ligament*), the third component of the inferior hypogastric plexus (*bladder nerve supply*) and the *distal ureter* inside the VU ligament (Fig. 1.3).

1.4.1.2 Exit lateral or medial to the IP ligaments at the pelvic brim

The *PR spaces* are two bilateral spaces located laterally to the rectum and the uterosacral ligaments, reaching the levator ani muscle. Ureter, covered by mesoureter (dependence of presacral fascia) divides the PR space into two regions, the *medial PR space (of Okabayashi)* and the *lateral PR space (of Latzko)*, located between the ureter and internal iliac vessels. It is bordered by the parametrium and paracervix, ventrally; by the piriformis muscle, dorsally; and by the anterior trunk of internal iliac artery, laterally. The medial PR space communicates with the retrorectal space, while lateral one with the presacral space.

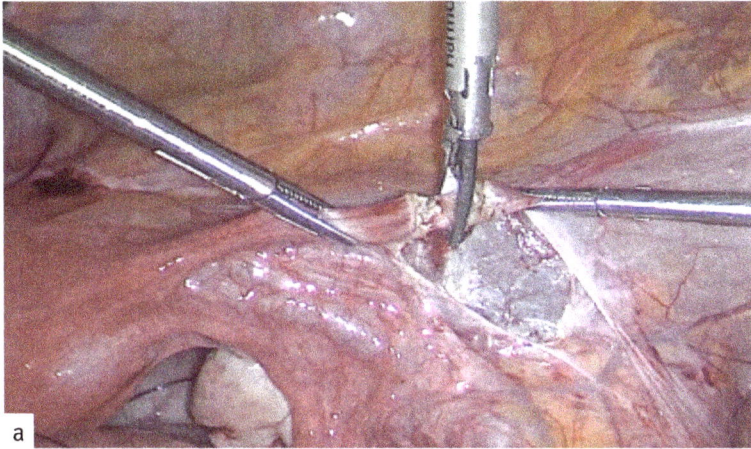

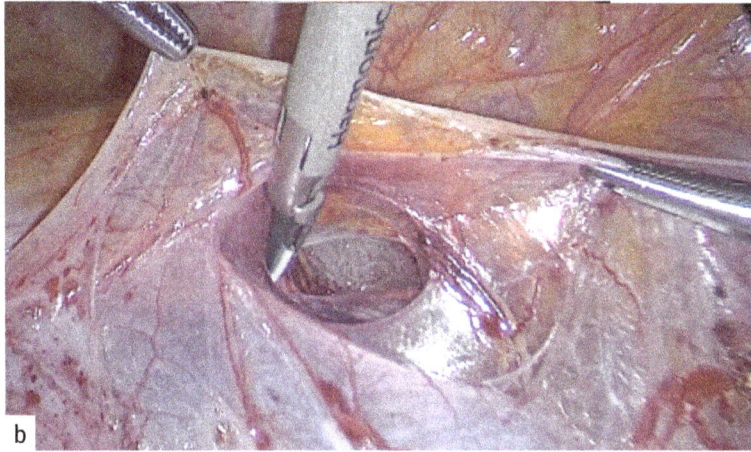

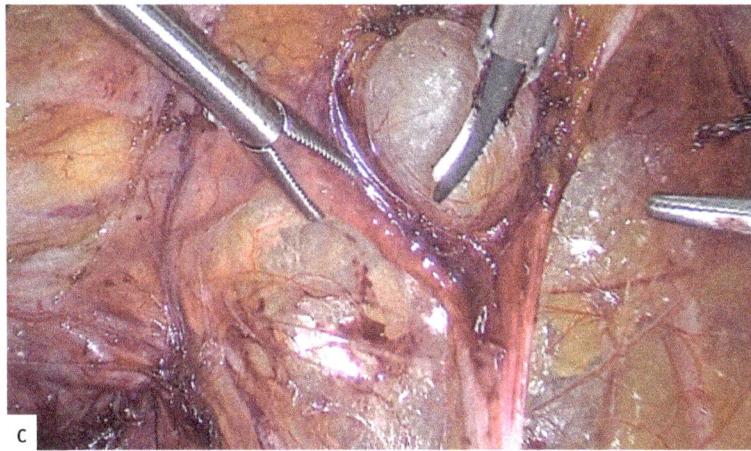

Fig. 1.3: (a, b) Opening of the round ligament exit (right side). (c) Developing of medial and lateral paravesical spaces, divided by obliterated umbilical artery.

To reach the medial PR space, it is preferred to start the peritoneal incision medially to the IP ligament at the pelvic brim. The dissection should be performed along the prehypogastric fascia to avoid unnecessary nerve dissection (Fig. 1.4).

To access the lateral PR space, it is useful to go lateral to IP ligament, pulling it medially and cephalically. In this way, it is possible to identify the *ureter* and internal and external iliac arteries. Going parallel to the lateral aspect of the ureter and following a cranio-caudal direction, the *uterine artery* and deep uterine vein can be revealed (Fig. 1.5).

The importance of these spaces is related to the presence of the iliac vessels with their collaterals and, from the functional point of view, of autonomic nervous system structures:

- The *HNs*, covered by the prehypogastric fascia (PHF), run approximately 5 mm to 20 mm below the course of the pelvic ureter in the upper part of the space, passing through the dorsolateral part of the uterosacral ligaments.
- The *pelvic splachnic nerves ("nervi erigenti")*, from the ventral sacral roots S2, S3, and S4, pierce the presacral fascia, follow the middle rectal artery, below the deep uterine vein, and join with the HN to form the inferior hypogastric plexus (or pelvic plexus).

1.4.1.3 Vesico-uterine exit

After pushing the uterus toward the promontory, the *vesico-uterine (VU) space* can be reached via the VU exit. After the peritoneal incision, the peritoneum and underlying

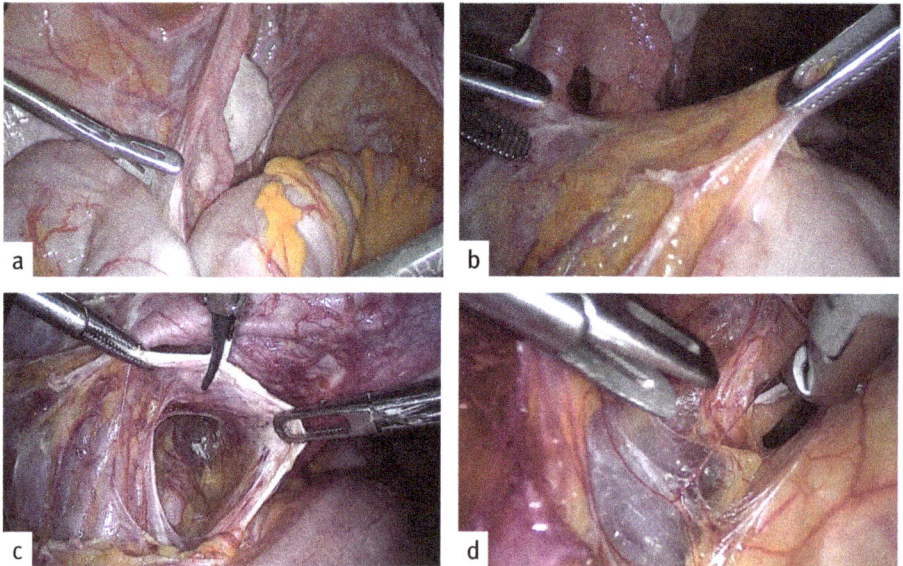

Fig. 1.4: (a, b) Opening of the exit door medial to the infundibulo-pelvic (IP) ligament and developing of the medial pararectal space (left side). (c) Ureter covered by the endopelvic fascia. (d) Hypogastric nerve and pelvic plexus covered by prehypogastric fascia and rectum covered by fascia propria recti.

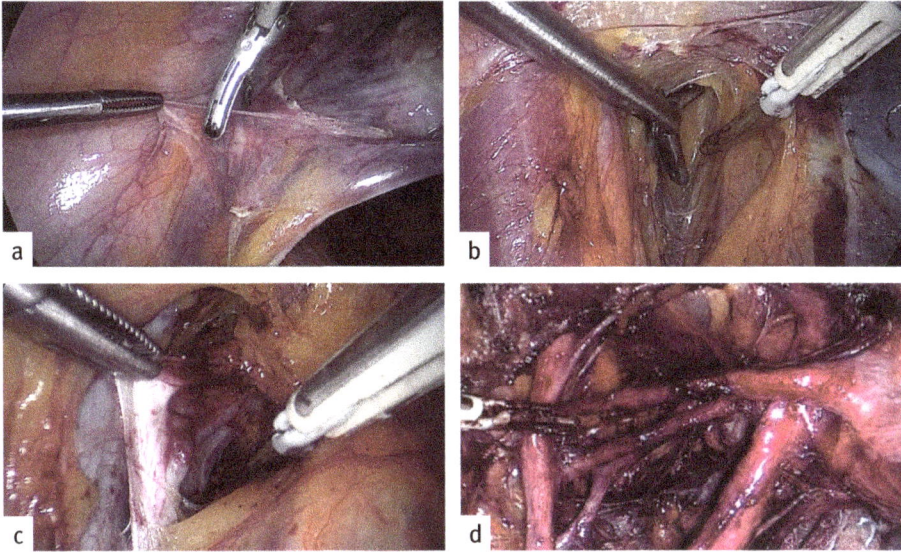

Fig. 1.5: (a, b) Opening of the exit door lateral to the infundibulo-pelvic (IP) ligament and developing of the lateral pararectal space (left side). (c) Ureteric tunnel below the uterine artery. (d) Accessory uterine artery passing below the ureter (anatomical variant).

bladder are pulled ventrally and caudally in order to expose the VU septum. The VU septum can be dissected through a mediolateral or lateromedial approach (preferred in case of adhesions or endometriotic implant) (Fig. 1.6).

The VU space is located between the posterior face of the bladder and the anterior face of the vagina and cervix, covered by Halban's pubo-cervical fascia. This fascia connects the anterior portion of the cervix and upper vagina to the posterior face of the pubic bones, diverging around the urethra. The lateral limits of the VU space are formed by the *VU ligaments (or anterior parametrium, bladder pillars)*, while caudal limit by the levator ani muscle and its fascia.

The cervix of the uterus is separated from the vesical bladder by a septum of loose connective tissue (*VU septum*), which allows the two organs to be easily dissected from each other during hysterectomy. The septum continues caudally, separating the bladder from the anterior fornix of the vagina, and it is crossed obliquely by the distal ureters and branches from the inferior hypogastric plexus. In the caudal part, the anterior face of the vagina is posterior to the urethra and vesical neck. At this point, the walls of the two organs are intimately attached, giving rise to the urethro-vaginal septum, which cannot be divided into two laminae.

1.4.1.4 Prevesical exit

Prevesical exit is located between the medial umbilical ligaments. Pulling dorsally and caudally the parietal peritoneum between the symphysis and the umbilicus, the

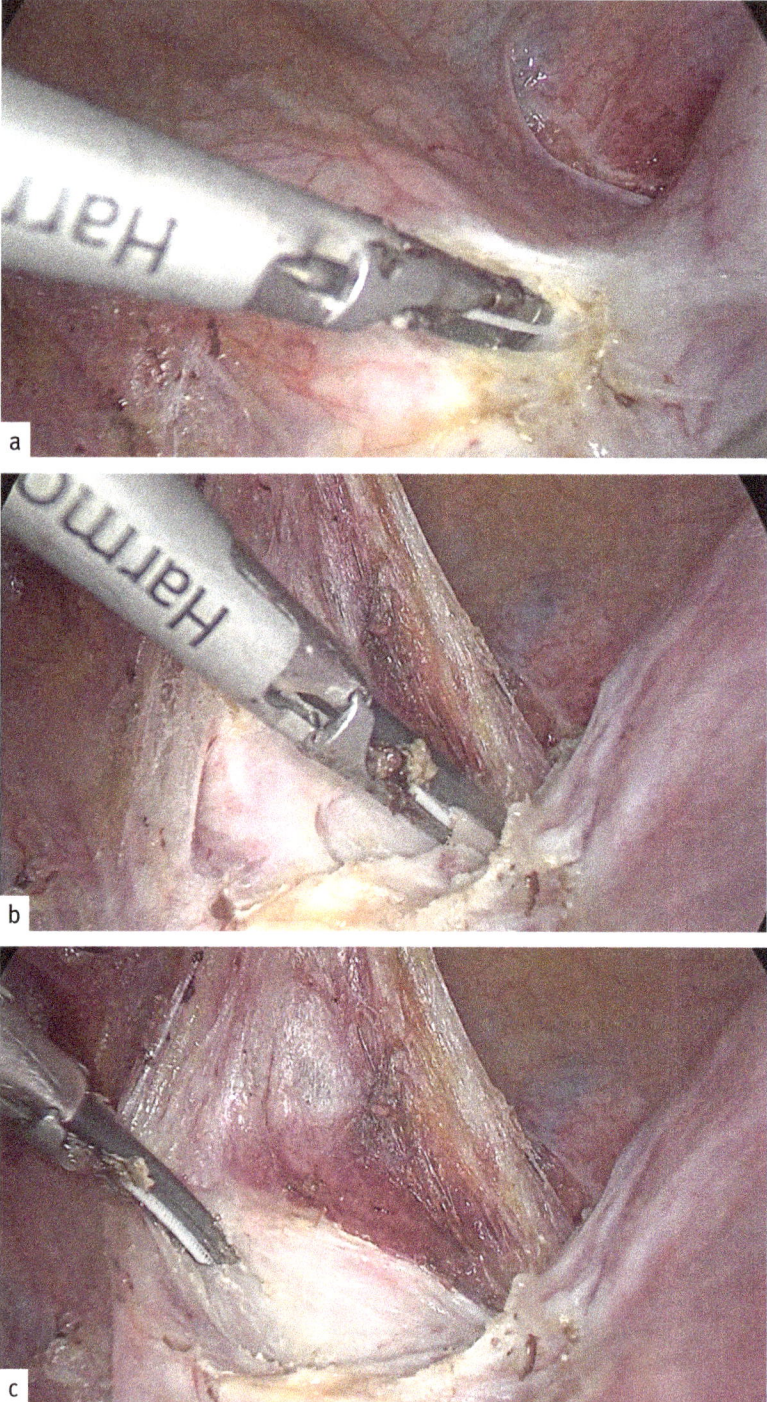

Fig. 1.6: (a–c) Opening of the vesico-uterine exit and developing of the vesico-uterine space.

peritoneal incision and the umbilico-vesical fascia division are performed to reach this space (Fig. 1.7).

The *prevesical (or retropubic or Retzius') space* extends from the pelvic floor to the umbilicus. In the pelvis, this space is horizontal and U shaped, with the concavity that wraps the vesical bladder. It communicates with the paravaginal (Yabuki's fourth space), medial PV and Bogros' (retroinguinal) spaces. Its posterior and cephalic limit is the *umbilico-vesical fascia*, a triangular fibrous tissue that extends from the

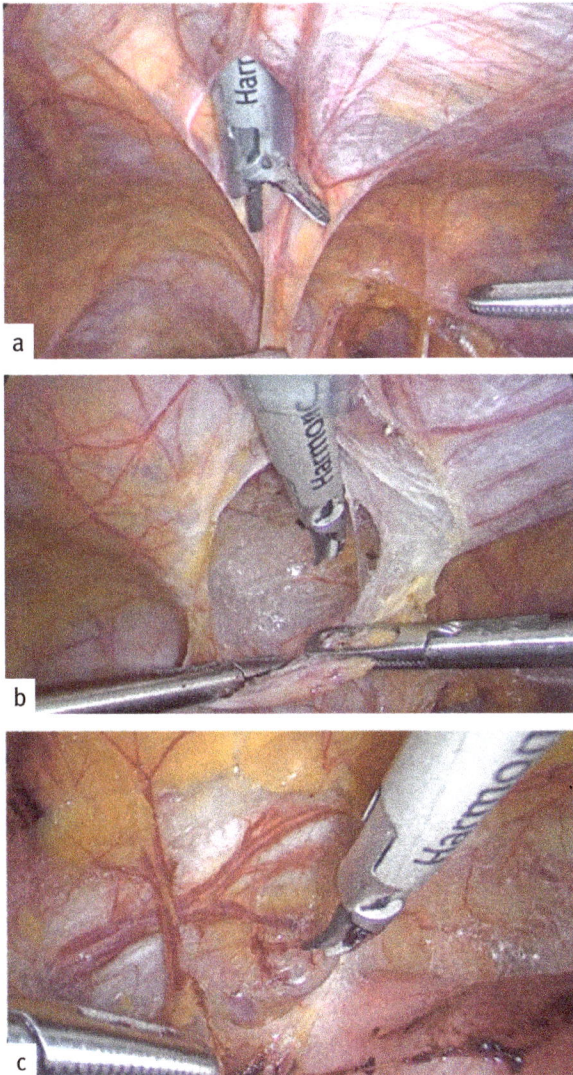

Fig. 1.7: (a–c) Opening of the prevesical exit and developing of the prevesical space.

superior part of the umbilicus to the pubo-vesical ligaments and the fascia of the internal obturator muscle. Anteriorly, this space is closed by the posterior layer of the rectus' sheath (covered by the fascia trasversalis up to Douglas' arcuate line), pubic bones, symphysis and Cooper's pectinate ligament. The floor of this space is made up by the pubo-vesical and pubo-urethral ligaments, the internal obturator, and levator ani muscles.

The prevesical space contains adipose tissue, lymph nodes, and the pelvic-vesical venous plexus, which receives the anterior vesical veins, the veins from the urethra and the dorsal vein of the clitoris, finally draining into the internal iliac veins [9–11].

1.4.1.5 Rectovaginal exit

Through the RV exit, between the insertion of distal part of uterosacral ligaments on torus uterinum, we can access the *RV space*. Anteverting the uterus and pulling the rectum cephalically and dorsally, a peritoneal incision is made at the level of RV pouch. The RV space can be developed via medio-lateral or latero-medial approach (preferred in case of adhesions or endometriotic implant).

The RV space is an avascular area located between the posterior wall of the vagina, covered by the cervico-vaginal fascia, and the anterior wall of the rectum, covered by the fascia propria recti. It extends caudally until the upper part of the perineal body and pelvic floor muscles. This space is separated from the retrorectal spaces by lateral rectal ligaments on both sides [17, 18] (Fig. 1.8).

Inside this space *Denonvilliers' fascia (or rectovaginal septum)*, a fusion of the vaginal fascia and fascia propria recti, is identified.

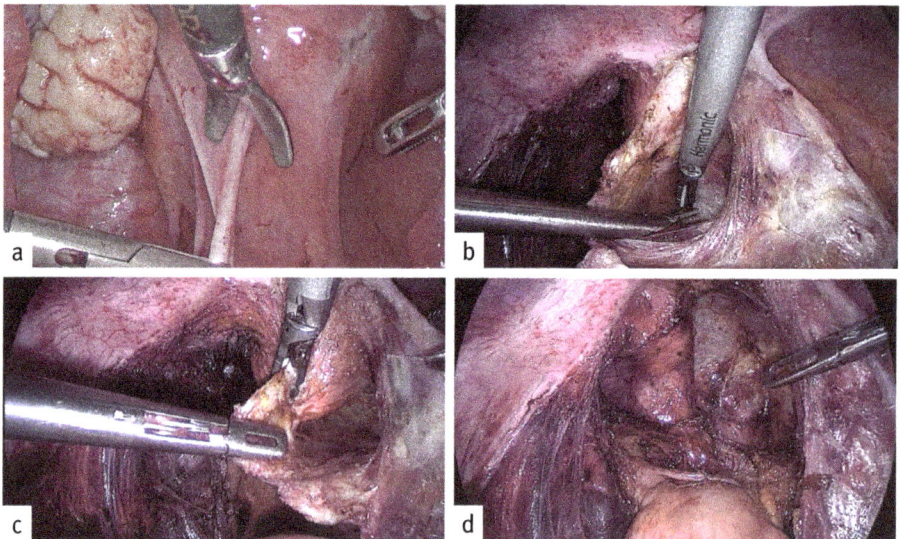

Fig. 1.8: (a–d) Opening of the rectovaginal exit and developing of the rectovaginal space.

Laterally, it is divided into several thin laminae *(RV ligaments)*; one of them extends dorsolaterally fusing with PHF and enveloping pelvic plexus. The RV septum is less prominent in females, thinning out with age and thickening in patients with transmural inflammation of the rectum (i.e., radiotherapy) [19]. In postmenopausal females and after childbirth, the connective tissue of the septum may atrophy, reducing the support of the rectal and vaginal walls. Moving caudally and laterally, it is possible to reach pubo-rectal and pubo-coccygeal muscles.

1.4.1.6 Retrorectal exit

Pulling laterally on the left side, cranially and ventrally the rectosigmoid tract, we can highlight the retrorectal exit in order to develop two spaces, divided by the prescral fascia (or Waldayer's fascia or fascia hypogastrica sacralis): retrorectal and prescral spaces.

Presacral fascia is a part of parietal pelvic fascia, pelvic continuation of the visceral abdominal fascia (Gerota fascia). This fascia is divided into (1) the fasciae enclosing the pelvic plexus together with PHF (see below); (2) the fasciae providing a posterior attachment for the levator ani muscle; and (3) the fasciae enclosing the sacral plexus and associated vessels [20].

Retrorectal space (Fig. 1.9):

The rectum has no mesentery and is surrounded by the mesorectum, enclosed within the *mesorectal fascia (or fascia propria recti)*, which lies ventrally to the

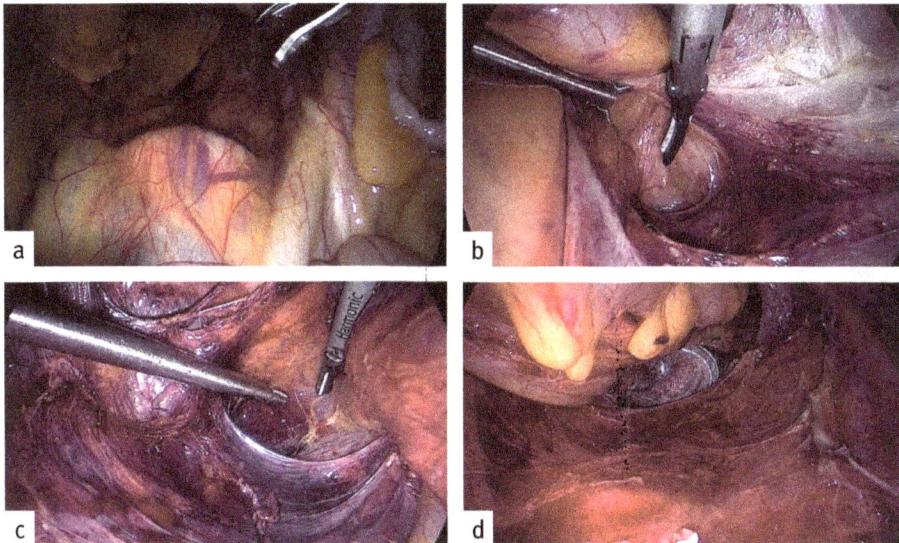

Fig. 1.9: (a, b) Developing of the retrorectal space through the retrorectal exit. (c) Left lateral ligament of the rectum and levator ani (rectosacral fascia transacted). (d) Retrorectal space between sacrum covered by presacral fascia and rectum enveloped by fascia propria recti.

presacral fascia. The median space between these two fasciae is named retro-rectal space, which continues laterally in the medial PR space on both sides.

The mesorectal fascia is connected to the parietal pelvic fascia by the two *lateral rectal "ligaments" (or rectal stalks or wings),* containing inconstant middle rectal vessels and rectal nerve branches from pelvic plexus, and the recto-sacral fascia, 3–5 cm above the anorectal junction [21]. Superiorly, this fascia blends with the sigmoid mesentery.

The mesorectal fascia is encircled by an avascular layer of loose areolar tissue, separating it from the posterior and lateral walls of the pelvis, along the sacral bone's concavity, called *"holy plane of Heald"* [22, 23].

A critical step during mobilization of the rectum is the separation of postero-lateral fasciae in order to avoid nerve injury, in particular of the *HN*. Dorsally to the rectum, the *PHF* is a ventral dependence of presacral fascia enveloping the HN and, more ventrally and caudally, the inferior hypogastric plexus. From this scheme, to avoid the risk of nerve injury, the ideal plane for rectal mobilization is between the fascia propria recti and the PHF [20]. Interestingly, the relationship between PHF and ureters varies according to the side: the left ureter runs dorsal to the PHF, while the right ureter runs ventral to it.

Presacral space (Fig. 1.10):

The presacral space is situated between the presacral fascia, ventrally, and the *anterior longitudinal ligament* of the sacrum and coccyx, dorsally. It begins just below the aortic bifurcation and extends inferiorly to the pelvic floor muscle. It communicates with the lateral PR space on both sides.

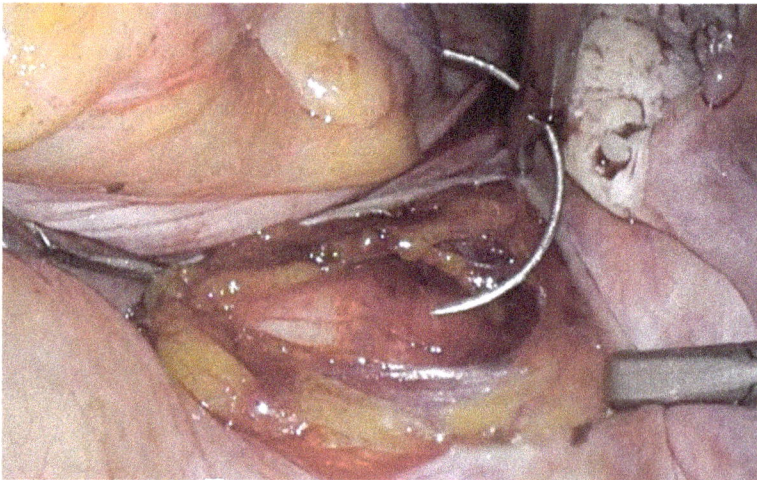

Fig. 1.10: Developing of the presacral space through the retrorectal exit and division of the presacral fascia.

The presacral space contains:
- *bifurcation of aorta and left common iliac vein*: the left common iliac vein can be located as close as 3 mm from the midline at the sacral promontory [24];
- *superior hypogastric plexus*: a reticular or band-like structure containing predominately sympathetic fibers and deriving from intermesenteric plexus and lumbar trunks;
- *median and lateral sacral vessels*: the lateral ones are variably found on either side of the sacral promontory's midline and can be source of important bleeding; and
- *ventral sacral roots and sacral sympathetic trunks*: they give birth to the sacral plexus lining up the *piriformis muscle* and give a contribute to the inferior hypogastric plexus through the parasympathetic splachnic pelvic nerves (or "nervi erigenti") [9–11].

References

[1] Lentz GM, Mandel LS, Lee D, et al. Testing surgical skills of obstetric and gynecologic residents in a bench laboratory setting: validity and reliability. Am J Obstet Gynecol 2001;184:1462–70.
[2] Arraez-Aybar LA, Sanchez-Montesinos I, Mirapeix RM, et al. Relevance of human anatomy in daily clinical practice. Ann Anat 2010;192:341–8.
[3] Waterston SW. Survey of clinicians' attitudes to the anatomical teaching and knowledge of medical students. Clin Anat 2005;18:330–84.
[4] Sgroi J, Abbott J. Surgical anatomy in obstetrics and gynecology: the trainees' perspective. Aust N Z J Obstet Gynaecol 2014 Apr;54(2):172–6.
[5] Cruikshank SH. Retroperitoneal dissection in gynecologic surgery for benign disease. South Med J 1987 Mar;80(3):296–300.
[6] Gingold JA, Falcone T. Retroperitoneal anatomy during excision of pelvic side wall endometriosis. J Endometr Pelvic Pain Disord 2016 Apr–Jun;8(2):62–6.
[7] Sharma N, Ganesh D, Srinivasan J, Jayakumar S, Mathew R. Retroperitoneal approach for dissection of inflamed pelvic viscera in acute pelvic inflammatory disease – case report. J Clin Diagn Res 2014 May;8(5):OD03–5.
[8] Ramanah R, Berger MB, Parratte BM, DeLancey JOL. Anatomy and histology of apical support: a literature review concerning cardinal and uterosacral ligaments. Int Urogynecol J 2012 Nov;23(11):1483–94.
[9] Standring S. Gray's anatomy, The Anatomical Basis of Clinical Practise. 41st ed. Elsevier; London, 2016.
[10] Testut L, Jacob O. Trattato di Anatomia Topografica con applicazioni medico-chirurgiche. Edra-Masson; Torino, 1998.
[11] Detton AJ. Grant's Dissector (International Edition). 16th ed. Lippincott Williams and Wilkins; Philadelphia, 2016.
[12] Ercoli A, Delmas V, Fanfani F, et al. Terminologia Anatomica versus unofficial descriptions and nomenclature of the fasciae and ligaments of the female pelvis: a dissection-based comparative study. Am J Obstet Gynecol 2005 Oct;193(4):1565–73. PubMed PMID: 16202758.
[13] International Anatomical Terminology/Federative Committee on Anatomical Terminology (FCAT). Terminologia Anatomica. Stuttgart/New York: Thieme; 1998.
[14] Yabuki Y, Sasaki H, Hatakeyama N, Murakami G. Discrepancies between classic anatomy and modern gynecologic surgery on pelvic connective tissue structure: harmonization of those concepts by collaborative cadaver dissection. Am J Obstet Gynecol 2005 Jul;193(1):7–15.

[15] Tamakawa M, Murakami G, Takashima K, Kato T, Hareyama M. Fascial structures and autonomic nerves in the female pelvis: a study using macroscopic slices and their corresponding histology. Anat Sci Int. 2003 Dec;78(4):228–42. PubMed PMID: 14686478.

[16] Darmanis S, Lewis A, Mansoor A, Bircher M. Corona mortis: an anatomical study with clinical implications in approaches to the pelvis and acetabulum. Clin Anat 2007 May;20(4):433–9.

[17] Herschorn S. Female pelvic floor anatomy: the pelvic floor, supporting structures, and pelvic organs. Rev Urol 2004; 6(Suppl 5):S2–10.

[18] Hinata N, Hieda K, Sasaki H, et al. Nerves and fasciae in and around the paracolpium or paravaginal tissue: an immunohistochemical study using elderly donated cadavers. Anat Cell Biol 2014;47(1):44–54.

[19] Church JM, Raudkivi PJ, Hill GL. The surgical anatomy of the rectum – a review with particular relevance to the hazards of rectal mobilisation. Int J Colorectal Dis 1987;2:158–66.

[20] Kinugasa Y, Murakami G, Suzuki D, Sugihara K. Histological identification of fascial structures postero-lateral to the rectum. Br J Surg 2007 May;94(5):620–6.

[21] Havenga K, DeRuiter MC, Enker WE, Welvaart K. Anatomical basis of autonomic nerve-preserving total mesorectal excision for rectal cancer. Br J Surg 1996;83:384–8.

[22] Ceccaroni M, Clarizia R, Bruni F, et al. Nerve-sparing laparoscopic eradication of deep endometriosis with segmental rectal and parametrial resection: the Negrar method. A single-center, prospective, clinical trial. Surg Endosc 2012 Jul;26(7):2029–45.

[23] Ceccaroni M, Clarizia R, Roviglione G, Ruffo G. Neuro-anatomy of the posterior parametrium and surgical considerations for a nerve-sparing approach in radical pelvic surgery. Surg Endosc 2013 Nov;27(11):4386–94.

[24] Flynn MK, Romero AA, Amundsen CL, Weidner AC. Vascular anatomy of the presacral space: a fresh tissue cadaver dissection. Am J Obstet Gynecol 2005 May;192(5):1501–5.

Elisabeth Bean and Davor Jurkovic

2 Preoperative imaging for minimally invasive surgery in gynecology

2.1 Introduction

Minimally invasive surgery has many advantages over traditional open procedures and has greatly improved the surgical care of women with a wide range of gynecological conditions such as ectopic pregnancy, benign ovarian cysts, endometriosis, and certain types of pelvic malignancies. Minimally invasive surgery, however, is not without limitations, and good selection of patients is critical both for its therapeutic efficacy and safety.

The selection of women for surgery is a complex process, which has to take into account many factors such as their general health, personal preferences, previous medical and surgical history, as well as their social circumstances. Clinical examination also provides invaluable information and is an essential part of this process. In modern clinical practice, however, preoperative selection can rarely be completed without detailed preoperative imaging. Ultrasound scanning is the most common clinical modality in gynecology and is routinely used in the initial assessment of women presenting with a wide range of gynecological conditions. It is widely available and relatively inexpensive compared to other imaging modalities. It avoids the use of ionizing radiation and contrast mediums, supporting its safety profile in pregnant women and for patients with allergies or systemic illness that prevent use of contrast. It is relatively quick, easy, reliable, and reproducible in performance.

Recent improvements in ultrasound technology have greatly increased our ability to examine pelvic anatomy with a high level of accuracy. In addition to providing detailed morphological analysis, transvaginal ultrasound (TVS) also allows assessment of mobility and tenderness of pelvic organs. Transrectal ultrasound provides an alternative method for detailed pelvic examination when TVS is contraindicated or transabdominal ultrasound is inadequate, e.g., women who have not previously been sexually active or women with vaginismus or vaginal atrophy.

Detailed preoperative gynecological ultrasound is valuable in selecting women for surgical treatment, planning operations, and deciding on the level of surgical expertise and techniques required to complete surgery safely and successfully. However, the accuracy and usefulness of ultrasound examination are highly dependent upon the skill and expertise of the operator [1]. This is particularly important in the assessment of women with ovarian tumors and pelvic endometriosis. The skill of the operator is also of critical importance in the diagnosis of ectopic pregnancy. This is an important limitation of this technique, and the skill of the operator needs to be taken into account when ultrasound findings are used for preoperative selection of patients.

https://doi.org/10.1515/9783110535204-002

2.2 Role of preoperative imaging in specific conditions

2.2.1 Pelvic adhesions

Ultrasound is a dynamic investigation, which can be used to assess the mobility of pelvic organs and for the presence of adhesions. Bimanual palpation of the uterus with gentle pressure on the cervix with the ultrasound probe and suprapubic pressure with one hand on the woman's lower abdomen can be used to assess for presence of adhesions in both anterior and posterior pelvic compartments [2]. Guerriero *et al.* found that the mobility of the ovary could be evaluated using TVS imaging. The positive predictive value (PPV) of TVS in diagnosing adhesions was reported as 81% [3]. Okaro *et al.* assessed ovarian mobility by applying pressure with the ultrasound probe. They reported a good correlation between ovarian mobility on TVS and at laparoscopy (kappa = 0.81). However, most of their patients had normal ovaries, which are much easier to assess for mobility than large pelvic tumors [4]. Yazbek *et al.* conducted a study involving preoperative ultrasound assessment of 137 women. The diagnosis of severe pelvic adhesions was made with a sensitivity of 44% (95% confidence interval [CI], 17–69), specificity of 98% (95% CI, 94–99), and a PPV of 67% (95% CI, 30–90) (Fig. 2.1). The presence of adhesions was particularly difficult to predict in obese patients and in those with large tumors [5].

2.2.2 Endometriosis

In modern practice, many women with endometriosis are managed conservatively and the final diagnosis is based on the results of gynecological imaging. TVS is an acceptable and noninvasive method of imaging the female pelvis. It has 94% accuracy for diagnosing women with moderate to severe endometriosis. Overall, there is a good level of agreement between ultrasound and laparoscopy in identifying moderate and severe disease [6].

It is widely acknowledged that the success of surgery for pelvic endometriosis is highly dependent on the expertise and training of the operating surgeon. Factors that increase the risk of conversion to laparotomy include severe pelvic adhesions and severe pelvic endometriosis. While mild to moderate endometriosis can be treated by medium-level laparoscopic surgeons, severe pelvic disease should be operated on by surgeons with significant laparoscopic expertise, particularly if the disease involves the rectovaginal septum [7–9]. In an attempt to optimize the treatment of severe pelvic endometriosis, tertiary referral endometriosis centers have been established in the UK. The capacity of these tertiary centers is limited; therefore, the ability to triage patients with severe disease for expert care is crucial. Ultrasound has the ability to diagnose severe disease with a high level of accuracy and therefore allows better triaging of women with pelvic endometriosis for referral to regional endometriosis centers.

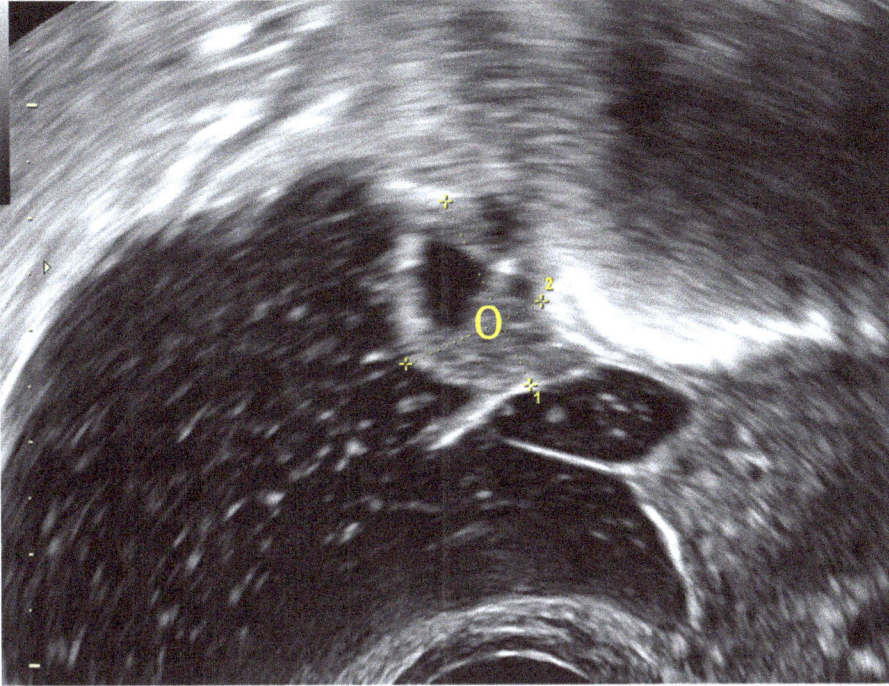

Fig. 2.1: Transverse section of the pelvis showing a large cystic structure (C) filled with moderately echogenic fluid. A normal ovary (O) is seen in the center of the image suspended in the fluid. These findings are typical of pelvic adhesions forming a large peritoneal pseudocyst.

Accurate assessment of bowel or urinary tract involvement allows appropriate counseling of patients regarding the risks associated with surgery and the likelihood of women requiring specialist urinary or bowel treatments, including diversion techniques (Fig. 2.2). Knowing the extent of disease enables preoperative involvement of specialist bowel or urological surgeons. The use of preoperative Gonadotropin-releasing hormone (GnRH) therapy, bowel preparation and ureteric stenting can be tailored to the individual patient.

Commonly, magnetic resonance imaging (MRI) is used for preoperative evaluation of deep infiltrating endometriosis (DIE), particularly in women with suspected urinary tract involvement. MRI and TVS have been shown to have equivalent accuracy scores in the preoperative assessment of bladder endometriosis. MRI, although very precise, is less versatile than TVS and less accurate in establishing the margins of lesions, probably due to the relatively low hemosiderin content [10]. Pateman *et al.* concluded that pelvic segments of normal ureters can be identified in almost all women on TVS examination and that visualization of the ureters could be integrated into the routine pelvic ultrasound examination. In their study of 245 consecutive women, the overall visualization rate of ureters was 96% and it was not significantly affected by the experience of the operator [11]. Although assessment of the urinary tract

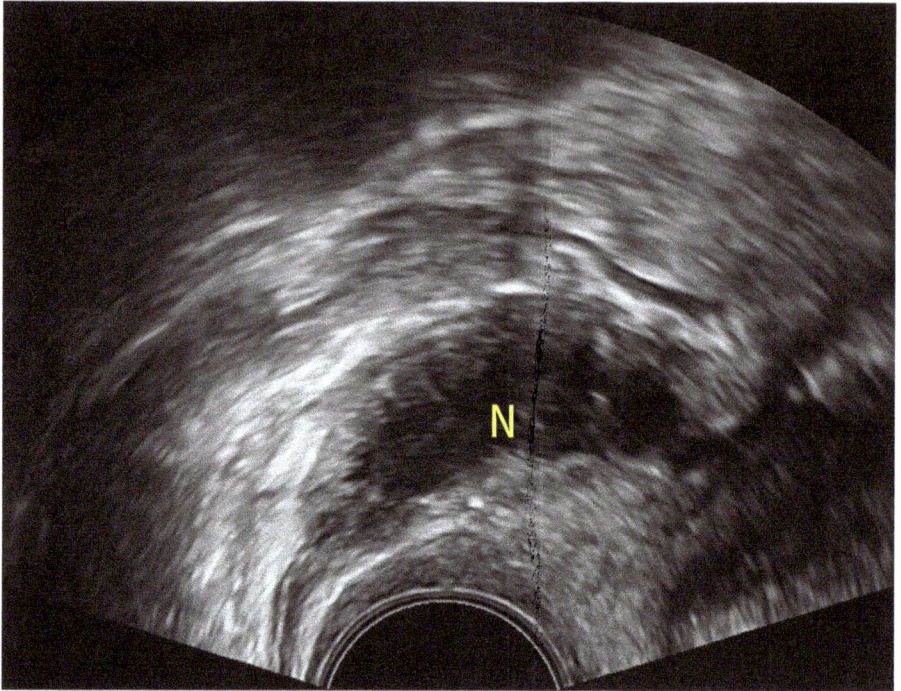

Fig 2.2: A large endometriotic nodule (N), which is located in the anterior wall of the rectosigmoid colon. The nodule measures 55 mm in length. These findings are typical of severe pelvic endometriosis.

is more traditionally achieved with MRI, it is now possible to establish the extent of involvement during routine pelvic ultrasound, providing a complete assessment at the time of a single investigation. MRI may become a superfluous investigation in the work-up of women with DIE, which is likely to have a positive impact on the patient's experience and financial costs to the health service.

2.2.3 Differential diagnosis of pelvic tumors

The role of ultrasound in the assessment of adnexal pathology is well established. However, accurate discrimination between benign and malignant adnexal tumors remains difficult due to the considerable overlap between the morphological features of benign and malignant tumors on all imaging modalities. When planning surgical treatment, it is crucial that malignant tumors are distinguished from benign pathology. The former warrant urgent management under the care of a specialist gynecological oncologist, whereas benign ovarian cysts may be managed conservatively using minimal-access surgery.

The more complex the appearance of a cyst is on ultrasound scan, the greater is the likelihood of malignancy (Fig. 2.3). Studies assessing ovarian morphology using

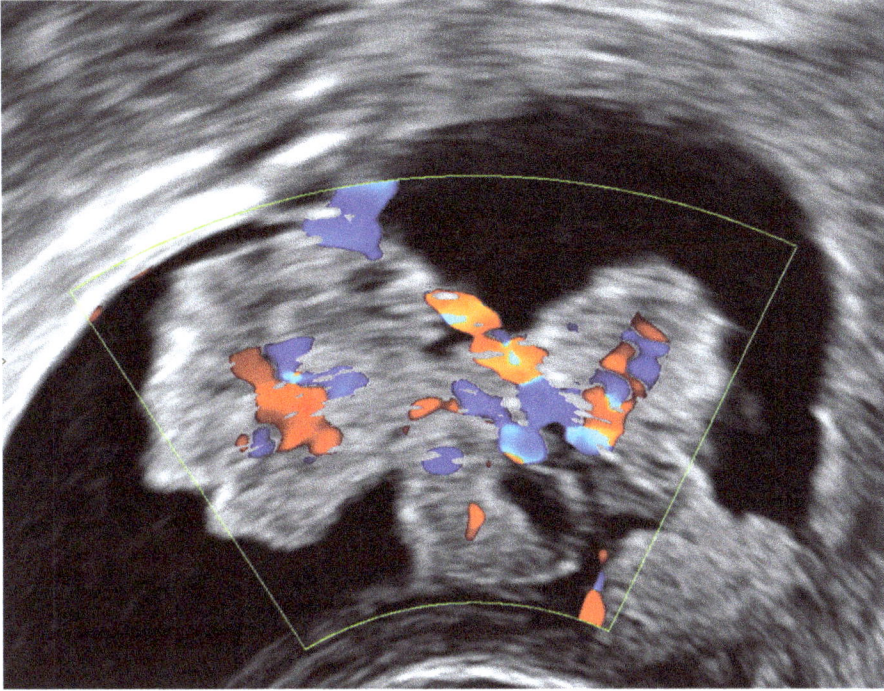

Fig 2.3: Transverse section of the right ovary. A large cystic structure with a prominent irregular solid component is seen. On Doppler examination, the tumor vascularity was increased. These findings are typical of an epithelial ovarian cancer.

B-mode grey-scale ultrasound showed that small unilocular simple cysts had a low probability of being malignant [12]. However, the presence of papillary projections and solid areas within the cyst increased the probability of ovarian malignancy [13]. Furthermore, the risk of malignancy increases with increasing locularity and size of the cyst. In order to improve the accuracy of ultrasound diagnosis, several morphological scoring systems have been designed. These systems assigned scores to each tumor depending on the presence or absence of certain morphological features on grey-scale ultrasound. It was hoped that with the advent of TVS color Doppler imaging, vascular changes within the ovary could be assessed and this would subsequently lead to better detection of malignant changes. However, significant variations exist in the reported results of color and pulsed Doppler studies in the assessment of adnexal masses [14–16]. Overall, the addition of color Doppler imaging has not been shown to improve the accuracy of the assessment significantly when compared with grey-scale morphology alone.

The most popular diagnostic model in routine clinical practice is the Risk of Malignancy Index (RMI). This remains the case despite several recent studies showing that the RMI has a relatively low specificity, which results in overdiagnosis of ovarian cancer and a large number of unnecessary surgical interventions [17]. More recent models developed by IOTA collaboration show promise, but they have not gained wider popularity and they are mainly seen as techniques in development, which have not been fully validated.

Pattern recognition is the use of grey-scale ultrasound morphology to characterize adnexal tumors and is superior to all other ultrasound methods, e.g., simple classification systems, scoring systems and mathematical models in discriminating between benign and malignant adnexal tumors. Grey-scale ultrasound images provide us with similar information that is obtained during surgery or on macroscopic pathological examination of surgical specimens. Many pelvic tumors have a typical macroscopic appearance that allows for a fairly confident diagnosis to be made based on their grey-scale ultrasound appearance alone. This is true of most dermoid cysts, endometriomas, corpora lutea, hydrosalpinges, peritoneal pseudocysts, para-ovarian cysts, and benign solid ovarian tumors. An expert ultrasound operator can confidently and correctly distinguish between benign and malignant adnexal masses by this method with or without the use of color Doppler ultrasound examination with a sensitivity ranging from 88% to 98% and specificity ranging from 89% to 96% [18, 19].

2.2.4 Uterine fibroids

Ultrasound is of utmost importance in the preoperative planning of minimally invasive surgery for fibroids. Ultrasound "mapping" of fibroids provides surgeons with information about their numbers, sizes, and locations within the uterus. This facilitates selection of women for hysteroscopic, laparoscopic, or open surgery. It also helps to determine whether preoperative treatment with GnRH analogues should be considered. Uterine sarcomas are very rare, but recently, there have been concerns about the risks associated with morcellation of undiagnosed leiomyosarcoma. Findings on preoperative ultrasound suggestive of uterine malignancy include irregularly shaped tumors, blurred margins, signs of necrosis, peritoneal deposits, and inability to visualize the endometrial cavity. Careful assessment of the morphology of uterine tumors facilitates preoperative detection of most uterine sarcomas. In a recent publication from our center, we showed that there were no cases of misdiagnosed uterine sarcomas among 514 women who underwent a laparoscopic myomectomy over a 10-year period [20].

2.2.5 Benign dermoid cysts

The composition of benign ovarian cysts is important in planning minimally invasive excision. Dermoid cysts are the most common tumor of the ovary and are varied in their morphology [21]. The improved quality of ultrasound equipment and increasing experience of operators have resulted in an increased accuracy of ultrasound diagnosis of dermoid cysts (Fig. 2.4). This increased confidence in diagnosis has largely eliminated the possibility of cancer as an indication for surgery in these cases. In the majority of cases, these cysts are diagnosed incidentally and are not the cause of the patient's presenting complaint, and yet their presence is often considered to be an indication for surgery. In asymptomatic women with a diagnosis of a dermoid cyst, the possible benefits of surgical intervention are not clear, and the risks and costs of surgery are hard to justify. Expectant management is a feasible option in this group of patients. Dermoid cysts have been shown to grow slowly over a period of time, with different studies reporting a similar mean cyst growth rate of up to 1.8 mm/year [22]. The tendency of dermoid cysts, however, to grow continuously may be used to justify surgery in younger women. Our recommendation is that expectant management is a feasible option in older, nulliparous women especially in those with a small unilateral cyst.

Correct preoperative identification of dermoid cysts prior to laparoscopic surgery is particularly important. The main risk associated with minimally invasive

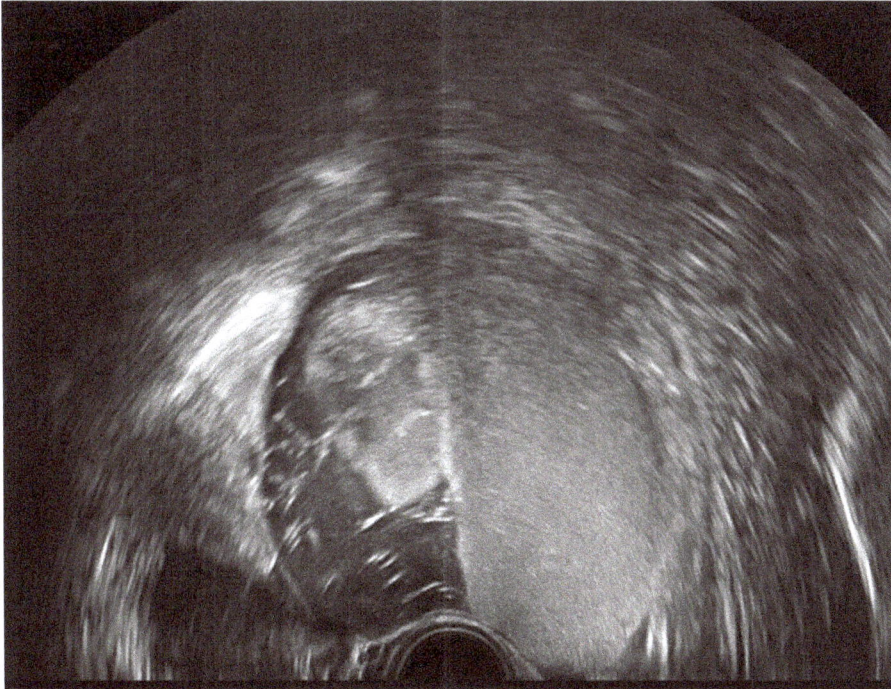

Fig. 2.4: An ultrasound image of the left ovary, which is enlarged by a complex cyst. The cyst contains hyperechoic fluid, typical of sebum and multiple thin echoes, representing hair. These features are typical of a benign dermoid cyst

excision of dermoid cysts is spillage of cyst content, which may result in peritoneal irritation or chemical peritonitis [23, 24]. Some authors advocate open surgery for all large dermoid cysts, with a mean diameter of greater than 10 cm, as they are difficult to remove from the abdominal cavity without rupture [25]. Preoperative assessment of cyst composition may encourage surgeons to prepare surgical bags in which to manoeuvre the cyst during surgical treatment, allowing a method to "catch" fluid leakage. For larger solid lesions, a mini-laparotomy may be preferable to laparoscopy and ultrasound can be used perioperatively to localize the incision directly above the cyst. A purse string suture can be used around the cyst capsule to contain any spillage, minimize blood loss and facilitate rapid surgical closure once cystectomy is complete.

2.2.6 Ectopic pregnancy

In modern clinical practice, TVS in conjunction with measurements of serum human chorionic gonadotrophin and progesterone enables accurate preoperative detection of most ectopic pregnancies. Imaging is also helpful in safely triaging women to either conservative or surgical management. It has been shown that approximately 30–40% of tubal ectopic pregnancies can be safely and successfully managed nonsurgically [26, 27]. In current practice, the role of laparoscopy for diagnosis of ectopic pregnancy is limited and it is now almost exclusively used for the treatment. Ultrasound examination can also be used to assess the amount of hemopertioneum, which is important in prioritizing women for surgery. It can also help to decide whether open surgery should be considered when highly skilled minimally invasive surgeons are not immediately available for emergency operations.

Preoperative ultrasound examination is also helpful in determining the exact location of ectopic pregnancy. This is particularly important in women with rare types of ectopic pregnancies such as interstitial, cornual, ovarian, and abdominal pregnancies (Fig. 2.5). Surgical treatment of these pregnancies is often technically more difficult compared to tubal ectopics and the correct preoperative diagnosis is vital for planning of surgical technique and ensuring availability of surgeons with expertise and skill to carry out advanced minimally invasive procedures.

2.3 Conclusion

Ultrasound has an invaluable role in surgical triage, identifying which women should be managed in a specialist center (endometriosis center or cancer center) or by a specialist team (multidisciplinary team approach). Ultrasound improves planning of type and site of surgical incisions and informs surgical teams what equipment may be required and the expected timing of surgery. Selection criteria

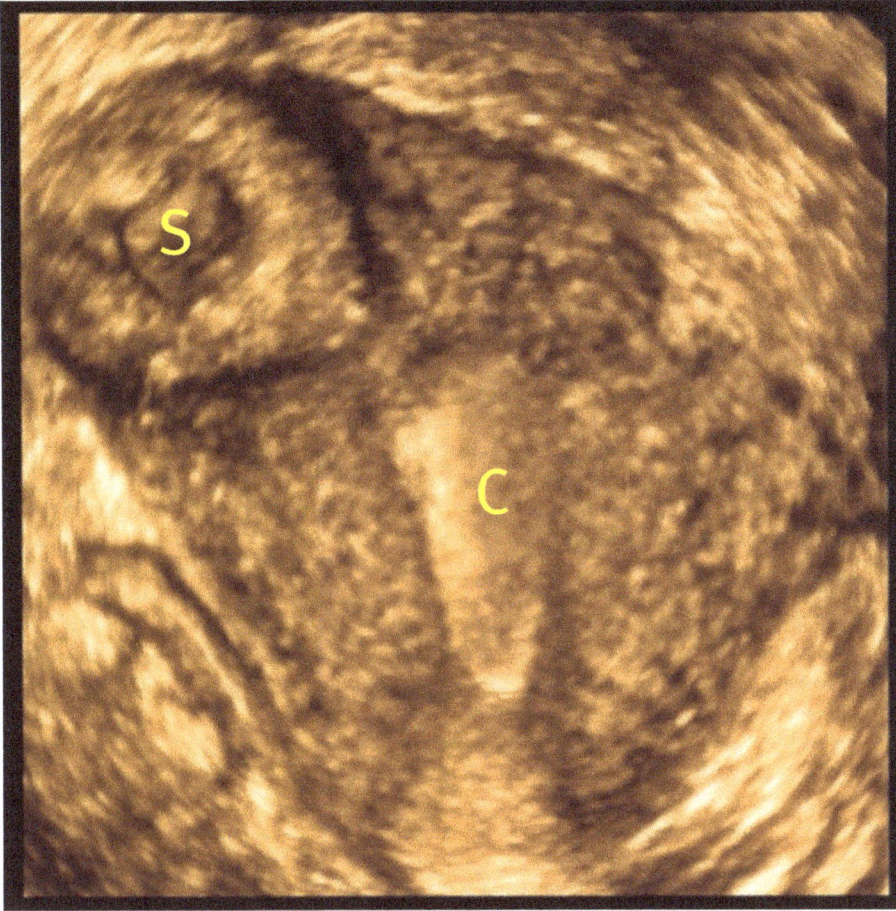

Fig. 2.5: A three-dimensional scan showing a coronal view of the uterus. A gestational sac (S) is seen within the right interstitial tube. These findings are typical of an interstitial ectopic pregnancy. Uterine cavity (C).

for performing laparoscopic surgery may be used to identify those women in whom the risk of conversion to laparotomy is low and are suitable for day case surgery and enhanced recovery programs.

Detailed preoperative TVS examination, performed by skilled and experience individuals, is helpful for assessing the feasibility of laparoscopic surgery in women with benign adnexal lesions. The assessment of tumor morphology and mobility helps counsel women about the specific risks associated with surgery, including conversion to laparotomy and their anticipated recovery. Ultrasound assessment of women with suspected endometriosis has greatly improved in recent years. The introduction of high-resolution TVS scanning combined with targeted palpation enables accurate diagnosis and staging of pelvic endometriosis. This has facilitated the referral of women to minimally invasive surgeons who are highly skilled in the management of severe pelvic endometriosis and the involvement of a specialist multidisciplinary approach. Adjuvant and perioperative methods have further enhanced the use of ultrasound in maximizing the role of minimally invasive surgery for management of women with both benign and malignant gynecological pathologies.

References

[1] Timmerman D, Schwärzler P, Collins WP, et al. Subjective assessment of adnexal masses with the use of ultrasonography: an analysis of interobserver variability and experience. Ultrasound Obstet Gynecol 1999;13:11–6.

[2] Guerriero S, Condous G, Van den Bosch T, et al. Systematic approach to sonographic evaluation of the pelvis in women with suspected endometriosis, including terms, definitions and measurements: a consensus opinion from the International Deep Endometriosis Analysis (IDEA) group. Ultrasound Obstet Gynecol 2016 Sep 1;48(3):318–32.

[3] Guerriero S, Ajossa S, Lai MP, Mais V, Paoletti AM, Melis GB. Transvaginal ultrasonography in the diagnosis of pelvic adhesions. Hum Reprod 1997;12:2649–53.

[4] Okaro E, Condous G, Khalid A, et al. The use of ultrasound-based 'soft markers' for the prediction of pelvic pathology in women with chronic pelvic pain—can we reduce the need for laparoscopy? BJOG 2006;113:251–6.

[5] Yazbek J, Helmy S, Ben-Nagi J, Holland T, Sawyer E, Jurkovic D. Value of preoperative ultrasound examination in the selection of women with adnexal masses for laparoscopic surgery. Ultrasound Obstet Gynecol 2007;30:883–8.

[6] Holland TK, Yazbek J, Cutner A, Saridogan E, Hoo WL, Jurkovic D. Value of transvaginal ultrasound in assessing severity of pelvic endometriosis. Ultrasound Obstet Gynecol 2010 Aug 1;36(2):241–8.

[7] Kennedy S, Bergqvist A, Chapron C, et al. ESHRE guideline for the diagnosis and treatment of endometriosis. Hum Reprod 2005;20:2698–704.

[8] Jacobson TZ, Barlow DH, Garry R, Koninckx P. Laparoscopic surgery for pelvic pain associated with endometriosis. Cochrane Database Syst Rev 2001:CD001300.

[9] Dunselman GA, Vermeulen N, Becker C, Calhaz-Jorge C, D'Hooghe T, De Bie B, Heikinheimo O, Horne AW, Kiesel L, Nap A et al. ESHRE guideline: management of women with endometriosis. Hum Reprod 2014;29:400–412.

[10] Fedele L, Bianchi S, Raffaelli R, Portuese A. Pre-operative assessment of bladder endometriosis. Hum Reprod 1997 Nov 1;12(11):2519–22.

[11] Pateman K, Mavrelos D, Hoo WL, Holland T, Naftalin J, Jurkovic D. Visualization of ureters on standard gynecological transvaginal scan: a feasibility study. Ultrasound Obstet Gynecol 2013 Jun 1;41(6):696–701.

[12] Granberg S, Wikland M, Jansson I. Macroscopic characterization of ovarian tumors and the relation to the histological diagnosis: criteria to be used for ultrasound evaluation. Gynecol Oncol 1989;35:139–44.

[13] Granberg S, Norstrom A, Wikland M. Tumors in the lower pelvis as imaged by vaginal sonography. Gynecol Oncol 1990;37:224–9.

[14] Rehn M, Lohmann K, Rempen A. Transvaginal ultrasonography of pelvic masses: Evaluation of B-mode technique and Doppler ultrasonography. Am J Obstet Gynecol 1996;175:97–104.

[15] Buy JN, Ghossain MA, Hugol D, et al. Characterization of adnexal masses: combination of color Doppler and conventional sonography compared with spectral Doppler analysis alone and conventional sonography alone. Am J Roentgenol 1996;166:385–93.

[16] Valentin L, Sladkevicius P, Marsal K. Limited contribution of Doppler velocimetry to the differential diagnosis of extrauterine pelvic tumors. Obstet Gynecol 1994;83:425–33.

[17] Nunes N, Foo X, Widschwendter M, Jurkovic D. A randomised controlled trial comparing surgical intervention rates between two protocols for the management of asymptomatic adnexal tumours in postmenopausal women. BMJ Open 2012 Jan 1;2(6):e002248.

[18] Valentin L, Hagen B, Tingulstad S, Eik-Nes S. Comparison of 'pattern recognition' and logistic regression models for discrimination between benign and malignant pelvic masses: a prospective cross validation. Ultrasound Obstet Gynecol 2001;18:357–65.

[19] Valentin L. Use of morphology to characterize and manage common adnexal masses. Best Pract Res Clin Obstet Gynaecol 2004;18:71–89.

[20] Bean EM, Cutner A, Holland T, Vashisht A, Jurkovic D, Saridogan E. Laparoscopic myomectomy: a single-centre retrospective review of 514 patients. J Minim Invasive Gynaecol 2017 Apr 30;24(3);485–93.

[21] Hasanzadeh MA, Tabare SH, Mirzaean S. Ovarian dermoid cyst. Professional Med J 2010 Jan 1;17(3):512–5.

[22] Caspi B, Appelman Z, Rabinerson D, Zalel Y, Tulandi T, Shoham Z. The growth pattern of ovarian dermoid cysts: a prospective study in premenopausal and postmenopausal women. Fertil Steril 1997 Sep 1;68(3):501–5.

[23] Huss M, Lafay-Pillet MC, Lecuru F, et al. Granulomatous peritonitis after laparoscopic surgery of an ovarian dermoid cyst. Diagnosis, management, prevention, a case report. J Gynecol Obstet Biol Reprod 1996;25(4):365–72.

[24] Coccia ME, Becattini C, Bracco GL, Scarselli G. Infertility: case report: acute abdomen following dermoid cyst rupture during transvaginal ultrasonographically guided retrieval of oocytes. Hum Reprod 1996 Sep 1;11(9):1897–9.

[25] Remorgida V, Magnasco A, Pizzorno V, Anserini P. Four year experience in laparoscopic dissection of intact ovarian dermoid cysts. J Am Coll Surg 1998 Nov 30;187(5):519–21.

[26] Elson J, Tailor A, Banerjee S, Salim R, Hillaby K, Jurkovic D. Expectant management of tubal ectopic pregnancy: prediction of successful outcome using decision tree analysis. Ultrasound Obstet Gynecol 2004 Jun 1;23(6):552–6.

[27] Mavrelos D, Memtsa M, Helmy S, Derdelis G, Jauniaux E, Jurkovic D. β-hCG resolution times during expectant management of tubal ectopic pregnancies. BMC Womens Health 2015 May 21;15(1):43.

Alexis McQuitty

3 Anesthetic considerations for minimally invasive surgery

3.1 Introduction

Three conditions uniquely alter the patient's physiology during laparoscopic procedures: increase in intraabdominal pressure (IAP) (pneumoperitoneum [PNP]), patient positioning, and use of carbon dioxide for insufflation [1]. These procedures are safe, and there are few consequences for healthy women; however, complications may occur during long or extensive surgeries or in those with coexisting medical conditions. Patients with increased intracranial pressure (ICP), glaucoma, severe uncorrected hypovolemia, and intracardiac shunts are poor candidates for many minimally invasive surgeries (MISs) [2, 3]. Caution should be used with renal or hepatic disease.

3.2 Consequences of CO_2 PNP

The physiologic response to CO_2 PNP is influenced by intravascular volume, preoperative medications, cardiopulmonary status, and anesthetic agents [4]. With proper management, many hemodynamic changes that occur with CO_2 PNP will be clinically insignificant.

Bradycardia may occur with high IAP [5]. This may be associated with high vagal tone or preoperative beta-blockade; slow insufflation may limit heart rate changes, and tachyphylaxis of this response occurs. Glycopyrrolate and atropine are rarely indicated.

A biphasic cardiac output (CO) response occurs with increasing IAP. Initially, due to higher preload, CO increases; then, as venous return decreases, CO may decrease [5]. Minimal effects may be seen in healthy individuals, and CO may decrease more with IAP > 15 mmHg. The mean arterial pressure (MAP), systemic vascular resistance, and central venous pressure (CVP) may all increase due to IAP and increasing sympathetic tone. Volatile anesthetic agents and judicious fluid management may mitigate many of these effects.

Significant hypercarbia may have detrimental effects on those unable to compensate (elderly, coronary artery disease); myocardial dysfunction and arrhythmias may develop if the respiratory acidosis is severe [6]. Caution should be used in those with pulmonary hypertension, as hybercarbia may exacerbate this condition and further strain the right ventricle. CO may decrease up to 60% after abdominal insufflation in patients with severe cardiac disease (valvular disorders, congestive heart failure), and inotropic support may be necessary [7]. CO_2 PNP should be used

https://doi.org/10.1515/9783110535204-003

cautiously in poorly compensated patients in the ICU, as it may further increase left ventricular afterload, decrease CO, and exacerbate the ill-effects of positive end-expiratory pressure (PEEP) [8].

With abdominal insufflation, the peak and plateau airway pressures increase. Pulmonary compliance and functional residual capacity decrease. These changes may be significant in those with obesity [9] or cardiopulmonary disease; without physiologic compensation or ventilator adjustments, hypercarbia and hypoxemia may occur. Although atelectasis occurs, it appears that redistribution of blood flow away from these collapsed regions limits pulmonary shunting (and hypoxemia) when hypercapnia is present [10].

Hypercarbia increases in response to higher IAP with CO_2 PNP, and Badawy *et al.* [11] reported an incidence of hypercapnia in 18% of 133 robotic hysterectomy patients. Insufflation time influences the uptake of CO_2; after 2 hours, there may be an end-tidal CO_2 ($EtCO_2$) increase of 2 kPa [12]. In healthy patients, the $EtCO_2$-$PaCO_2$ gradient is <5, and $EtCO_2$ can be used to monitor hypercarbia. Patients with pulmonary disease may have a higher gradient, and this gradient increases with long insufflation times, age, and obesity [13, 14].

With constant $EtCO_2$ and MAP, cerebral blood flow and ICP increase as a direct result of higher IAP [15]. Hypercapnia may worsen these effects. Obese patients have chronically elevated IAP and ICP, although usually clinically insignificant. Compared to nonobese patients, these patients will have higher elevations of ICP with PNP [16]. The elevated ICP and subsequent slight decrease in cerebral perfusion pressure should not affect the outcome and have little clinical relevance in healthy women [17].

Alterations in renal and splanchnic perfusion are proportional to the pressure and length of time of PNP. Renal and hepatic flow is significantly compromised with increasing IAP; this should be a consideration in patients with existing disease when determining suitability for MIS [2]. Insufflation pressures >20 mmHg reduce gastrointestinal blood flow, and metabolic acidosis will ensue if high IAP is sustained. Both impaired CO and mechanical compression of renal arteries reduce renal blood flow and increase renin release. Patients with chronic kidney disease may develop acute or chronic kidney injury, as higher IAP also decreases glomerular filtration rate and urine output [5]. PNP can cause an increase in antidiuretic levels [4], with resultant oliguria (also influenced by positioning and pooling of urine in the bladder).

3.3 Consequences of patient positioning

Positioning in steep Trendelenburg (sTb) may contribute to the physiologic consequences of PNP. Cephalad movement of the diaphragm can further increase peak airway pressures, requiring ventilator adjustments. Obese patients with higher visceral versus subcutaneous fat will have higher peak airway pressures with positioning. Higher amounts of intraabdominal fat correlate with pulmonary intolerance in sTb, and the degree of tilt may need to be limited [18]. As higher IAP may decrease CO, sTb may increase preload and slightly improve CO (to compensate for the decrease seen with PNP). Higher cardiac filling pressures may be worrisome for those with systolic and diastolic dysfunction. It should be noted that hypotension due to decreased venous return may occur with the head-up position, which is rarely used for gynecologic MIS.

Although most develop facial edema, it is unlikely to reflect airway edema, which would delay extubation [11]. Airway resistance due to edema may persist into the postoperative period, even in those without chronic obstructive pulmonary disease (COPD); this resistance begins to improve in the first 2 hours after return to the 30-degree head-up position [19]. Endobronchial (mainstem) migration of the endotracheal tube (ETT) may occur and should be suspected with high airway pressures. As it may be difficult to replace the ETT in sTb, a bronchoscope can assist with the ETT positioning.

There can be many neurologic sequelae to the positioning of the patient for MIS. These include both cerebral effects and peripheral nerve injuries. There can be further increases in ICP with sTb. Younger patients have better cerebral autoregulation; however, cerebral edema is still a concern with lengthy procedures [20]. At 3 hours of sTb, cerebral oxygenation is maintained (although postoperative cerebral complications with very lengthy sTb have occurred) [21].

Patients should be examined preoperatively for any preexisting neuropathy, especially those with higher risk conditions: obesity, diabetes mellitus, peripheral vascular disease, heavy alcohol intake, and expected lengthy surgery [22, 23]. Although most positioning nerve injuries are mild and resolve (e.g., foot numbness), the incidence of these injuries may approach 2% [24, 25]. sTb with shoulder braces may result in varying degrees of brachial plexus neuropathies, and incorrectly tucking the arms or robotic arm compression may cause upper extremity nerve injury. Extreme flexion of the hip can cause nerve damage by stretch (sciatic, obturator) or by pressure (femoral nerve under the inguinal ligament). Compression injury may occur in the distal lower extremities with positioning devices; the common peroneal and saphenous nerves are at risk [26].

In the lithotomy position, calf compression (by boot devices) and hip flexion (in conjunction with PNP) predispose the patient to venous thromboembolism and compartment syndrome. Patients in the lithotomy position for >5 hours are at high risk [2, 26]. Lower elevation of the legs and the time limitation of this position lower the risk. Ankle sling supports or intermittent return to the supine position may be considered for prolonged procedures.

Studies have shown that prolonged sTb results in a significant increase in intraocular pressure (IOP) and decrease in ocular perfusion pressure [20, 27], which returns to baseline postoperatively [28]. This transient increase in IOP does not appear to affect healthy eyes, and vision loss is very rare. Eyes with preexisting disease may not tolerate the increase in IOP, and those with glaucoma may experience higher elevations in IOP, a risk factor for vision impairment.

3.4 Anesthetic management

The preoperative evaluation includes a thorough history and physical examination with emphasis on cardiac and pulmonary conditions. With adequate exercise tolerance, no further testing is usually indicated. Consultation may be needed for optimization of higher-risk populations: elderly, morbidly obese, ischemic heart disease, cardiac murmurs, COPD, heavy tobacco use, and neurosurgery history/ventriculoperitoneal shunts [29]. Several published guidelines offer algorithms for preoperative management of patients with cardiac disease for noncardiac surgery (acc.org, escardio.org). Dyspnea may be cardiac or noncardiac in origin, and a cause should be elicited (e.g., decompensated heart failure versus ascites due to ovarian cancer).

The type of anesthetic is dictated by hospital costs and physician preference. Management includes perioperative thromboprophylaxis, especially for obese and oncology patients [30]. To avoid hypovolemia, oral hydration is encouraged until 2 hours prior to surgery (per many anesthesia guidelines). Those at risk for aspiration may receive H_2 antagonists or nonparticulate antacids.

Enhanced recovery pathways involve the coordination of many care teams. Implementation of these guidelines can improve patient pain scores and decrease hospital costs, opioid use, and length of stay [31]. Many of these recommendations are beneficial for anesthetic care, including the following: patient optimization (e.g., stop smoking); correction of anemia preoperatively; adequate preoperative hydration, avoid benzodiazepines if possible, use thromboembolism prophylaxis, use short-acting anesthetic agents and protective lung strategies for ventilation (e.g., 5–7 cc/kg TV), multimodal agents for nausea and pain control (limit narcotics), maintain normothermia, avoid liberal fluid regimes (helpful for sTb cases) and maintain euvolemia (using advance hemodynamic monitors as needed) [32]. These guidelines may assist with early ambulation.

MIS can be completed using general (GA), regional (RA), or a combined anesthetic. GA may assist with the patient work of breathing (avoid fatigue) and ensure a secure airway with robotic surgeries (the airway may not be easily accessible). GA with an ETT can provide patient comfort, controlled ventilation to correct hypercarbia, muscle relaxation, airway protection from regurgitation due to higher IAP and gastric tube placement (higher gastric pressure with insufflation) [33]. GA with volatile anesthetic agents can be utilized to control elevation of blood pressure [34]. Adequate anesthesia depth and analgesia are needed; patient movement is dangerous when the robotic trocars are fixed in place [17]. Although GA may be the safe and conservative approach, RA (epidural, spinal) as the sole anesthetic can be used; this requires a lower IAP, patient cooperation, and minimal Trendelenburg angle and can be considered in women with severe pulmonary disease. With many MISs for neoplasm, a combined GA/epidural anesthetic results in overall reduced amount of anesthetic, hemodynamic stability, good postoperative analgesia, and reduced recovery time [35].

The usual standard monitoring for GA is needed for MIS, including temperature and frequent documentation of the positioning. The peak and plateau ventilator pressures should be recorded. Urine output and pulse oximetry should also be monitored postoperatively until values return to normal. Obese women with obstructive sleep apnea may require longer monitoring; immediately after surgery, continuous positive airway pressure may decrease atelectasis, hypercapnia, and reintubation [36].

As most MISs are low-risk procedures, invasive monitoring is rare; the positioning and IAP requirements are usually tolerated in older and more debilitated patients [6]. Invasive monitoring can be used for prolonged operative times in higher-risk patients; arterial lines can be used for blood analysis and assist with hemodynamic monitoring of cardiopulmonary disease patients. Blood pressure cuffs may be too small and the $EtCO_2$-$PaCO_2$ gradient may be higher in obese patients. Although MIS can be safe in obesity with proper monitoring, there is higher perioperative morbidity [37].

CVP may be a poor indicator of preload and misleading to guide fluid management, as IAP and intrathoracic pressure are increased. Pulse pressure variation (PPV) can be measured during mechanical ventilation and used to guide fluid therapy [38]. As a measure of volume responsiveness available with arterial blood pressure monitoring systems, PPV allows for early detection of hypovolemia and avoidance of fluid overload. Significant fluid shifts may occur during some advanced oncologic surgeries [31]. Fluid management may be optimized using goal-directed algorithms, invasive monitoring, or many of the less invasive CO monitors available (e.g., esophageal Doppler).

As an alternative to an ETT, many MIS centers have shown the efficacy and safety of supraglottic airway devices (SADs) with PNP; however, there is no guaranteed protection against pulmonary aspiration [39, 40]. Many of the published case studies involve limited Trendelenburg (not steep) or reverse Trendelenburg, lower insufflation pressures and short operative times. In healthy patients (e.g., no obesity, diabetes, or gastroesophageal reflux), a SAD can be used safely if the PNP time and the degree of sTb (<15 degrees) are limited [41]. In this population, a maximum incidence of regurgitation was 2.5% when utilizing a ProSeal device (Teleflex, USA).

Anesthesia management during surgery involves avoidance of hypoxemia and significant hypercapnia. Both pressure control (PCV) and volume control can be used, and spontaneous ventilation may be inadequate to compensate for hypercarbia in the sTb position. In patients with cardiopulmonary or restrictive lung disease due to morbid obesity, PCV may offer some advantages: lower peak airway pressures and higher intraoperative lung compliance [42]. The $EtCO_2$, $PaCO_2$ and pH can remain within physiologic range by increasing minute ventilation (usually by ⇧ respiratory rate). Hyperventilation (with hypocapnia) and large tidal volumes should be avoided [43, 44].

Application of PEEP (up to 10 cmH$_2$0) during PNP may improve oxygenation, ventilation (limiting respiratory acidosis), compliance, and perioperative stress response (reduced cortisol rise postoperatively) [45]. Although PEEP can improve gas exchange and decrease atelectasis [46], it should be used cautiously in those with marginal cardiac function, hypovolemia, or emphysema. In normovolemic patients without cardiac disease, PEEP applied after PNP will have minimal effects on CO and may prevent caval collapse induced by higher IAP [47].

Proper positioning is critical for the surgical team; without it, surgical times can be long and complications may occur. Higher positioning injuries may be seen with extremes of weight, diabetes, elderly, peripheral vascular disease and preexisting neuropathy [25]. With PNP and hip flexion, there is a reduction in femoral venous flows and a higher risk for venous thrombosis [48]. Sequential pneumatic compression of the lower extremities is recommended for prolonged laparoscopic procedures, and this can be combined with pharmacologic prophylaxis (e.g., subcutaneous heparin).

Many strategies may prevent injury: protective padding of joints, no shoulder braces, blood pressure cuffs placed above the antecubital fossa, antiskid foam mattresses with gel pads to prevent sliding and pressure on shoulders [25, 49]. A patient consent regarding the positioning risk and assessment of any limitation before surgery is recommended [26]. An intermittent return to supine or head-up position can improve IOP and airway edema [27]; moving the legs from lithotomy every 2 hours can also improve circulation and help prevent injury [26].

3.5 Pain control

For the prevention of postoperative pain, a wide range of treatment options exists (www.jpain.com). Despite small incisions, many require postoperative opioids [2]. A multimodal pain regimen with less opioid may limit the hospital stay, improve return of bowel function, and allow for early ambulation.

Postoperative infiltration of bupivacaine can significantly reduce pain at the trocar sites [50], and intraperitoneal spray with local anesthetic has been used. Various peripheral nerve blocks (including transverse abdominis plane and paravertebral) can be combined with intravenous (IV) or oral medication.

Preemptive use of low-dose ketamine (<.5 mg/kg) may allow for hemodynamic stability and improved pain control, especially in women with chronic pain conditions. This low dose avoids the psychomimetic effects [51].

Preoperative gabapentin may reduce pain and nausea [52]. Intraoperative acetaminophen and ketorolac are also beneficial. Magnesium or dexmedetomidine infusions can ameliorate operative pain responses [53]. These anesthetic adjuncts, without opioids, can assist with the avoidance of respiratory depression in pulmonary disease.

3.6 Management of complications

Most anesthetic complications are minor, and preparation will help prevent serious complications. For MIS with limited access to the patient, it is important to strongly secure the ETT, use extension IV tubing, and place an extra peripheral IV before positioning the patient. Vigilance is needed to prevent airway, ocular, and extremity positioning injuries. Corneal abrasions may occur in up to 3% of robotic cases. This may be a direct mechanical injury (robot arms) or can occur due to desiccation, as edema may open the eyelids and expose the cornea. A key to prevention is the use of an ocular lubricant and transparent film dressing.

A multimodal antiemetic regimen is recommended for gynecologic MIS. There are many strategies to reduce the risk of nausea/vomiting: avoid inhalation agents for patients with history of postoperative emesis, use propofol infusions, avoid nitrous oxide, minimize opioids, and provide adequate hydration [52]. The choice of medications is based on history and the intraoperative course. These medications include 5-HT3 rc antagonists, NK-1 rc antagonists, and dexamethasone (one dose at induction, may avoid in diabetics). Antihistamines and anticholinergics (transdermal scopalamine) can be considered.

Hemodynamic emergencies are rare and related to medical comorbidities, patient anatomy, IAP and length of PNP, and the skill of the physicians. Using low to moderate insufflation pressure (<12 mmHg), low gas flows and shorter periods of PNP may limit the associated physiologic perturbations [6]. Subcutaneous emphysema, while not life-threatening, may occur with extraperitoneal insufflation and should be suspected with significantly increasing $EtCO_2$ [5]. This may also be associated with capnothorax, which is treated conservatively (remove PNP, provide oxygen). Major complications include CO_2 embolus, pneumothorax (can occur with high peak airway pressure) and pneumomediastinum. Small CO_2 emboli may cause an increase in $EtCO_2$ with minimal hemodynamic changes, while a large embolus results in a decrease in $EtCO_2$ and CO [54]. In the event of an emergency, the laparoscopic arms must be disengaged prior to cardiopulmonary resuscitation [55].

3.7 Summary

Anesthetic complications due to prolonged periods of PNP and steep Trendelenburg positioning are rare [11]. With adequate preparation and a team approach to management, MIS may be safely performed in many patients, including the morbidly obese, the elderly, and those with cardiopulmonary conditions.

References

[1] Henny CP, Hofland J. Laparoscopic surgery: pitfalls due to anesthesia, positioning, and pneumoperitoneum. Surg Endosc 2005;19:1163–71.

[2] Hayden P, Cowman S. Anaesthesia for laparoscopic surgery: Table 1. Contin Educ Anaesth Crit Care 2011;11:177–80.

[3] Hoshikawa Y, Tsutsumi N, Ohkoshi K, et al. The effect of steep Trendelenburg positioning on intraocular pressure and visual function during robotic-assisted radical prostatectomy. Br J Ophthalmol 2014;98:305–8.

[4] O'Malley C, Cunningham A. Physiologic changes during laparoscopy. Anesthesiol Clin 2001;19:1–19.

[5] Atkinson TM, Giraud GD, Togioka BM, Jones DB, Cigarroa JE. Cardiovascular and ventilatory consequences of laparoscopic surgery. Circulation 2017;135:700–10.

[6] Gutt CN, Oniu T, Mehrabi A, et al. Circulatory and respiratory complications of carbon dioxide insufflation. Dig Surg 2004;21:95–105.

[7] Tillman Hein H, Joshi G, Ramsay M, et al. Hemodynamic Changes during laparoscopic cholecystectomy in patients with severe cardiac disease. J Clin Anesth 1997;9:261–5.

[8] Moffa SM, Quinn JV, Slotman GJ. Hemodynamic effects of carbon dioxide pneumoperitoneum during mechanical ventilation and positive end-expiratory pressure. J Trauma Injury Infect Crit Care 1993;35:613–8.

[9] Tomescu DR, Popescu M, Dima SO, Bacalbasa N, Bubenek-Turconi S. Obesity is associated with decreased lung compliance and hypercapnia during robotic assisted surgery. J Clin Monit Comput 2017;31:85–92.

[10] Ketabchi F, Egemnazarov B, Schermuly RT, et al. Effects of hypercapnia with and without acidosis on hypoxic pulmonary vasoconstriction. Am J Physiol Lung Cell Mol Physiol 2009;297:L977–83.

[11] Badawy M, Beique F, Al-Halal H, et al. Anesthesia considerations for robotic surgery in gynecologic oncology. J Robot Surg 2011;5:235–9.

[12] Kendall A, Bhatt S, Oh T. Pulmonary consequences of carbon dioxide insufflation for laparoscopic cholecystectomies. Anaesthesia 1995;50:286–9.

[13] Satoh K, Chikuda M, Ohashi A, et al. Arterial and end-tidal carbon dioxide in supine obese patients during general anesthesia. Open J Anesthesiol 2015;05:79–84.

[14] Choi DK, Lee IG, Hwang JH. Arterial to end-tidal carbon dioxide pressure gradient increases with age in the steep Trendelenburg position with pneumoperitoneum. Korean J Anesthesiol 2012;63:209–15.

[15] Kamine TH, Elmadhun NY, Kasper EM, Papavassiliou E, Schneider BE. Abdominal insufflation for laparoscopy increases intracranial and intrathoracic pressure in human subjects. Surg Endosc 2016;30:4029–32.

[16] Dip F, Nguyen D, Sasson M, et al. The relationship between intracranial pressure and obesity: an ultrasonographic evaluation of the optic nerve. Surg Endosc 2016;30:2321–5.

[17] Irwin M, Wong S. Anaesthesia and minimally invasive surgery. Anaesth Intensive Care Med 2015;16:17–20.

[18] Abdelbadee AY, Paspulati RM, McFarland HD, et al. Computed tomography morphometrics and pulmonary intolerance in endometrial cancer robotic surgery. J Minim Invasive Gynecol 2016;23:1075–82.

[19] Kilic OF, Borgers A, Kohne W, et al. Effects of steep Trendelenburg position for robotic-assisted prostatectomies on intra- and extrathoracic airways in patients with or without chronic obstructive pulmonary disease. Br J Anaesth 2015;114:70–6.

[20] Blecha S, Harth M, Schlachetzki F, et al. Changes in intraocular pressure and optic nerve sheath diameter in patients undergoing robotic-assisted laparoscopic prostatectomy in steep 45° Trendelenburg position. BMC Anesthesiol 2017;17:40.

[21] Closhen D, Treiber AH, Berres M, et al. Robotic assisted prostatic surgery in the Trendelenburg position does not impair cerebral oxygenation measured using two different monitors: a clinical observational study. Eur J Anaesthesiol 2014;31:104–9.

[22] Abdalmageed OS, Bedaiwy MA, Falcone T. Nerve Injuries in gynecologic laparoscopy. J Minim Invasive Gynecol 2017;24:16–27.

[23] Sukhu T, Krupski TL. Patient positioning and prevention of injuries in patients undergoing laparoscopic and robot-assisted urologic procedures. Curr Urol Rep 2014;15:398.

[24] Maerz DA, Beck LN, Sim AJ, Gainsburg DM. Complications of robotic-assisted laparoscopic surgery distant from the surgical site. Br J Anaesth 2017;118:492–503.

[25] Fleisch MC, Bremerich D, Schulte-Mattler W, et al. The prevention of positioning injuries during gynecologic operations. Guideline of DGGG (S1-Level, AWMF Registry No. 015/077, February 2015). Geburtshilfe Frauenheilkd 2015;75:792–807.

[26] Knight DJW, Mahajan RP. Patient positioning in anaesthesia. Contin Educ Anaesth Crit Care Pain 2004;4:160–3.

[27] Borahay MA, Patel PR, Walsh TM, et al. Intraocular pressure and steep Trendelenburg during minimally invasive gynecologic surgery: is there a risk? J Minim Invasive Gynecol 2013;20:819–24.

[28] Ozcan MF, Akbulut Z, Gurdal C, et al. Does steep Trendelenburg positioning effect the ocular hemodynamics and intraocular pressure in patients undergoing robotic cystectomy and robotic prostatectomy? Int Urol Nephrol 2017;49:55–60.

[29] Cobianchi L, Dominioni T, Filisetti C, et al. Ventriculoperitoneal shunt and the need to remove a gallbladder: Time to definitely overcome the feeling that laparoscopic surgery is contraindicated. Ann Med Surg (Lond) 2014;3:65–7.

[30] Morosan M, Popham P. Anaesthesia for gynaecological oncological surgery. Contin Educ Anaesth Crit Care 2014;14:63–8.

[31] Chapman JS, Roddy E, Ueda S, et al. Enhanced recovery pathways for improving outcomes after minimally invasive gynecologic oncology surgery. Obstet Gynecol 2016;128:138–44.

[32] Nelson G, Altman AD, Nick A, et al. Guidelines for pre- and intra-operative care in gynecologic/oncology surgery: Enhanced Recovery After Surgery (ERAS(R)) Society recommendations—part I. Gynecol Oncol 2016;140:313–22.

[33] Minimally invasive surgery fundamentals. In: Hoffman BL, Schorge JO, Bradshaw KD, Halvorson LM, Schaffer JI, Corton MM, eds. Williams Gynecology. 3rd ed. New York, NY: McGraw-Hill Education; 2016.

[34] Makwana D, Patil P, Kerketta C, Ghoghari D, Patel B. A Comparison of EtCO2 and PaCO2 in laparoscopic surgery during general anaesthesia. GCSMC J Med Sci 2014;III:12–5.

[35] Xu Q, Zhang H, Zhu Y-M, Shi N-J. Effects of combined general/epidural anesthesia on hemodynamics, respiratory function, and stress hormone levels in patients with ovarian neoplasm undergoing laparoscopy. Med Sci Monit 2016;22:4238–46.

[36] De Jong A, Chanques G, Jaber S. Mechanical ventilation in obese ICU patients: from intubation to extubation. Crit Care 2017;21:63.

[37] Khoury W, Kiran RP, Jessie T, Geisler D, Remzi FH. Is the laparoscopic approach to colectomy safe for the morbidly obese? Surg Endosc 2010;24:1336–40.

[38] Bliacheriene F MS, Fonseca EB, Otsuke D, Auler JO Jr, Michard F. Pulse pressure variation as a tool to detect hypovolaemia during pneumoperitoneum. Acta Anaethesiol Scand 2007;51:1268–72.

[39] Subramanian S, Divya S. Supraglottic devices in laparoscopic surgery—a review of literature. J Anesth Clin Care 2016;3.

[40] Chen BZ, Tan L, Zhang L, Shang YC. Is muscle relaxant necessary in patients undergoing laparoscopic gynecological surgery with a ProSeal LMA? J Clin Anesth 2013;25:32–5.

[41] Lemos J, De Oliveira GS Jr, de Pereira Cardoso HE, et al. Gastric regurgitation in patients undergoing gynecological laparoscopy with a laryngeal mask airway: a prospective observational study. J Clin Anesth 2017;36:32–5.

[42] Liao CC, Kau YC, Ting PC, Tsai SC, Wang CJ. The Effects of volume-controlled and pressure-controlled ventilation on lung mechanics, oxidative stress, and recovery in gynecologic laparoscopic surgery. J Minim Invasive Gynecol 2016;23:410–7.

[43] Amato M, Barbas C, Medeiros D, et al. Effect of a protective-ventilation strategy on mortality in the acute respiratory distress syndrome. N Engl J Med 1998;338:347–54.

[44] Way M, Hill GE. Intraoperative end-tidal carbon dioxide concentrations: what is the target? Anesthesiol Res Pract 2011;2011:271539.

[45] Sen O, Erdogan Doventas Y. Effects of different levels of end-expiratory pressure on hemodynamic, respiratory mechanics and systemic stress response during laparoscopic cholecystectomy. Braz J Anesthesiol 2017;67:28–34.

[46] Kim JY, Shin CS, Kim HS, Jung WS, Kwak HJ. Positive end-expiratory pressure in pressure-controlled ventilation improves ventilatory and oxygenation parameters during laparoscopic cholecystectomy. Surg Endosc 2010;24:1099–103.

[47] Bernard D, Brandely A, Scatton O, et al. Positive end-expiratory pressure does not decrease cardiac output during laparoscopic liver surgery: a prospective observational evaluation. HPB (Oxford) 2017;19:36–41.

[48] Millard J, Hill B, Cook P, Fenoglio M, Stahlgren L. Intermittent sequential pneumatic compression in prevention of venous stasis associated with pneumoperitoneum during laparoscopic cholecystectomy. Arch Surg 1993;128:914–9.

[49] Practice advisory for the prevention of perioperative peripheral neuropathies 2018: an updated report by the American Society of Anesthesiologists Task Force on Prevention of Perioperative Peripheral Neuropathies. Anesthesiology 2018;128:11–26.

[50] Einarsson JI, Sun J, Orav J, Young AE. Local analgesia in laparoscopy: a randomized trial. Obstet Gynecol 2004;104:1335–9.

[51] Atashkhoyi S, Negargar S, Hatami-Marandi P. Effects of the addition of low-dose ketamine to propofol-fentanyl anaesthesia during diagnostic gynaecological laparoscopy. Eur J Obstet Gynecol Reprod Biol 2013;170:247–50.

[52] Gan TJ, Diemunsch P, Habib AS, et al. Consensus guidelines for the management of postoperative nausea and vomiting. Anesth Anal 2014;118:85–113.

[53] Zarif P, Abdelaal Ahmed Mahmoud A, Abdelhaq MM, Mikhail HM, Farag A. Dexmedetomidine versus magnesium sulfate as adjunct during anesthesia for laparoscopic colectomy. Anesthesiol Res Pract 2016;2016:7172920.

[54] Schoeffer P. Anaesthesia for Gynecological Endoscopy. Geneva Switzerland: Geneva Foundation for Medical Education and Research, 2017.

[55] Hsu R, Kaye A, Urman R. Anesthetic challenges in robotic-assisted urologic surgery. Rev Urol 2013;15:178–84.

Mohsen El-Sayed and Ertan Sarıdoğan

4 Principles and safe use of electrosurgery in minimally invasive surgery

The development of surgical energy sources has revolutionized minimally invasive surgery and facilitated the performance of more complex procedures. Electricity is the most commonly used type of energy in both open and endoscopic surgery due to its lower cost, availability and versatility. The use of Bovie generator by Cushing in 1926 was the turning point that paved the way for the modern applications of electrosurgery [1]. However, electrosurgery can cause serious complications, which can be attributed to the surgical technique or inherent flaws in the device design [2]. It is essential for the practicing surgeons to have a good understanding of the principles and safe use of electrosurgery.

4.1 Applied physics

Electrosurgery is the use of high-frequency alternating current in surgery to achieve the thermal tissue effects of cutting, desiccation, and coagulation. It is not a synonym for electrocautery, which is the passive transfer of heat to the tissue with no current passing through it. Electrosurgery uses high-frequency current to avoid the Faradic effect of nerve and muscle stimulation, which ceases at frequencies above 100 KHz. The electrosurgical circuit includes a generator, two electrodes, and the patient. Electrosurgical instruments may be monopolar or bipolar. The main difference between them is where the two electrodes are placed. The monopolar instrument has the active electrode, whereas the dispersive electrode is placed on the patient away from the active electrode. In contrast, the bipolar instrument has the two electrodes at its tip with no need for a dispersive electrode (Fig. 4.1). Table 4.1 summarizes the various electrical terms and their formulae. The generator or electrosurgical unit (ESU) converts the mains low frequency alternating current of 50–60 Hz to higher frequencies of 500 KHz–3 MHz. It also controls the wattage (power), voltage and duty cycle of the current [3].

4.2 Thermal tissue effects

Application of high-frequency current to the tissue results in friction of the oscillating intracellular ions, which leads to heat production. The resultant heat will cause various electrosurgical tissue effects. If the temperature rises rapidly to more than 100 °C, vaporization of intracellular water leads to cellular explosion. This results in a cutting effect. A gradual rise in temperature between 60 and 95 °C leads to

https://doi.org/10.1515/9783110535204-004

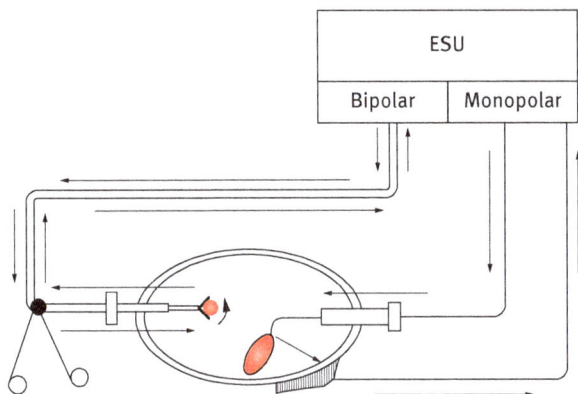

Fig. 4.1: Electrosurgical circuit with monopolar and bipolar devices. ESU, Electrosurgical unit.

Tab. 4.1: Essential terminology and formulae for electrosurgery

Electrical term	Definition/Formula	Unit
Current (I)	The rate of flow of electric charge in a circuit $I = V/R$ (Ohm's law)	Ampere (Amp) Coulomb/second
Current density (J)	The electric current per unit cross-sectional area of a conductor $J = I/A$ (current/area)	Amp/m^2
Voltage (V)	The electromotive force that pushes electrons along a circuit $V = I \times R$	Volt (V) Joule/Coulomb
Resistance (R)	The opposition to current flow in a circuit $R = V/I$	Ohm (Ω)
Power (P)	The rate at which energy (work) is transferred or changed $P = Q/T = V \times I$	Watt (W) Joule/second
Energy (Q) (Thermal)	The capacity for doing work $Q = P \times T = (I/A)^2 \times R \times T$ (Joule's first law)	Joule (j) Watt second
Duty cycle	The fraction of one on-and-off cycle in which the signal is on	Ratio or percentage (%)
Frequency	The number of waves per second	Hertz (Hz)
Waveform	The pattern of voltage changes over time as seen on an oscilloscope	
Circuit	The route of the flow of electric current	

A = area, T = time.

simultaneous tissue desiccation and coagulation. Fulguration is a type of coagulation where the current with high voltage is only on for 6% of the time. It is non-contact where electrical arcs hit the tissue to produce a superficial layer of black coagulation that insulates deeper tissue and reduces lateral thermal spread. It is ideal to deal with a wide oozing surface [3].

4.3 Monopolar devices

Monopolar instruments are the most common energy devices. They are versatile and produce tissue effects of cutting, coagulation, fulguration, and small vessel sealing. All these tissue effects are best achieved with the cut waveform except the fulguration that is best achieved with the coagulation waveform.

4.4 Factors modifying electrosurgical tissue effects

1. Waveform
The generator produces two main electrical waveforms with different tissue effects. A continuous sinusoidal waveform with a high current and low voltage raises the temperature to more than 100 °C and results in tissue cutting. An interrupted waveform with a low current and high voltage raises the temperature gradually to less than 100 °C that leads to tissue desiccation and coagulation. These two waveforms are inaccurately known as "cut" (yellow coded) and "coagulation" (blue coded) modes, respectively. Blend waveform is a modulated cut waveform with a variable duty cycle, current, and voltage to cause variable degrees of combined cutting and coagulation. Any of the above waveforms can produce both cutting and coagulation by altering the factors that influence the tissue effect (Fig. 4.2).

2. Power output
As complications are associated with higher power output, surgeons should use the lowest effective power setting. Generally, for effective cut mode, a power setting of

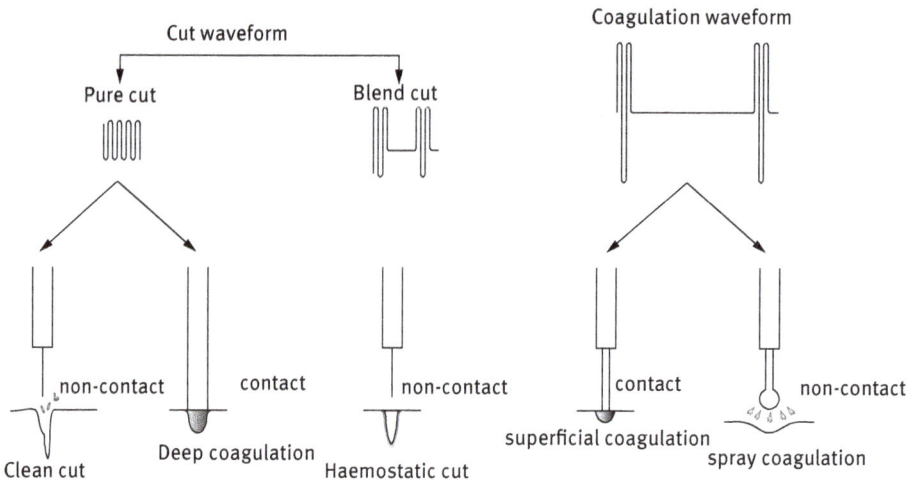

Fig. 4.2: Different electrosurgical tissue effects.

50–80 W is recommended, whereas 30–50 W is recommended for effective coagulation mode [4].

3. *Electrode surface area*
The smaller the electrode, the higher the current density and the higher the resulting heat is. Surgeons can use the narrow edge of the electrode to produce more heat and the wide side to produce less heat without changing the power output [5].

4. *Activation time*
Longer activation increases tissue damage, whereas too short application may not produce the intended tissue effect [4].

5. *Tissue contact*
In the cut and fulguration modes, current sparks from the active electrode to the tissue without contact. Coagulation and desiccation occur when there is contact between the active electrode and the tissue [3].

6. *Tissue impedance*
Thermal change is directly proportional to tissue impedance. Tissues with high water content as muscles and skin have low impedance. Conversely, scarred tissue and fat have high impedance. Surgeons can modify their technique to increase tissue impedance by removing blood, compressing arteries or stretching tissue. This leads to increased thermal effect without increasing the power output [5].

7. *Eschar*
As it has high impedance, surgeons are advised to clean the active electrode by removing eschar as this reduces impedance and produces the intended thermal effect.

4.5 Conventional bipolar devices

Bipolar devices were developed to overcome the inherent problems and associated complications of monopolar instruments. They are designed with two electrodes situated at the tip of the instrument. There is no need for a dispersive electrode as current passes through the grasped tissue between the two electrodes. They use continuous low-voltage waveform. Their vessel-sealing effect is achieved by the combined effect of desiccation, coagulation, and the mechanical compression of the vessel by the tines of the bipolar forceps. Surgeons rely on visual clues as vapor bubbles and color changes to assess the thermal tissue effects. Although they are generally safer than monopolar instruments, lateral thermal spread still occurs beyond the tines of the forceps, especially with a longer application (mushroom effect). Hence, surgeons must be careful when using bipolar instruments close to important structures. They also have to avoid overcompression of the bipolar tines as they can touch leading to electrical bypass and inadequate coagulation [6].

4.6 Advanced bipolar devices

The introduction of advanced bipolar devices was driven by the limitations of their conventional counterparts and the need for reliable hemostasis to undertake complex laparoscopic procedures. These devices can seal vessels up to 7 mm in diameter through mechanical compression and coagulation. Their generators have feedback mechanisms to monitor tissue impedance continually and adjust the delivered voltage and current accordingly so as to achieve the intended tissue effects with less thermal spread, charring, and smoke. Their generators produce a specific audio signal to indicate that vessel sealing is complete. They use less voltage than conventional bipolar devices and deliver current intermittently to give the tissue time to cool down [3]. Advanced design of such devices can allow dissection, vessel sealing, and cutting, which reduces instrument traffic and operative time. Several studies indicate that advanced bipolar devices provide better outcomes in terms of operative time, blood loss, complications, postoperative pain, and hospital stay [7].

4.7 Combination energy devices

Advanced technology has resulted in the combination of electrosurgery and ultrasound energy in a single device where one button activates advanced bipolar and ultrasonic outputs simultaneously to achieve sealing and transection of vessels up to 7 mm in diameter. The second button activates advanced bipolar output only. Such devices have the potential of reducing the multiple exchanges of instruments.

4.8 Complications

Laparoscopic electrosurgical injuries occur in two to five per thousand procedures. Most such injuries are not detected during surgery. This delayed diagnosis can lead to increased morbidity and mortality. As a result, guidelines were released to address the safe use of electrosurgery [8].

4.8.1 Lateral thermal spread

This injury results from the spread of heat to tissues close to the active instrument. It is the most common electrosurgical injury with possible damage to the bowel, ureter, or blood vessels. It can occur with monopolar, bipolar, ultrasonic, and laser devices. Monopolar coagulation causes more lateral thermal spread than the others [9]. Higher

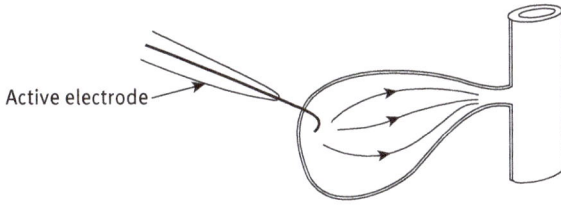

Fig. 4.3: Pedicle effect.

voltage and wattage increase are associated with increased lateral thermal spread. It is recommended to avoid using electrosurgical energy in close proximity of vital structures such as bowel, ureter, and blood vessels. Shorter intermittent activation is recommended to minimize the lateral thermal spread.

4.8.2 Pedicle effect

Pedicle effect happens when a monopolar device is activated on a structure with a narrow pedicle or adhesion. The unintended burn takes place remotely at the narrow pedicle or adhesion where the current density is higher (Fig. 4.3) [3].

4.8.3 Inadvertent activation

This can result in unintended burns. It is good practice to remove the energy device from the patient when not in use and to place it in a dry rigid plastic holder with no other instruments. Also, switching on the activation tone would alert the surgical team to that problem.

4.8.4 Residual heat

Energy devices can retain the heat for a variable time after deactivation. Ultrasonic devices have higher residual heat than their electrosurgical counterparts. Surgeons should avoid touching vital structures with the tip of an electrosurgical device immediately after deactivation. If you inadvertently touch the bowel with a hot device, examine it for blanching and consider suturing it to avoid delayed perforation [3].

4.8.5 Insulation failure

This is due to the breach of the insulation layer of the active electrode. It can affect about 20% of reusable instruments and 3% of single-use devices. It commonly affects the distal third of the device. Its possible causes include wear and tear, repeated cleaning, and sterilization, as well as the use of high-voltage current. Although it is recommended to examine the instrument for defects before use, most of such defects are not easily seen. The smaller the defect, the higher is the stray current concentration with increased risk of catastrophic burns. Electrical scans and porosity detectors can identify the defects already present before surgery, but not those that might develop during the surgery. Active electrode monitoring (AEM) technology prevents burns from insulation failure [2].

4.8.6 Direct coupling

Direct coupling occurs when the active electrode touches another metal instrument where current flows from the active electrode to the second instrument and to any tissue touching it. This can lead to unintended burns. It is related to the surgical technique; hence, surgeons should keep the active electrode and other metal instruments in a panoramic view and not activate energy unless the instrument tip is in view [3].

4.8.7 Capacitive coupling

Capacitative coupling is the transfer of electric current through the intact insulation of the active electrode to adjacent conductive materials (Fig. 4.4). It happens on passing the active electrode down a metal suction irrigator, an operative laparoscope, or a hybrid cannula. Also, the active electrode can induce a current in a nearby cold instrument or in a tissue that is in contact with the intact insulation of the active electrode.

Capacitive coupling can be minimized by avoiding high wattage, open activation, hybrid cannulas and activation close to metal instruments. In addition, use of the "cut" rather than "coag" mod for coagulation with short interrupted activations can reduce this complication. [10]. Adaptive electrosurgical technology that monitors tissue impedance to vary the output voltage accordingly can reduce capacitive coupling whereas AEM technology eliminates it [2].

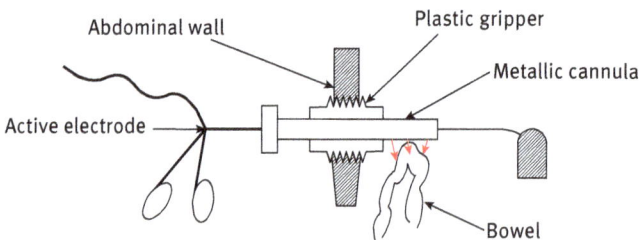

Fig. 4.4: Capacitive coupling.

4.8.8 Antenna coupling

The active electrode cord emits electromagnetic energy in the air, which is captured by a nearby inactive cord or wire such as the camera cord or electrocardiogram (ECG) wires. This can result in unintended burns. Separating the laparoscopy stack from ESU and avoiding parallel arrangement of cords reduce such risk [11].

4.9 Technological developments and safe electrosurgery

4.9.1 Isolated generators and return electrode monitoring technology

The introduction of these technologies mostly eliminated alternate site burns at ground points and return electrodes, which were the most common complications of electrosurgery during its early use in open surgery.

4.9.2 Active electrode monitoring

Electrosurgery in laparoscopic surgery has created a new pattern of alternate site burns (insulation failure and capacitive coupling). Such burns, in contrast to their earlier counterparts in open surgery, are internal, mostly undetected intraoperatively and possibly fatal. AEM technology was introduced to prevent burns due to insulation failure and capacitive coupling. The AEM instrument has two extra layers: a conductive shield and extra insulation layer (Fig. 4.5). The AEM monitor fitted to the ESU continuously monitors the conductive shield for stray currents. When the AEM monitor identifies a high level of stray current, it stops the ESU to prevent any tissue burns [2]. The three technological innovations of isolated ESUs, return electrode monitoring (REM) and AEM systems have addressed the design flaws in electrosurgery and significantly reduced most electrosurgical burns. Training programs for surgeons and relevant staff in safe electrosurgery would complement such technologies.

4.10 Electrosurgery in single incision laparoscopic surgery

Such surgery where multiple instruments are passed through one incision has intensified the risks of monopolar instrumentation (insulation failure, direct coupling, and capacitive coupling) [12]. This is because of the proximity and crossing of instruments as well as their longer zone 2 (Fig. 4.6). To reduce such risks, AEM monopolar, bipolar, or ultrasonic devices should be used.

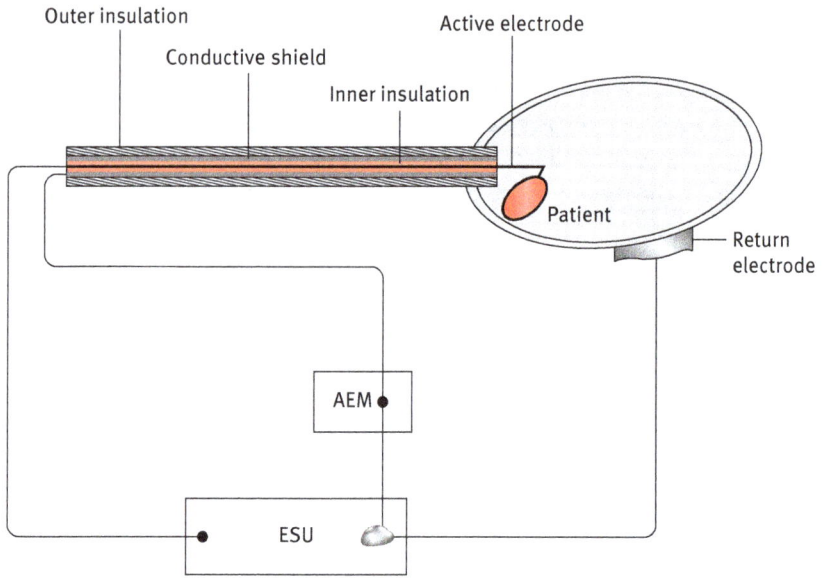

Fig. 4.5: Active electrode monitoring (AEM) instrument and circuit. ESU, Electrosurgical unit.

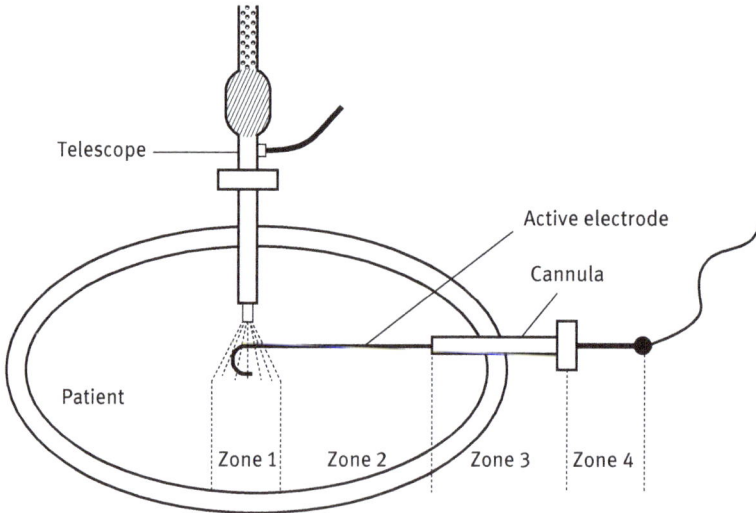

Fig. 4.6: The four zones of laparoscopic instrument.

4.11 Electrosurgery in hysteroscopic surgery

Electrosurgical devices (monopolar and bipolar) can be used for the hysteroscopic treatment of submucous fibroids, endometrial polyps, intrauterine synechiae, and uterine septae. Monopolar hysteroscopic devices require nonconductive distension media such as 1.5% glycine or 3% Sorbitol, which are hypo-osmolar. Bipolar devices work in conductive iso-osmolar media such as 0.9 % saline or lactated ringer's solution. Complications such as electrolyte imbalance and its consequences are more common with hypo-osmolar distension media, hence bipolar systems are considered to be safer compared to monopolar devices. In addition, the bipolar uses less voltage with less chance of unintended electrical injury. Bipolar hysteroscopic devices are somewhat different than the conventional bipolar device, as in the hysteroscopic counterpart only the active electrode touches the tissue and the nearby return electrode drains the current through the conductive medium. Fluid management systems are recommended to reduce fluid overload hazards associated with hysteroscopic surgery with both monopolar and bipolar systems.

4.12 Electrosurgery and electromagnetic interference

Electrosurgical devices can interfere with active implants such as permanent pacemakers (PPMs), implantable cardioverter defibrillator (ICD), and neurologic stimulators. This can damage or inhibit such implants, burn the myocardium or cause arrhythmias and asystole [13].

The following prevention strategies can be used to avoid these problems:
- Get advice from the manufacturer or cardiology team before surgery.
- In patients highly dependent on the implant, use bipolar or ultrasonic devices.
- When using monopolar:
  - Place the dispersive electrode away from the implant.
  - Avoid capacitively coupled return electrode.
  - Use low power, cut mode to coagulate with short activation.
  - Avoid current vector crossing the implant.
  - Use ECG to monitor PPM during surgery and reprogram it, if required, posoperatively.
  - Deactivate ICD preoperatively then activate it after surgery. A magnet can be used in an emergency when cardiology input is not available.

4.13 Surgical smoke

Surgical smoke is a by-product of surgical energy use. It lowers laparoscopic visibility with its potential risk of complications. Its harmful gases and chemicals can cause ocular and upper respiratory tract irritation in theatre staff. In addition, it contains viruses and bacteria that can pose an infection risk. While regular surgical masks are not protective against smoke risks, standard smoke evacuation systems are recommended to reduce such risks [3].

4.14 Key points for safe electrosurgical use

4.14.1 Monopolar instruments

- Use the lowest effective wattage (power).
- Avoid bony prominences, metal prosthesis, scar tissue, hairy skin, or pressure areas for the dispersive electrode.
- Use the narrow edge of the active electrode to increase tissue effects without increasing the wattage.
- Use the cut rather than the coagulation mode to achieve good coagulation with low voltage.
- Avoid prolonged activation.
- Do not use open activation.
- Do not activate the device near or in contact with another metal instrument.
- Use REM dispersive electrode and AEM instruments.

4.14.2 Bipolar instruments

- Take extra caution near vital structures due to lateral thermal spread.
- Avoid tissue tension during activation as it affects coagulation. In structures with anatomical tension, do few overlapping applications.
- To produce the desired tissue effect, always keep the instrument jaws clean by using a wet swab.
- To prevent tissue charring, do short intermittent activations and release the tissue at the vapor phase just before switching the instrument off.
- If the instrument jaws are stuck to the tissue, reapproximate the jaws, and reactivate before opening them. Irrigate the jaws and tissue with fluid before reactivation if needed.
- Never use in tissues with metal clips or staples.
- Do not over-compress the grasped tissue to prevent the bypass effect and do not include a big tissue bundle in the instrument jaws to achieve a good seal. Skeletonize vessels before application to produce an adequate seal.
- In patients with possible abnormal vessels due to liver cirrhosis, prolonged steroid use, atherosclerosis, aneurysm, diabetes, malnutrition, and collagen diseases take extra caution and consider alternative hemostatic methods.

References

[1] Sutton C, Abbott J. History of power sources in endoscopic surgery. J Minim Invasive Gynecol 2013;20:271–8.
[2] Odell RC. Surgical complications specific to monopolar electrosurgical energy: engineering changes that have made electrosurgery safer. J Minim Invasive Gynecol 2013;20:288–98.

[3] El-Sayed MM, Mohamed SA, Saridogan E. Safe use of electrosurgery in gynaecological laparoscopic surgery. The Obstetrician & Gynaecologist 2020;22:9–20.

[4] Wang K, Advincula AP. "Current thoughts" in electrosurgery. Int J Gynaecol Obstet 2007;97:245–50.

[5] Voyles CR. The art and science of monopolar electrosurgery. In: Feldman LS, Fuchshuber PR, Jones DB, eds. The SAGES Manual on the Fundamental Use of Surgical Energy (FUSE). New York: Springer; 2012:81–91.

[6] Brill AI. Bipolar electrosurgery: convention and innovation. Clin Obstet Gynecol 2008;51:153–8.

[7] Jaiswal A, Huang KG. Energy devices in gynaecological laparoscopy—Archaic to modern era. Gynecol Minim Invasive Ther 2017;6:147–51.

[8] Rey JF, Beilenhoff U, Neumann CS, Dumonceau JM. European Society of Gastrointestinal Endoscopy (ESGE) guideline: the use of electrosurgical units. Endoscopy 2010;42:764–72.

[9] Sutton PA, Awad S, Perkins AC, Lobo DN. Comparison of lateral thermal spread using monopolar and bipolar diathermy, the Harmonic Scalpel™ and the Ligasure™. Br J Surg 2010;97:383–90.

[10] Robinson TN, Pavlovsky KR, Looney H, Stiegmann GV, McGreevy FT. Surgeon-controlled factors that reduce monopolar electrosurgery capacitive coupling during laparoscopy. Surg Laparosc Endosc Percutan Tech 2010;20:317–20.

[11] Robinson TN, Barnes KS, Govekar HR, Stiegmann GV, Dunn CL, McGreevy FT. Antenna coupling-a novel mechanism of radiofrequency electrosurgery complication: practical implications. Ann Surg 2012;256:213–8.

[12] Abu-Rafea B, Vilos GA, Al-Obeed O, AlSheikh A, Vilos AG, Al-Mandeel H. Monopolar electrosurgery through single-port laparoscopy: a potential hidden hazard for bowel burns. Minim Invasive Gynecol 2011;18:734–40.

[13] Siddaiah-Subramanya M, Tiang KW, Nyandowe M. Complications, implications, and prevention of electrosurgical injuries: Cornerstone of diathermy use for junior surgical trainees. Surg J 2017;3:148–53.

Nisse V. Clark and Jon I. Einarsson

5 Laparoscopic entry techniques

5.1 Introduction

While laparoscopic surgery is generally safe and offers many advantages over open surgery, a small minority of patients suffer life-threatening complications, including major vascular or visceral injury [1, 2]. Nearly half of these complications occur while accessing the peritoneal cavity, making initial entry one of the most dangerous steps in laparoscopy [2, 3]. The incidence of major vascular injury during entry is estimated at 0.2 per 1000 procedures, and the incidence of bowel injury during entry is estimated at 0.4 per 1000 procedures [4]. While rare, these injuries incur serious morbidity and mortality, particularly in the case of major vascular injury or unrecognized bowel injury [3, 5]. Other complications that can also occur include carbon dioxide embolism, small vessel injury, extraperitoneal insufflation, or failed entry.

Opinion is divided as to the safest entry technique, with many gynecologists using a closed entry method and other surgical specialties routinely using an open entry method [6, 7]. There are risks regardless of the technique, and high-quality evidence supporting one approach over another is generally lacking [8]. This chapter will review and compare laparoscopic entry techniques, including methods, entry site, and other considerations.

5.2 Techniques

Laparoscopic entry techniques can be broadly classified into closed or open methods. Closed methods include the Veres needle, direct trocar, and direct vision entry. Open methods include the Hasson technique and single-incision laparoscopy.

5.2.1 General principles

A few principles hold true for all entry methods. The bladder should be drained with a Foley catheter and the stomach decompressed with an orogastric or nasogastric tube, especially if a left upper quadrant entry is planned. Primary entry should take place with the patient flat in the horizontal position as the Trendelenburg position may distort the anatomy and result in inadvertent injury.

First entry is typically at the base of the umbilicus, where the fascial layers fuse and the abdominal wall is thinnest. A vertical or curvilinear skin incision is made at the deepest part of the umbilicus, with the size depending on the ultimate trocar diameter. Instruments such as Allis clamps can be used to evert the umbilicus and

https://doi.org/10.1515/9783110535204-005

facilitate making an incision at the base. Care should be taken not to stab through the entire abdominal wall, which may cause injury to underlying structures.

Once an incision is made, the fascia is grasped with an instrument such as a Kocher or piercing towel clip to elevate the abdominal wall. This increases the space between the umbilicus and the great vessels, a distance that can be as little as 2 cm in a thin patient [9]. Of note, grabbing only the skin by hand may increase the risk of failed entry [10].

5.2.2 Veres needle

The Veres needle technique is a closed entry method that uses a small-bore needle to insufflate the peritoneal cavity prior to trocar placement. The technique was named after Janos Veres, who originally used the needle to alleviate pneumothorax in patients with tuberculosis [11]. The instrument popularized in laparoscopic surgery in the 1970s and is now the primary entry method used by gynecologists (Fig. 5.1) [6, 7, 12].

The Veres needle is 2 mm in diameter and has a sharp outer sheath that pierces tissue as well as a spring-loaded inner cannula that springs forward once inside a low-pressure cavity. The instrument can be inserted at several different entry sites, although is frequently used at the umbilicus. Prior to insertion, the needle should be checked for proper spring-loading action and free flow of carbon dioxide gas. It is advisable to attach the gas tubing prior to insertion so the needle does not become dislodged once positioned. After a skin incision is made and the fascia elevated, the Veres needle is inserted at a 90-degree angle until the fascia is reached. The needle tip is then either maintained at a 90-degree angle or reoriented slightly caudad if

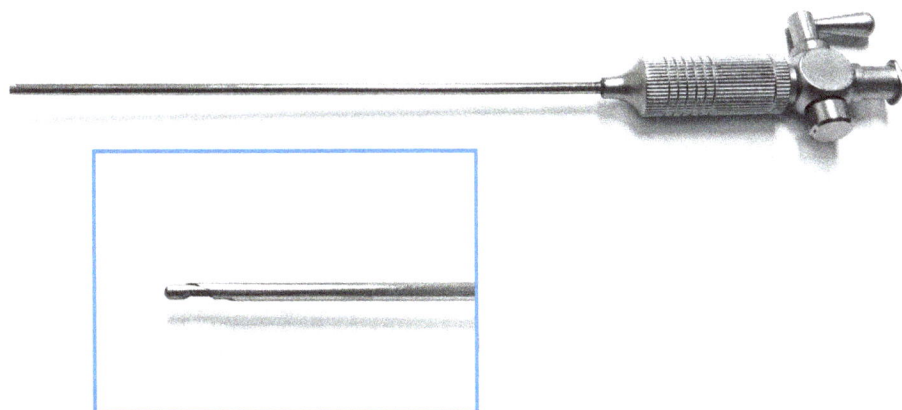

Fig. 5.1: Veres needle.

the patient is very thin. During insertion, the needle itself should be grasped and constant gentle pressure used to introduce the needle in a controlled fashion. At the umbilicus, two "pops" are often felt—one as the fascia is entered and the other as the peritoneum is entered; however, these are not always distinct.

To assess for proper placement, the gas should be turned on and a low insufflation pressure documented as gas flows freely into the nondistended peritoneal cavity. The pressure should register less than 10 mmHg and is usually less than 5 mmHg unless the patient is obese or has a less distensible abdomen, such as following an abdominoplasty. Other ways to assess intraperitoneal placement include the inability to aspirate injected saline or a positive saline drop test, although neither test is as reliable as a low opening pressure [13].

Pneumoperitoneum is obtained while evaluating for uniform abdominal distension and tympany. A primary port is then placed, typically in the same location as the Veres needle. This can be done with or without direct vision using the laparoscope in an optical trocar.

The risk of failed entry with the Veres needle is up to 11.6% on the first attempt and 3.0% on the second attempt [14]. Failed attempts often result in preperitoneal insufflation, which is estimated to occur 2% of the time [8, 14]. Most experts advise choosing an alternate entry site if Veres needle placement fails after three attempts [15, 16].

5.2.3 Direct trocar

Direct trocar entry involves blindly inserting a trocar without prior peritoneal insufflation. The technique was first described by Dingfelder in 1978 and is thought to avoid complications related to the Veres needle, including extraperitoneal insufflation, omental injury, or failed entry [17, 18].

Following an incision, typically at the base of the umbilicus, the abdominal wall is elevated and a trocar is introduced directly toward the hollow of the pelvis. On removal of the trocar, the laparoscope is inserted to confirm appropriate placement. Pneumopertioneum is obtained through the trocar and the abdomen is surveyed for entry-related trauma. Sharp and pointed trocars are recommended to minimize penetration force; however, unshielded bladed trocars should be avoided for direct trocar entry [16, 19].

5.2.4 Direct vision

Primary trocar insertion under direct vision is a potentially safer alternative to direct trocar entry that uses visual guidance to insert a trocar prior to insufflation. Direct vision entry requires an optical trocar with a pointed transparent tip and a 0-degree laparoscope placed inside to observe passage of the abdominal wall layers. Unlike direct trocar entry, this technique relies on visualization rather than feel. At the umbilicus, one can expect to see subcutaneous fat, fascia, preperitoneal fat and peritoneum before entering the peritoneal cavity. The technique can also be used when placing the primary port after prior insufflation with the Veres needle.

5.2.5 Hasson technique

The open Hasson technique, named after Harrith Hasson, is the most common method of laparoscopic entry used by general surgeons [20]. The technique involves directly inserting a trocar into an open peritoneal incision and is therefore considered less "blind" than other methods. Open entry is advocated in patients with suspected adhesions as well as in very thin or pregnant patients where blind entry may pose greater risks.

The Hasson technique uses making a curvilinear incision along the base of the umbilicus or a vertical incision in the depth of the umbilicus. The incision is typically 12 mm, although the technique has also been described with a 5-mm incision [21]. The subcutaneous tissue is then dissected down to the fascia and the fascia is grasped with a Kocher clamp. The fascia is incised with a scalpel to expose the preperitoneal fat and peritoneum. At this point, the fascia can be tagged with stay sutures to secure the port to the fascia and assist with eventual closure. The peritoneum is then entered sharply, sweeping the underside of the abdominal wall with a finger to open the incision and assess for adhesions. The blunt-tip trocar (e.g., Hasson trocar) is placed in the incision and the stay sutures are tied to the trocar to secure it. Pneumoperitoneum can then be achieved through this port (Fig. 5.2).

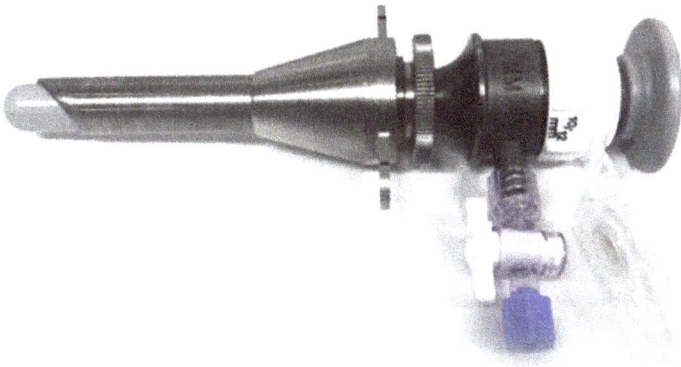

Fig. 5.2: Hasson trocar.

5.2.6 Single-incision laparoscopy

Single-incision laparoscopic surgery uses an open technique for primary entry similar to the Hasson method. Once an initial trocar is placed through an open peritoneal incision and pneumoperitoneum is established, second and third trocars are placed adjacent to the first trocar, either in the same fascial incision or leaving a small bridge of fascia between them to avoid gas leakage. The suggested benefits of this technique include reduced postoperative pain and improved cosmesis [22].

5.3 Choosing a technique

A Cochrane review of 46 randomized controlled trials including 13 laparoscopic entry techniques and 7389 procedures found no evidence of an advantage for any single technique in preventing major vascular or visceral complications [8]. The studies reviewed are generally recognized as low quality due to inadequate numbers and poor reporting of study methods. Of note, all studies were underpowered to identify a preferred entry method, a task that is estimated to require an analysis of over 800,000 procedures [23].

It has been suggested that open techniques are safer than closed techniques as open entry avoids blind insertion of a needle or trocar [6, 7]. While small observational studies have drawn this conclusion, the Cochrane review found no difference in major complications when comparing open and closed entry methods [8]. The only advantage identified in the Cochrane review was a reduction in failed entry compared with the closed methods [8]. Single-incision laparoscopy also does not reduce major complications and has been shown to prolong operative time [8].

Comparing closed entry techniques, the Cochrane review reported reduced vascular injury and failed entry with the direct trocar compared to the Veres needle technique, although these data are noted as being of very low quality [8]. Some studies also show a higher risk of minor complications with Veres needle entry, including extraperitoneal insufflation and omental injury [24, 25]. Direct vision entry may confer an advantage over direct trocar entry, although these methods have not been compared in a randomized fashion. Of note, injury with either direct trocar or direct vision entry may be more catastrophic than Veres needle entry given the trocar size. Conversely, bowel injuries from the 2-mm Veres needle are thought to be self-limited and require no treatment.

Surgeons should use the technique with which they have the most experience while being familiar with the other techniques. Choosing an entry method also requires consideration of the patient's anatomy, surgical history, and planned intervention. For example, if a minilaparotomy is going to be performed for specimen extraction, this can be created at the procedure outset using an open entry technique. As another example, if there is concern for umbilical adhesions and ipsilateral ports are planned, direct entry in the left upper quadrant also creates a functional port site.

5.4 Alternative entry sites

5.4.1 Left upper quadrant

Primary entry in the left upper quadrant is a feasible alternative to umbilical entry and should be considered in patients with a prior midline laparotomy, a massively enlarged uterus, pregnancy or multiple failed attempts at umbilical entry [26, 27]. It may also be advantageous in very thin or morbidly obese women, where umbilical entry is less reliable and could pose an increased risk of vascular injury [28].

The classic left upper quadrant access site is Palmer's point, located 3 cm below the left costal margin in the midclavicular line [12]. The abdominal wall layers at Palmer's point include the skin, subcutaneous fat, anterior fascia, external oblique muscle, internal oblique muscle, transversus abdominis muscle, posterior fascia, pre-peritoneal fat, and peritoneum (Fig. 5.3). Entry at Palmer's point is typically obtained using a closed entry technique. If a Veres needle is used, three distinct "pops" may be felt as the two layers of fascia and peritoneum are entered. If a direct optical trocar is used, a muscular layer is seen between two layers of white fascia before traversing the peritoneum and entering the abdominal cavity.

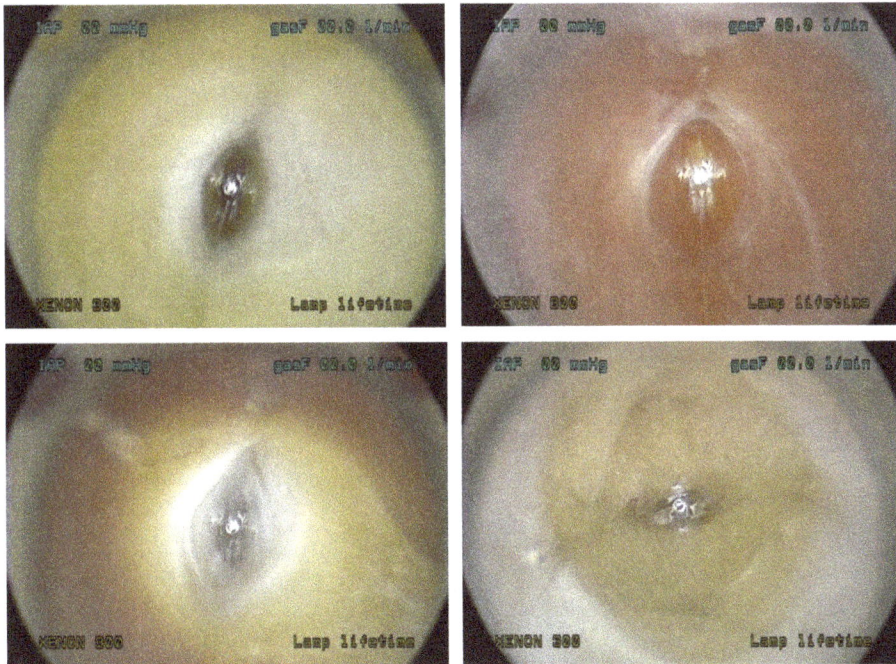

Fig. 5.3: Abdominal wall layers with direct vision entry in the left upper quadrant. From left to right, bottom to top, the anterior fascia, muscle, posterior fascia, and peritoneum are shown.

Depending on the patient's anatomy, Palmer's point may be located too far ceph-alad or medial for pelvic surgery, and an entry site in the left mid abdomen may be preferred. A point at the level of the umbilicus and 2.5 cm medial to the anterior supe-rior iliac spine has been described as a modification of Palmer's point for gynecologic procedures [29].

When using the left upper or mid quadrant for primary access, it is important to decompress the stomach with an orogastric or nasogastric tube beforehand. As with all entry sites, consideration of the underlying anatomy is critical. Patients with splenomegaly, hepatomegaly, portal hypertension, gastric, or pancreatic masses or a history of splenic or gastric surgery are not good candidates for left upper quadrant entry.

5.4.2 Other entry sites

Several other abdominal entry sites have been reported in the literature, including the left or right costal margins, the left ninth intercostal space and the hypogastrium [30–33]. The posterior cul-de-sac and uterine fundus have also been trialed for Veres needle insufflation, especially in obese women, where abdominal entry may be more challenging [34, 35]. Similar to choosing an entry technique, selecting an entry site depends on the patient's anatomy, the procedure and the likelihood of underlying adhesions. In general, surgeons should be flexible in their approach and comfortable with more than one primary access site (Fig. 5.4).

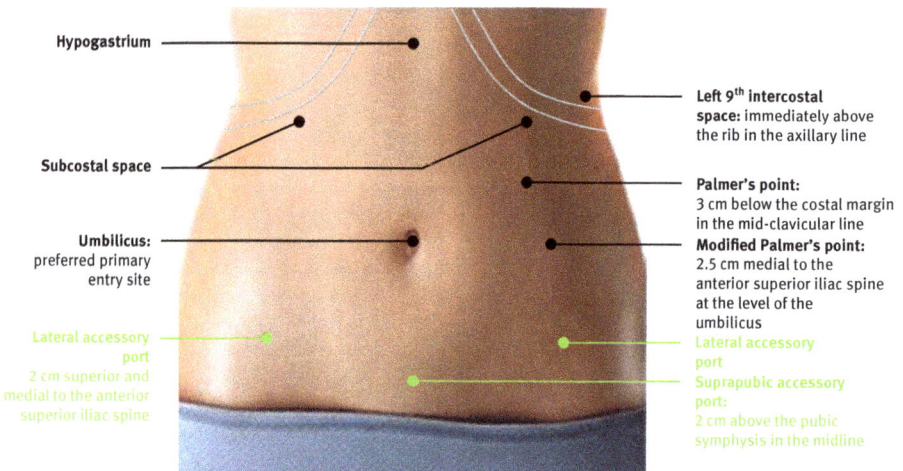

Fig. 5.4: Entry sites. Primary entry is typically at the umbilicus. Alternate primary entry sites are shown in black. Common accessory port sites are shown in green.

5.5 Considerations

5.5.1 Prior surgery

Patients with prior abdominal surgery are at an increased risk of entry-related complications. A prior midline laparotomy confers a 51.7% to 59% risk of umbilical adhesions, prompting many surgeons to enter in the left upper quadrant [36–38]. The risk of umbilical adhesions ranges from 19.8% to 28% in the setting of a prior low transverse laparotomy and 1.6% to 21.2% in the setting of a prior umbilical incision from laparoscopy [38, 39]. The likelihood of severe umbilical adhesions that risk visceral injury with a low transverse laparotomy or umbilical laparoscopy is likely lower and does not preclude first entry at the umbilicus. Regardless, clinical judgment is advised as multiple prior surgeries or a history of abdominal or pelvic infection can increase the risk of adhesions.

5.5.2 Morbidly obese patients

Morbidly obese patients present several challenges during laparoscopic entry due to a loss of anatomic landmarks, caudal deviation of the umbilicus and increased abdominal wall thickness. This can result in unsuccessful entry, preperitoneal insufflation and an increased risk of severe complications. Most experts recommend closed entry given poor visualization with an open technique [15]. Veres needle insertion at the umbilicus should be performed at a 90-degree angle to minimize abdominal wall thickness. Moreover, the umbilicus is displaced caudally in obese patients and no longer overlies the great vessels [28]. A long Veres needle may be necessary in the case of left upper quadrant entry. Alternative techniques include inserting the Veres needle through the uterine fundus or posterior vaginal fornix or shifting the obese pannus cranially to assist with umbilical entry [34, 35, 40].

5.5.3 Very thin patients

In extremely thin patients, the distance between the anterior abdominal wall and the retroperitoneum is sometimes less than 2 cm, placing these patients at an increased risk of injury during umbilical entry [9]. If umbilical entry with the Veres needle is used, it is advised to direct the needle 45 degrees caudad to avoid vascular injury [9]. Other experts suggest manually pulling the umbilicus caudad during Veres needle insertion [16]. Although there are limited quantitative data comparing different entry techniques in very thin patients, an open technique at the umbilicus or a closed technique in the left upper quadrant is favored by many experts [15].

5.5.4 Pregnancy and the large uterus

Laparoscopic entry in the second or third trimester of pregnancy should be adapted to the height of the uterine fundus. Both closed and open methods can be used, although closed entry in the left upper quadrant is likely to reduce the risk of uterine injury [41]. In the case of a massively enlarged, nongravid uterus, left upper quadrant entry may also be beneficial. Gas insufflation of 15 mmHg can be used during pregnancy with no reported adverse outcomes to the fetus [41].

5.6 Conclusion

Primary entry is a critical step in laparoscopy, during which a patient is vulnerable to serious injury. Several entry techniques exist, each with advantages and disadvantages that must be weighed together with the surgeon's preference, the patient's anatomy, and the surgery at hand. No one technique or tool is superior for all patients; therefore, surgeons should use their preferred approach when possible and alternate methods as clinically necessary.

References

[1] Jansen FW, Kapiteyn K, Trimbos-Kemper T, Hermans J, Trimbos JB. Complications of laparoscopy: a prospective multicenter observational study. Br J Obstet Gynaecol 1997;104:595–600.

[2] Jansen FW, Kolkman W, Bakkum EA, de Kroon CD, Trimbos-Kemper TC, Trimbos JB. Complications of laparoscopy: an inquiry about closed- versus open-entry technique. Am J Obstet Gynecol 2004;190:634–8.

[3] Fuller J, Ashar BS, Carey-Corrado J. Trocar-associated injuries and fatalities: an analysis of 1399 reports to the FDA. J Minim Invasive Gynecol 2005;12:302–7.

[4] Varma R, Gupta JK. Laparoscopic entry techniques: clinical guideline, national survey, and medicolegal ramifications. Surg Endosc 2008;22:2686–97.

[5] Llarena NC, Shah AB, Milad MP. Bowel injury in gynecologic laparoscopy: a systematic review. Obstet Gynecol 2015;125:1407–17.

[6] Molloy D, Kaloo PD, Cooper M, Nguyen TV. Laparoscopic entry: a literature review and analysis of techniques and complications of primary port entry. Aust N Z J Obstet Gynaecol 2002;42:246–54.

[7] Vilos GA, Ternamian A, Dempster J, Laberge PY. No. 193-Laparoscopic entry: a review of techniques, technologies, and complications. J Obstet Gynaecol Can 2017;39:e69–84.

[8] Ahmad G, Gent D, Henderson D, O'Flynn H, Phillips K, Watson A. Laparoscopic entry techniques. Cochrane Database Syst Rev 2015;8:CD006583.

[9] Hurd WW, Bude RO, DeLancey JO, Pearl ML. The relationship of the umbilicus to the aortic bifurcation: implications for laparoscopic technique. Obstet Gynecol 1992;80:48–51.

[10] Briel JW, Plaisier PW, Meijer WS, Lange JF. Is it necessary to lift the abdominal wall when preparing pneumoperitoneum? A randomized study. Surg Endosc 2000;14:862–4.

[11] Szabo I, Laszio A. Veres needle: in memoriam of the 100th birthday anniversary of Dr Janos Veres, the inventor. Am J Obstet Gynecol 2004;191:352–3.

[12] Palmer R. Safety in laparoscopy. J Reprod Med 1974;13:1–15.

[13] Teoh B, Sen R, Abbott J. An evaluation of four tests used to ascertain Veres needle placement at closed laparoscopy. J Minim Invasive Gynecol 2005;12:153–8.

[14] Azevedo JL, Azevedo OC, Miyahira SA, et al. Injuries caused by Veress needle insertion for creation of pneumoperitoneum: a systematic literature review. Surg Endosc 2009;1428–32.

[15] la Chapelle CF, Bemelam WA, Rademaker BM, van Barneveld TA, Jansen FW. A multidisciplinary evidence-based guideline for minimally invasive surgery: Part 1. Entry techniques and the pneumoperitoneum. Gynecol Surg 2012;9:271–82.

[16] Taskforce for Abdominal Entry. Principles of safe laparoscopic entry. Eur J Obstet Gynecol Reprod Biol 2016;201:179–88.

[17] Dingfelder JR. Direct laparoscope trocar insertion without prior pneumoperitoneum. J Reprod Med 1978;31:45–7.

[18] Agresta F, Mazzarolo G, Bedin N. Direct trocar insertion for laparoscopy. JSLS 2012;16:255–9.

[19] Antoniou SA, Antoniou GA, Kock OO, Pointner R, Granderath FA. Blunt versus bladed trocars in laparoscopic surgery: a systematic review and meta-analysis of randomized trials. Surg Endosc 2013;27:2312–20.

[20] Hasson HM. A modified instrument and method for laparoscopy. Am J Obstet Gynecol 1971;110:886–7.

[21] Pryor KP, Hurd WW. Modified open laparoscopy using a 5-mm laparoscope. Obstet Gynecol 2016;127:535–8.

[22] Tsimoyiannis EC, Tsimogiannis KE, Pappas-Gogos G, et al. Different pain scores in single transumbilical incision laparoscopic cholecystectomy versus classic laparoscopic cholecystectomy: a randomized controlled trial. Surg Endosc 2010;24:1842–8.

[23] Garry R. Surgeons may continue to use their chosen entry technique. Gynecol Surg 2009;87–92.

[24] Jiang X, Anderson C, Schnatz PF. The safety of direct trocar versus Veress needle for laparoscopic entry: a meta-analysis of randomized clinical trials. J Laparoendosc Adv Surg Tech A 2012;22:362–70.

[25] Angioli R, Terranova C, De Cicco Nardone C, et al. A comparison of three different entry techniques in gynecologic laparoscopic surgery: a randomized prospective trial. Eur J Obstet Gynecol Reprod Biol 2013;171:339–42.

[26] Lam KW, Pun TC. Left upper quadrant approach in gynecologic laparoscopic surgery using reusable instruments. J Am Assoc Gynecol Laparosc 2002;9:199–203.

[27] Ngu SF, Cheung VY, Pun TC. Left upper quadrant approach in gynecologic laparoscopic surgery. Acta Obstet Gynecol Scand 2011;90:1406–9.

[28] Hurd WH, Bude RO, DeLancey JO, Gauvin JM, Aisen AM. Abdominal wall characterization with magnetic resonance imaging and computed tomography. The effect of obesity on the laparoscopic approach. J Reprod Med 1991;36:473–6.

[29] Jain N, Sareen S, Kanawa S, Jain V, Mann S. Jain point: A new safe portal for laparoscopic entry in previous surgery cases. J Hum Reprod Sci 2016;9:9–17.

[30] Tulikangas PK, Robinson DS, Falcone T. Left upper quadrant cannula insertion. Fertil Steril 2003;79:411–2.

[31] Ellatif ME, Ghnnam WM, Abbas A, Basheer M, Dawoud I, Ellaithy R. Latif's point: a new point for Veress needle insertion for pneumoperitoneum in difficult laparoscopy. Asian J Endosc Surg 2017 (ahead of print).

[32] Agarwala N, Liu CY. Safe entry techniques during laparoscopy: left upper quadrant entry using the ninth intercostal space—a review of 918 procedures. J Minim Invasive Gynecol 2005;12:55–61.

[33] Lee CL, Huang KG, Jain S, Wang CJ, Yen CF, Soong YK. A new portal for gynecologic laparoscopy. J Am Assoc Gynecol Laparosc 2001;8:147–50.

[34] van Lith DA, van Schie KJ, Beekhuizen W, du Plessis M. Int J Gynaecol Obstet 1980;17:375–8.

[35] Santala M, Jarvela I, Kauppila A. Transfundal insertion of a Veress needle in laparoscopy of obese subjects: a practical alternative. Hum Reprod 1999;14:2277–8.

[36] Brill AI, Nezhat F, Nezhat CH, Nezhat C. The incidence of adhesions after prior laparotomy: a laparoscopic appraisal. Obstet Gynecol 1995;85:269–72.

[37] Levrant SG, Bieber EJ, Barnes RB. Anterior abdominal wall adhesions after laparotomy or laparoscopy. J Am Assoc Gynecol Laparosc 1997;4:353–6.

[38] Audebert AJ, Gomel V. Role of microlaparoscopy in the diagnosis of peritoneal and visceral adhesions and in the prevention of bowel injury associated with blind trocar insertion. Fertil Steril 2000;73:631–5.

[39] Sepilian V, Ku L, Wong H, Liu CY, Phelps JY. Prevalence of infraumbilical adhesions in women with previous laparoscopy. JSLS 2007;11:41–4.

[40] Pelosi MA 3rd, Pelosi MA. Alignment of the umbilical axis: an effective maneuver for laparoscopic entry in the obese patient. Obstet Gynecol 1998;92:869–72.

[41] Pearl J, Price R, Richardson W, Fanelli R. Society of American Gastrointestinal Endoscopic Surgeons. Guidelines for diagnosis, treatment, and use of laparoscopy for surgical problems during pregnancy. Surg Endosc 2011;25:3479–92.

Ibrahim Alkatout

6 Principles of laparoscopic suturing and alternatives

6.1 Introduction

Ligatures and suturing techniques represent a safe and, in many cases, the only method of hemostasis in endoscopic surgery and are often better suited than thermal methods. Various suture materials, applicators and needle holders have been developed for this purpose.

Laparoscopic intracorporeal knot tying in minimally invasive surgery requires great manual dexterity. There is a difference between laparoscopic suturing and open or robotic-assisted suturing. Given a skill score of 10 for various surgical modalities, conventional laparotomy requires a score of 2; microsurgery, a score of 4; laparoscopy, a score of 6; and laparoscopic suturing, a score of 8, while robotic laparoscopic suturing returns to the skill level of general laparoscopic surgery with a score of 6. This is due to the limited movement abilities of laparoscopic instruments compared to open and robotic surgery. Furthermore, there is a variety of alternatives including bipolar and ultrasound-based sealing instruments that have replaced intracorporeal ligatures and needle handling. Therefore, the art of suturing also includes the art of proper selection [1, 2].

The lesson is clear: Never underestimate the art of laparoscopic suturing, never get too frustrated and understand that laparoscopic suturing requires repeated training [3].

6.2 Sutures and suture technique

6.2.1 Suture material

Sutures are either monofilament or polyfilament/braided and they are either absorbable or nonabsorbable depending on whether the body will naturally degrade and absorb the suture material over time. The resorption process includes hydrolysis and proteolytic enzymatic degradation. Depending on the material, the process can take from 10 days to 8 weeks. The suture holds the body tissues together long enough to allow healing, but it will disintegrate so that no foreign material is left. Initially, there is a transient foreign body reaction to the material. After complete resorption, only connective tissue remains. Nonabsorbable sutures are made of special silk or

https://doi.org/10.1515/9783110535204-006

synthetics. These sutures are used either on skin wound closure if the sutures can be removed after a few weeks or in stressful internal environments where absorbable sutures will not suffice. Nonabsorbable sutures mostly cause less scarring because they do not provoke immune responses.

Monofilament sutures: These sutures are rigid and the knots are not well positioned on the wound.

Braided sutures: These have a capillary effect and high friction resistance. For an overview on suture materials see Tab. 6.1 [4, 5].

6.2.2 Thread thickness/suture sizes

Suture sizes are defined by the United States Pharmacopeia and are shown in Tab. 6.2.

6.2.3 Barbed sutures

To avoid the time-consuming knotting process but still create reliable and fixed sutures, barbed suture threads have been invented. These sutures have small barbs that allow traction in one direction only, thereby preventing the thread from being drawn back. Barbed sutures are used for myomectomy, vaginal cuff closure and also for bowel or bladder surgery. Nevertheless, a higher rate of bowel irritation and infection has been described in some cases in the literature. Furthermore, barbed sutures have a higher price than normal absorbable suture materials. Nevertheless, the existing data and metaanalysis describe the use of barbed sutures as a safe procedure to reduce time and surgical difficulty compared to conventional sutures in vaginal cuff closure. The comparison of barbed suture versus conventional suturing is shown in Tab. 6.3 [6, 7].

Tab. 6.1: Examples of suture materials.

Absorbable		Nonabsorbable	
Monofilamental	Braided	Monofilamental	Braided
PDS (PD)	Vicryl (G/L)	Ethilon (PA)	Ethibond (POE)
Maxon (PGS)	Dexon (G/L)	Prolene (PP)	Mersilene (POE)
G/L = Glycolid/Lactid		POE = Polyester	
PD = Polydiaxanon		PP = Polypropylene	
PGS = Polygylcol acid		PA = Polyamid	

Tab. 6.2: Suture sizes, defined by the United States Pharmacopeia.

USO designation	Synthetic absorbable diameter (mm)	Nonabsorbable diameter (mm)
11-0		0.01
10-0	0.02	0.02
9-0	0.03	0.03
8-0	0.04	0.04
7-0	0.05	0.05
6-0	0.07	0.07
5-0	0.1	0.1
4-0	0.15	0.15
3-0	0.2	0.2
2-0	0.3	0.3
0	0.35	0.35
1	0.4	0.4
2	0.5	0.5
3	0.6	0.6
4	0.6	0.6
5	0.7	0.7
6		0.8
7		

Tab. 6.3: Comparison of barbed suture versus conventional suture material.

Barbed suture vs. conventional suture	
Less operative time	Higher costs
Less suturing time	Higher rate of bowel obstructions
Lower degree of suturing difficulty/technically less demanding	
Similar patient outcome	
Similar duration of hospital stay	
Preferred method based on surgeon's preference	

6.2.4 Surgical needles

Needles can be reusable (eyed needles). Reusable needles have holes (eyes) and are supplied separately from their suture thread, which must be threaded on site. The advantage of these needles is that any thread and needle combination is possible. Needles with integrated thread are used in laparoscopy. They have less traumatic tissue effects and are time efficient but more expensive. Needles may also be classified by their point geometry: taper, cutting, reverse cutting, trocar point, or blunt points.

There are several shapes of surgical needles. These are listed in Tab. 6.4.

Tab. 6.4: Surgical needle types and variations.

Straight
1/4 circle
3/8 circle
1/2 circle: subtypes include from larger to smaller: CT, CT-1, CT-2 and CT-3
5/8 circle
Compound curve
Half curved (ski needle)
Half curved at both ends of a straight segment (canoe needle)

The correct selection of the appropriate suture is essential. Each surgical procedure requires specific needle configurations and needle-suture combinations.

The following suture exercises describe in easy steps:

(a) Two extracorporeal knotting techniques, the Roeder and the von Leffern knot (Figs. 6.1 and 6.2).
(b) The step-by-step procedure of intracorporeal knotting using the common techniques of knot tying (Figs. 6.3 and 6.4).

The primary role of the needle holder/driver is handling the needle, although suturing and tissue grasping are also part of its function. The preferred shape of the tip is a slightly spooning curvature. For grasping tissue and looping suture, the tip must be able to reach in almost any direction. The jaws should be finely engineered to grasp fine sutures without slipping and have rounded edges to avoid accidental cutting of the suture as traction is applied. The dominant needle holder should have a lock that the surgeon can activate or inactivate at will. It should be strong and preferably have one moving jaw to reduce suture snagging. The lock on the nondominant needle holder should preferably be inactivated.

6.3 Tips and tricks

6.3.1 Loading the needle

First, grasp the thread about an inch from the needle with the assisting grasper. Dangle it in a fashion so that the tip of the needle touches the tissue surface. The needle is rotated and pivoted until it lines up in the direction required. It is then grasped with the contralateral needle driver. The needle is loaded up at the junction of middle and proximal third of the shaft of the needle and at the very end of the needle driver.

Optimal conditions for good suturing include a needle holding angle of 90 degrees and an angle of needle insertion into tissue of 80–100 degrees. This can be guaranteed only if the contralateral hand is flipping the targeted tissue over the needle.

von Leffern Knot

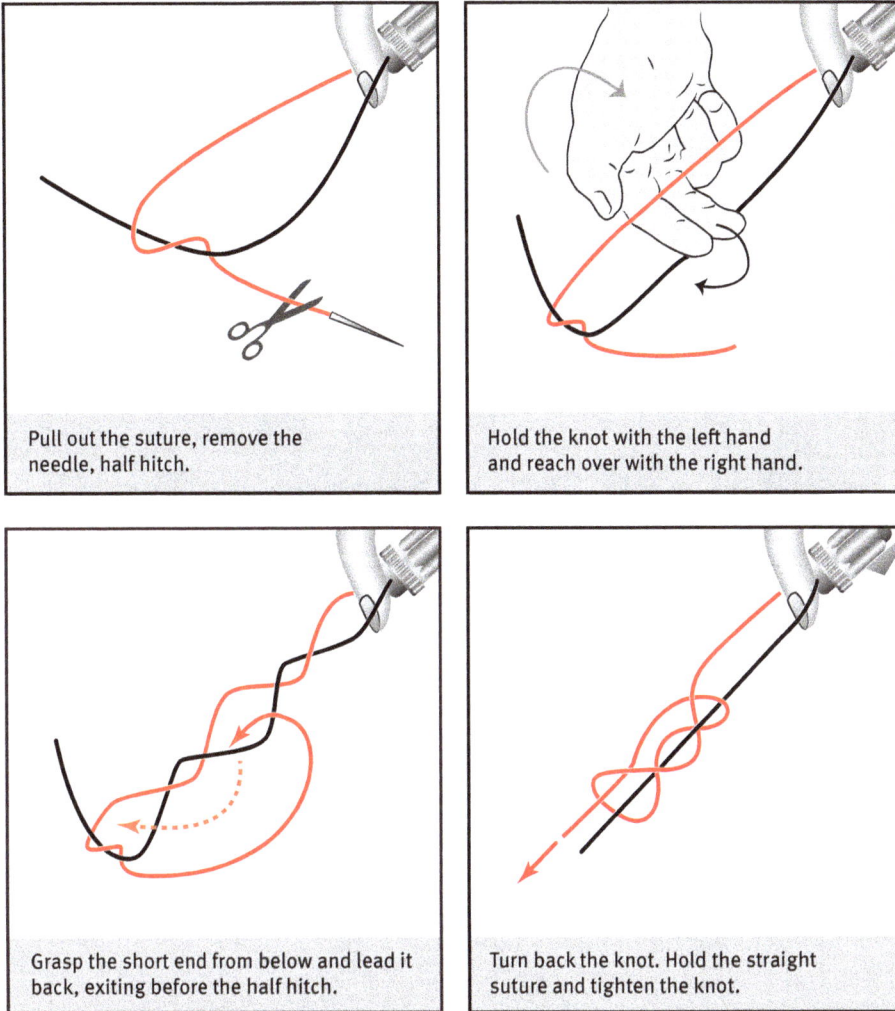

Pull out the suture, remove the needle, half hitch.

Hold the knot with the left hand and reach over with the right hand.

Grasp the short end from below and lead it back, exiting before the half hitch.

Turn back the knot. Hold the straight suture and tighten the knot.

Fig. 6.1: Von Leffern Knot: a half hitch is performed. The index and middle fingers then twist from below in between the sutures and grasp the short end, which is led back, exiting before the half hitch. Both ends are pulled on gently so that the knot does not slip over but tightens smoothly. Finally, the knot pusher can push the knot onto the leading suture line in the operating field.

6.3.2 Adjusting the needle

Adjusting the needle requires good coordination between the left and the right hand. After having grasped the needle at about the middle of the needle rounding, it is held very lightly. The other hand can then readjust by manipulating close to the tip in very deliberate movements.

Roeder Knot

Pull out the suture, remove the needle. Half hitch around the post strand.	Throw three loops around both strands. Maintain tension.
Half hitch around the post strand (red). Push the knot together.	Shorten the suture to approx. 2–3 cm and perform intraabdominal safety knot.

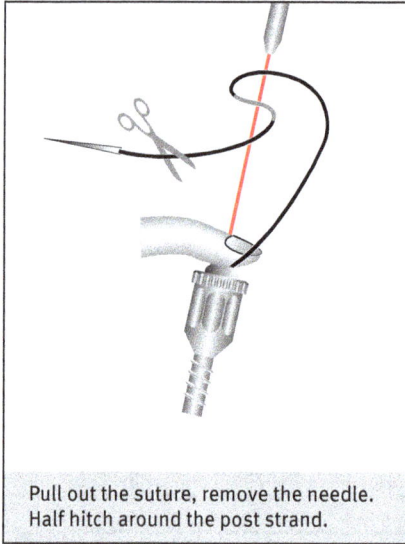

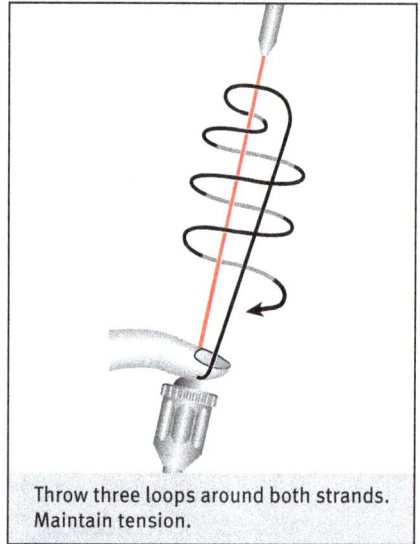

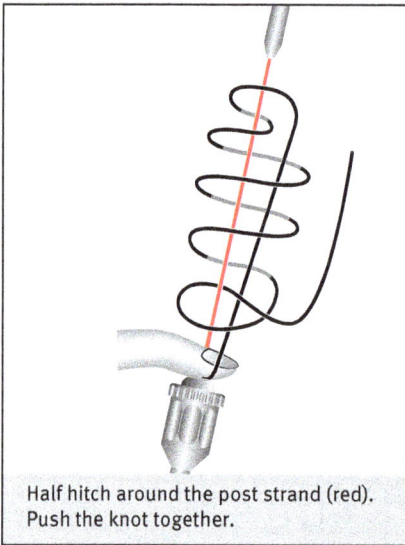

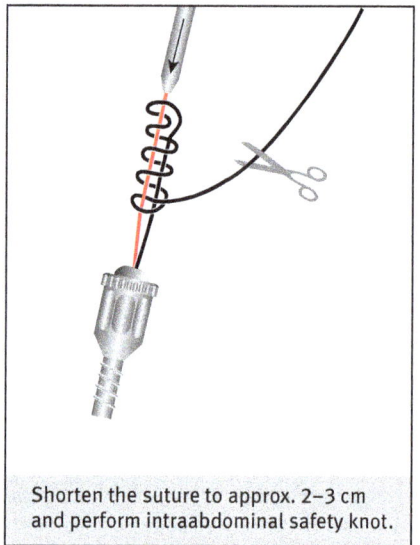

Fig. 6.2: Roeder knot: The shorter suture is looped three times around both sutures. The fourth time, it is looped only halfway and then pulled through the post strand. Both ends are pulled on gently that the knot does not slip over but tightens smoothly. Finally, the knot pusher can push the knot onto the leading suture line in the operating field.

Alternatively, the needle can be adjusted by holding the suture near the swaged end of the needle and maneuvering it until the needle is aligned perpendicular to the jaws. The other needle holder can then either grasp the needle in the estimated location or

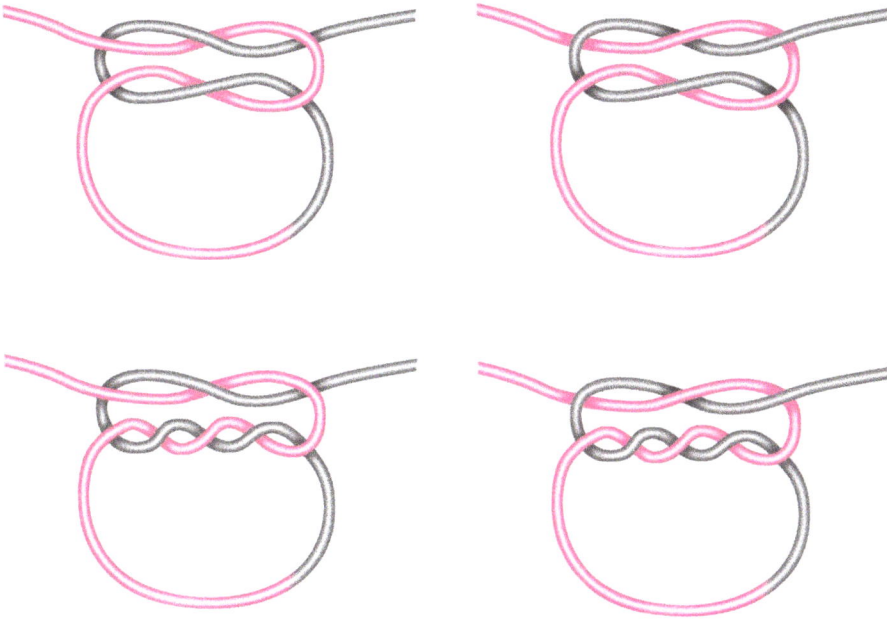

Fig. 6.3: The upper left drawing shows the classical square knot and the lower left drawing the surgical square knot. The upper right drawing depicts the classical granny knot and the lower right drawing the surgical granny knot.

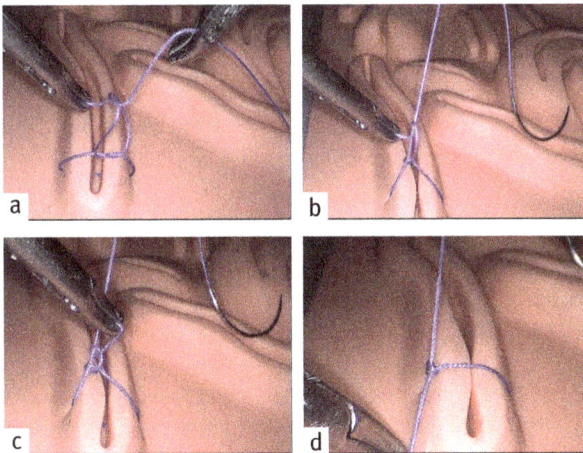

Fig. 6.4: Sliding knot. (a) After performing a normal half hitch, the initial knot lies directly on the wound. The second hitch is performed in exactly the same manner. (b) It is not essential that the lower knot lies deep in the tissue. The second knot is not straight but torqued. (c) As soon as the right instrument smoothly pulls the thread, the two knots, which are not yet tightened, will twist around the suture line that is being pulled on. (d) It is then possible to slide the complete double knot down to the tissue.

the needle is placed on the tissue so that it cannot squeeze out once the free needle holder takes over.

After the ideal position has been reached, the grip on the needle is tightened to lock it into position. Most important for stitching in the right position is that the targeted tissue is pushed over the needle tip at the exact location required. By this means, the limited degrees of freedom of movement in laparoscopy can be overcome even in challenging situations. Nevertheless, these are the steps that require the most time in training.

6.3.3 Tying the knot

The thread can be held in the right position by either adjusting the needle or the thread itself. It is most important that the thread runs as parallel as possible to the free and rotating needle holder. Rotating then becomes easy in both directions. Tying the knot is easier if the short end is really short (about 3 cm) and if the rotating needle holder grasps the thread at the very end before pulling it out of the loop smoothly using light rotating movements. For the second and the blocking knot, it is important to pull on the long end only so that there is enough thread for the following knots; however, the thread should not be longer than necessary [8].

Intracorporeal knotting techniques are shown in Figs. 6.3 and 6.4.

6.4 Conclusions

Laparoscopic suturing courses from beginner to expert for vertical and horizontal suturing, including hands-on training, are offered today all around the world. The advice of our teacher Kurt Semm, that laparoscopic suturing is essential, has been accepted by the endoscopic surgical community. Technical innovations have led to a number of alternatives including bipolar, monopolar, or ultrasound-guided energy. Nevertheless, for each individual situation, the right type of treatment needs to be selected, and therefore, it is obligatory that the experienced surgeon is conversant with all types of devices and is able to perform laparoscopic suturing. Otherwise, each surgery can become a jeopardy for both the patient and the surgeon [8, 9].

References

[1] Alkatout I, Mettler L, Maass N, Noe GK, Elessawy M. Abdominal anatomy in the context of port placement and trocars. J Turk Ger Gynecol Assoc 2015;16(4):241–51.
[2] Alkatout I, Mettler L, Maass N, Ackermann J. Robotic surgery in gynecology. J Turk Ger Gynecol Assoc 2016;17(4):224–32.
[3] Alkatout I. Complications of laparoscopy in connection with entry techniques. J Gynecol Surg 2017;33(3):81–91.

[4] Alkatout I, Mettler L. Hysterectomy—A Comprehensive Surgical Approach. Cham, Switzerland, Springer Science; 2017. 1639 p.

[5] Mettler L, Alkatout I, Keckstein J, Meinhold-Heerlein I. Endometriosis—A Concise Practical Guide to Current Diagnosis and Treatment. 1st ed. Tuttlingen: Endo Press; 2017.

[6] Bogliolo S, Musacchi V, Dominoni M, et al. Barbed suture in minimally invasive hysterectomy: a systematic review and meta-analysis. Arch Gynecol Obstet 2015;292(3):489–97.

[7] Kim JH, Byun SW, Song JY, et al. Barbed versus conventional 2-layer continuous running sutures for laparoscopic vaginal cuff closure. Medicine 2016;95(39):e4981.

[8] Alkatout I, Mettler L, Gunther V, et al. Safety and economical innovations regarding surgical treatment of fibroids. Minim Invasive Ther Allied Technol 2016;25(6):301–13.

[9] Alkatout I. [Communicative and ethical aspects of physician-patient relationship in extreme situations]. Wiener Medizinische Wochenschrift (1946) 2015;165(23–24):491–8.

Meghan McMahon and Mostafa A. Borahay

7 Challenges in minimally invasive surgery

Advances in the technology and expertise in minimally invasive surgery (MIS) enabled its expansion from diagnostic and minor operative procedures to more complex cases. While this extends the well-known benefits of MIS to complex and challenging cases (Box 7.1), it poses up to an eightfold increase of serious complications, including bowel, bladder, ureteral injuries, bleeding, and infection [1, 2]. In addition, the risk of conversion to laparotomy can be up to 45-fold higher in complex procedures [1]. These major complications and failed laparoscopy are most commonly attributed to obese patients and those with prior abdominal surgery [1]. In this chapter, we will discuss strategies for the safe management of these challenging cases.

7.1 Obesity

Obesity has increasingly become more common and currently affects more than one third of adults in the United States [3]. Unfortunately, obesity increases the risk of multiple gynecologic disorders. For example, obesity can exacerbate pelvic organ prolapse and urinary incontinence, while the associated sex steroid imbalance is associated with endometrial hyperplasia and cancer [4]. Therefore, obese women are more likely to require gynecologic surgery. Thus, it appears that obese women are double hit by an increased need for surgery and higher surgical complication rates. Although laparoscopic surgery in obese patients is associated with higher complication rates compared to non-obese patients such as estimated blood loss (EBL) and length of hospital stays; laparoscopic surgery can be successfully and safely completed in the majority of obese women [5, 6]. Obesity alone presents several challenges for surgery

Box 7.1: Examples of challenges in minimally invasive surgery.

- Obesity
- History of prior surgeries
- Endometriosis
- Cancer
- Radiation
- Tubo-ovarian abscess
- Pelvic inflammatory disease
- Large pelvic mass
- Large uterus
- Difficult entry

https://doi.org/10.1515/9783110535204-007

such as positioning, nerve injury, and trocar placement. In addition, obesity is often associated with comorbidities such as hypertension, type 2 diabetes, sleep apnea, and venous thromboembolism that make anesthesia, insufflation, wound healing, and recovery more risky.

7.1.1 Physiology

Obesity causes several cardiovascular, pulmonary, and gastrointestinal physiologic changes that impact surgical management. Cardiovascular changes include increased cardiac output, larger stroke volume, and decreased vascular resistance due to increased metabolic demands. These changes can lead to hypertension and cardiomegaly, placing patients at higher risk for arrhythmias and risk of sudden death. Obese patients also have decreased functional residual pulmonary volume secondary to reduced lung compliance. This is exacerbated with anesthesia and Trendelenburg position and therefore placing patients at risk for airway closure and hypoxemia. Obese patients are also suspected of having large gastric volumes and slower gastric emptying that can increase their risk for aspiration [7, 8].

7.1.2 Positioning

Obese patients are more likely to have nerve injury (Box 7.2) and pressure-related complications following laparoscopic surgery secondary to longer operating room times and more compressive forces [7]. Therefore, proper positioning and equipment are essential for prevention. Appropriate stirrups should be used in dorsal lithotomy position to accommodate the weight of the patient. Padding should be used generously in areas at risk, including the knees, calves, hips, and arms. Ideally, for both the surgeon and the patient, the arms should be tucked in military position, which may require bed extenders or sleds. Steep Trendelenburg position during surgery can lead to downward drifting of the patient, which is exacerbated with obesity and can cause brachial plexus stretch injuries. Therefore, egg crate, gel pad, or other materials should be placed underneath the patient for prevention [9].

Box 7.2: Common nerve injuries.

- *Peroneal*: foot drop
- *Femoral*: decreased knee extension, hip flexion, and sensation to anterior thigh
- *Obturator*: decreased adduction and sensation to medial thigh
- *Sciatic*: loss of sensation calf/foot and hamstring/calf weakness with loss of flexion
- *Ulnar*: numbness/tingling of fourth and fifth fingers. Weakening of grip
- *Brachial plexus*: numbness and weakness in hand, arm, and shoulder

---

7.1.3 Instruments

In preparation for the surgery, it is important to have the appropriate instruments, including longer Veress needle and trocars (120 to 150 mm) and instruments to retract bowel. Surgeons may also consider robotic surgery secondary to surgeon fatigue, better fluid movements with the articulated wrists and less torque of the instruments [7].

7.1.4 Trendelenburg and intraabdominal pressure

Trendelenburg position and pneumoperitoneum are required for successful laparoscopy. As mentioned above, obese patients have lower functional residual volume that can cause airway closure of dependent portions in the lung, resulting in perfusion/ventilation mismatch. It is known that supine positioning and anesthesia further decrease functional residual capacity (FRC) by approximately 25 and 20%, respectively [8]. However, positioning into Trendelenburg does not have a significant additional impact [8]. Morbidly obese patients have increased intraabdominal pressure that may require more pneumoperitoneum. This can lead to increased systemic absorption of CO_2, venous stasis, decreased urine output, lower respiratory compliance, decreased preload, and impaired cardiac function. However, proper ventilation adjustments, sequential compression devices, and intravascular volume monitoring and resuscitation can minimize these complications [10].

Most studies show that if patients tolerate the induction of anesthesia and supine positioning, they are likely to tolerate pneumoperitoneum and Trendelenburg position. However, it is recommended, once the patient is intubated and positioned, to perform the "Tilt Test." The patient is placed in steep Trendelenburg position for 2 to 5 minutes, while the cardiac and respiratory function is observed. These tests should also be performed for cephalad sliding of the patient. This is repeated after insufflation of pneumoperitoneum. If the patient remains normotensive and has inspiratory pressure of 30 to 40 mmHg before and after insufflation, the patient will likely tolerate laparoscopic surgery [8].

7.1.5 Entry

In the nonobese, entry into the abdomen is at the level of the umbilicus at a 45-degree angle and accessory trocar sites are placed in relationship to anatomical landmarks, such as the anterior superior iliac spines. However, abdominal entry in the morbidly obese poses challenges to this approach with increased subcutaneous tissue, preperitoneal fat and skewed anatomical landmarks. For example, the umbilicus is typically caudal (can be up to 6 cm) to the aortic bifurcation, anterior iliac spines can be difficult to palpate, and there is suboptimal visualization of the inferior epigastric vessels. Recommendations for safe entry include a supraumbilical approach, entering at a 90-degree angle to prevent tracking along the subcutaneous tissue (Fig. 7.1) and accessory trocar sites placed more lateral and cephalad [7, 8].

One Cochrane review reported that in the obese population, the Veress technique is associated with higher rates of false entry [11]. Therefore, other methods of entry can be considered such as the open Hasson technique, direct visualization with an optical trocar or the left upper quadrant (LUQ) approach (Palmer's point).

7.1.6 Closure

Due to increased intraabdominal pressure, obese patients are at higher risk of herniation through the trocar sites. Closure of any port size greater than or equal to

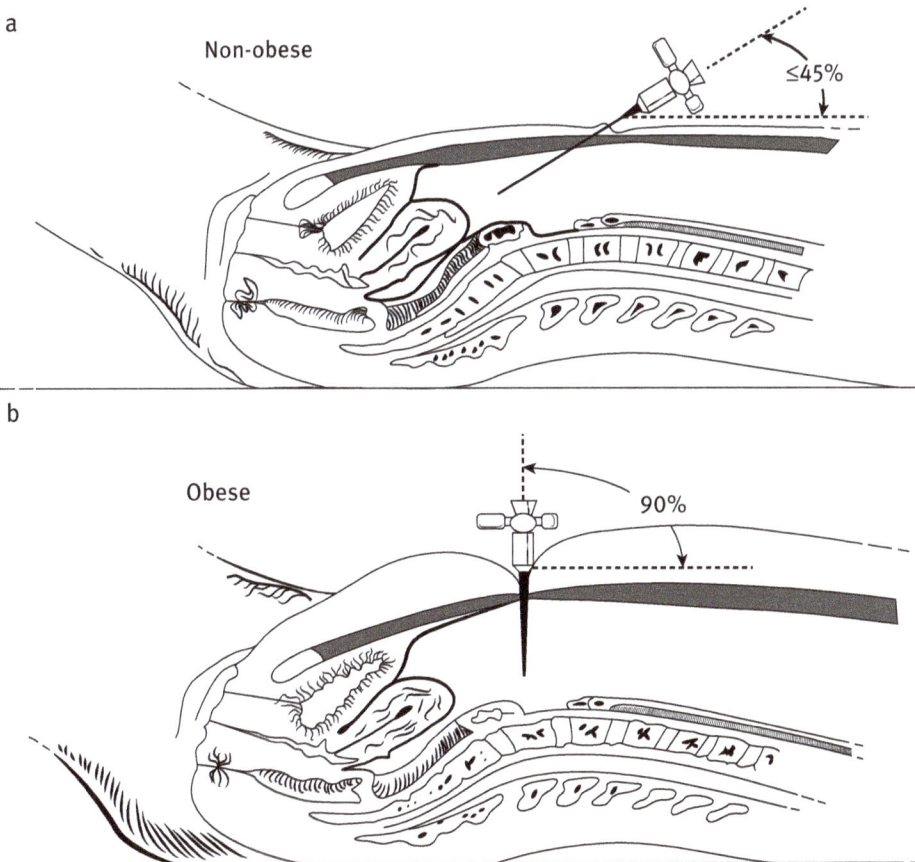

Fig. 7.1: An illustration showing the recommended angle of peritoneal entry by Veress needle in (a) the nonobese with an angle of 45 degrees and in (b) the obese with an angle of 90 degrees.

10 mm is essential. However, this closure can be very challenging secondary to large subcutaneous fat, and closure devices may be required.

7.1.7 Postoperative challenges

Common postoperative complications in obese patients include hypoxemia and pulmonary emboli. Consequently, aggressive pulmonary toilet with incentive spirometry, coughing exercises, deep breathing, and semirecumbent position are imperative. In addition, early ambulation, sequential compression devices, and prophylactic subcutaneous anticoagulation help prevent life-threatening complications.

7.2 Frozen pelvis

"No surgeon can expect surgical outcomes better than their dissection skills" [21].

A "frozen pelvis" is described as one in which normal anatomy and dissection planes are distorted by extensive adhesive disease and scarring. This can arise from several etiologies, including (1) prior surgery, (2) infections (pelvic inflammatory disease, tubo-ovarian abscess), (3) benign growths (endometriosis, adenomyosis, and leiomyomas), (4) cancer, and (5) radiation therapy [12].

Prior surgeries are one of the biggest risk factors for the development of adhesions. The risk for adhesions is related to the type of previous surgery and incision location. The risk of postoperative adhesions in all abdominal surgery is approximately 54% [13]. Specifically, in obstetrics and gynecologic surgery, it is estimated at 51% [13]. The risk of subsequent adhesion formation can be further broken down by type of incision: midline incision (57%), Pfannenstiel (27%), and all other incisions (22%) [13].

Preoperative management is extremely important when significant adhesive disease is suspected. The following steps should be taken to optimize a successful surgery [12]:

1. Determine risk factors—surgical, infectious, and medical history to see which of the above-mentioned etiologies the patient may be at risk for.
2. Physical examination—to determine the size of the mass or uterus and whether the structure is fixed or mobile. Rectovaginal examination is essential to provide information on the mobility of the posterior cul-de-sac.
3. Consider preoperative imaging studies in selected cases—pelvic ultrasound, computed tomography, or magnetic resonance imaging (MRI). These may yield information regarding involvement of other organs or structures (side walls, ureters, adnexa, bowel, bladder, etc.).

4. Intraoperative planning—cystoscopy, sigmoidoscopy, ureteral stent placement prior to surgery, preparing blood products.
5. Consultation of other specialties.

Once in the operating room, approximately 50% of complications related to laparoscopic surgery occur during the initial entry [14]. There are several different entry techniques, including closed (Veress), open (Hasson), direct visualized trocar entry, and more. Please refer to Chapter 6 ("Laparoscopic entry techniques") for more details. In general, it is advantageous to enter at virginal areas of the abdomen or nonclassical incisions in order to decrease injury. These entry points include the LUQ at Palmer's point or supraumbilical.

Two principles are critical for safe laparoscopic surgery, particularly with adhesive disease: knowledge of relevant anatomy and sound surgical technique.

Upon entry, identify landmarks and their relationships within the pelvis. At this time, the extent of adhesions and distortion of the anatomy can be assessed and adhesiolysis may be required. Principles of adhesiolysis include following natural tissue planes, traction-countertraction, and using blunt and sharp dissection over energy to avoid thermal injury [15]. Dissection should be performed millimeter by millimeter; this allows for good orientation, control of instruments, and technique, time to evaluate, quick control of bleeding and early identification of injury. Good surgical dissection utilizes the following techniques: (1) grasp and tent—elevates tissue away from vital structures; (2) push-spread—thins out tissue to visualize structures; (3) gentle wiping/teasing—further thins out tissue; and even (4) hydrodissection—helps dissect into potential spaces [16].

In a difficult frozen pelvis, it may be useful to also consider robotic technology, which has advantages such as improved ergonomics, three-dimensional visualization, improved dexterity and range of motion, and tremor filtration [17].

In cases with frozen pelvis, the retroperitoneal approach can be key to success where major vessels and the ureters can be identified. Entry includes isolating and transecting the round ligament to develop the retroperitoneal space while proceeding cephalad parallel to the infundibulopelvic ligament. It is then imperative to understand the retroperitoneal spaces (Box 7.3 and Fig. 7.2) [12, 16, 17]:

- The *paravesical* space is bordered anteriorly by the pubic bone, medially by the bladder, laterally by the fascia of the obturator internus muscle and posteriorly by the cardinal ligament/parametrium with the uterine artery. It includes important landmarks such as the external iliac vessels, obturator space, and nerve and the hypogastric nerve.
- The *pararectal* space has the ureter and rectum as the medial border and the internal iliac arteries as the lateral border. The sacrum is inferior, while the cardinal ligament separates it from the paravesical space anteriorly. The space contains the uterosacral ligament.

Box 7.3: Pelvic retroperitoneal spaces.

Lateral:	Midline:
− Paravesical	− Retropubic
− Pararectal	− Vesicovaginal
− Okabayashi	− Rectovaginal
	− Presacral

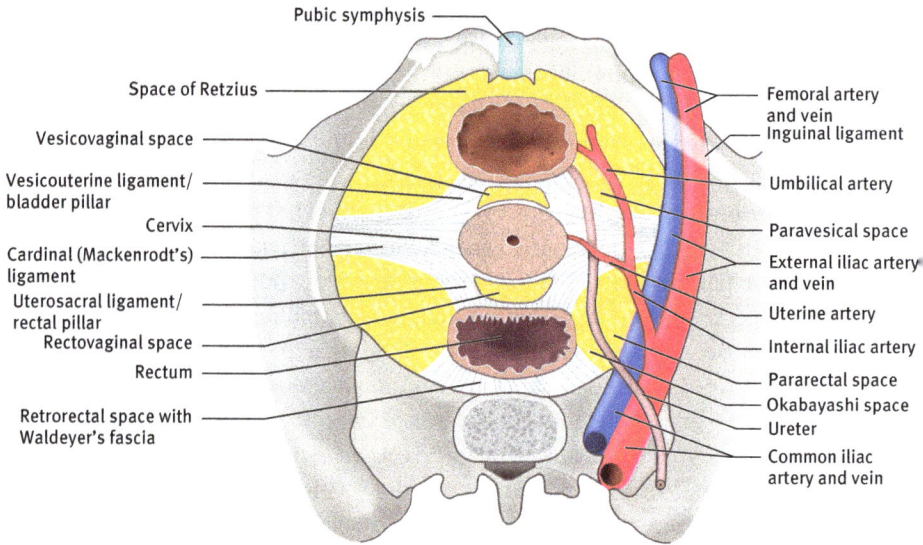

Fig. 7.2: An illustration demonstrating the pelvic retroperitoneal spaces and relevant anatomical landmarks. Please refer to text for further details.

- The *Okabayashi* space is created after dissecting the peritoneum from the ureter and mobilizing the peritoneum medially toward the rectum. The space is then bounded by the ureter laterally and the peritoneum medially. This space includes the hypogastric nerve to be identified and preserved in nerve-sparing radical hysterectomy.
- The *rectopubic* space of Retzius is located behind the pubic symphysis and in front the bladder.
- The *vesicovaginal* space is a potential avascular space between the posterior aspect of the bladder and the anterior aspect of the vagina. The bladder pillars are located laterally, where the vesical arteries, veins, nerves, and ureters pass on the anterolateral surface of the upper vagina. Development of the vesicovaginal space allows direct access to the bladder, cervix, vagina, and distal ureters.

- The *rectovaginal* space is bounded by the cul-de-sac peritoneum and the utero-sacral ligaments superiorly and the peritoneal body inferiorly. The iliococcygeus muscles are the lateral borders.
- The *presacral* space boundaries include the rectum, sacrum, uterosacral ligaments, and levator ani muscle. The right lateral border is the common iliac artery and ureter and the left lateral border is the common iliac vein and left ureter. This space contains the middle sacral artery and veins, sacral venous plexus, and hypogastric nerve plexus.

Last, our aim should be adhesion prevention whenever possible. Surgical techniques to limit adhesion formation include gentle tissue handling, meticulous hemostasis, irrigation, minimal use of energy, avoidance of excessive suturing, and less foreign materials. Other adjunct treatments include drugs to decrease the adhesion producing inflammatory cascade and barrier agents that separate the serosal surfaces during wound healing [16, 18]. Please refer to Chapter 9 ("Adhesions after laparoscopic and hysteroscopic surgery, prevention, and treatment") for additional information.

7.3 Large uterus or pelvic mass

The decision for laparoscopic versus open approach for a large uterus or pelvic mass depends on factors including the size and shape. However, there are no definite cut-offs. Several reviews and case reports suggest that MIS can be successfully adopted by experienced surgeons for virtually any mass size. Potential challenges include limited range of motion, obstructed field of view, impeded access to uterine vascular pedicles and other adjacent structures, and difficult extraction.

To increase success, the following recommendations should be followed. First, one may consider obtaining an MRI to better assess the size, the number, and the location of fibroids if present. Second, primary entry may not be feasible at the level of the umbilicus and a supraumbilical or LUQ approach may be required. The size and shape of the large uterus or mass should also be taken into account for accessory port placement. Third, using a 30-degree angle scope over 0 degrees can improve visualization around the corners of the pathology. Fourth, the use of a myoma spiral and robust uterine manipulator increases maneuverability. Fifth, to help decrease blood loss, one could ligate the uterine pedicle as the first step of the hysterectomy [19, 20]. The last challenge in these cases is removal of the large uterus and/or pelvic mass. This can be performed vaginally versus abdominally with morcellation, typically using a contained tissue extraction system. Please see Chapter 11 for more details on morcellation.

7.4 Difficult insufflation and positioning

Gynecologic laparoscopic surgery requires pneumoperitoneum and Trendelenburg positioning for visualization and exposure, safe trocar placement, and adequate space to perform the procedure at hand.

Pneumoperitoneum is obtained with insufflation of gas, usually CO_2, with pressures of 15 to 20 mmHg into the peritoneal cavity. The result of this increased abdominal pressure causes compression of vessels (including the inferior vena cava) and organs in the abdomen, leading to a reduction in venous return with subsequent decreased cardiac output and increased systemic vascular resistance. Also, the increased intraabdominal pressure triggers elevation of the diaphragm, which impedes expansion of the lungs, leading to decreased functional residual volume. This can produce atelectasis in the basal areas of the lungs, which then become underventilated, resulting in hypoxemia [21]. Pneumoperitoneum also induces hypercapnia by systemic absorption of the carbon dioxide [21, 22].

Trendelenburg positioning can also have unfavorable outcomes. Steep positioning can decrease venous return from the head, causing increased intracranial and intraocular pressures [21, 23]. In terms of pulmonary adverse effects, Trendelenburg exacerbates the already decreased functional residual volume, lung volumes, and lung compliance [21].

Cardiovascular and respiratory complications secondary to insufflation and positioning include arrhythmias, subcutaneous emphysema, pneumothorax, gas emboli, and even cardiac arrest [21, 22]. In these situations, it is imperative for the surgeon and anesthesiologist to work in collaboration to achieve an optimal outcome. More recent data suggest the utility of a low pressure pneumoperitoneum without any significant difference in visualization, operative time, estimated blood loss, or intraoperative complications, including conversion to laparotomy [24]. In addition, successful laparoscopic surgery can be achieved at a decreased Trendelenburg angle [25].

7.5 Conclusion

MIS is now the standard of care in gynecology due to its proven benefits. However, increasingly challenging cases require highly trained surgeons, possible only through adequate operating room training and simulation exercises. With the limited number of surgeries, residency programs should incorporate more simulation-based curricula. Furthermore, there is evidence that the current trainees may be different from past trainee due to factors including video and computer games [26, 27]. There is also evidence that laparoscopic and robotic simulation skills training cross over [28]. Multiple studies have proven that simulation training leads to significant improvements in the operating room [29–31]. Unfortunately, some data suggest that only 60–70% of programs teach laparoscopic skills and only 59% were satisfied with their training [32]. This is a huge area for improvement as the field of minimally invasive gynecologic surgery continues to grow.

References

[1] Fuentes MN, Rodríguez-Oliver A, Naveiro Rilo JC, et al. Complications of laparoscopic gynecologic surgery. J Soc Laparoendosc Surg 2014;18(3):e2014.00058. http://doi.org/10.4293/JSLS.2014.00058

[2] Magrina JF. Complications of laparoscopic surgery. Clin Obstet Gynecol 2002;45(2):469–80.

[3] Adult obesity Fact. Center for Disease Control and Prevention website. https://www.cdc.gov/obesity/data/adult.html. Updated August 29, 2017. Accessed November 20, 2017.

[4] Pandey S, Bhattacharya S. Impact of obesity on gynecology. Womens Health (Lond) 2010;6(1):107–17. doi:10.2217/whe.09.77.

[5] Papadia A, Ragni N, Salom EM. The impact of obesity on surgery in gynecological oncology: a review. Int J Gynecol Cancer 2006;16(2):944–52.

[6] Heinberg EM, Crawford BL 3rd, Weitzen SH, Bonilla DJ. Total laparoscopic hysterectomy in obese versus nonobese patients. Obstet Gynecol 2004;103(4):674–80.

[7] Scheib SA, Tanner E 3rd, Green IC, Fader AN. Laparoscopy in the morbidly obese: physiologic considerations and surgical techniques to optimize success. J Minim Invasive Gynecol 2014;21(2):182–95. doi:10.1016/j.jmig.2013.09.009.

[8] Lamvu G, Zolnoun D, Boggess J, Steege JF. Obesity: physiologic changes and challenges during laparoscopy. Am J Obstet Gynecol 2004;191:669–74.

[9] Bradshaw AD, Advincula AP. Postoperative neuropathy in gynecologic surgery. Obstet Gynecol Clin North Am 2010;37(3):451–9.

[10] Nguyen NT, Wolfe BM. The physiologic effects of pneumoperitoneum in the morbidly obese. Ann Surg 2005 Feb;241(2):219–26.

[11] Ahmad G, O'Flynn H, Duffy JM, Phillips K, Watson A. Laparoscopic entry techniques. Cochrane Database Syst Rev 2012;15(2).

[12] Goldstein D. Surgical strategies to untangle a frozen pelvis. OBG Manag 2007;19(3):62–70.

[13] Okabayashi K, Ashrafian H, Zacharakis E, et al. Adhesions after abdominal surgery: a systematic review of the incidence, distribution and severity. Surg Today 2014;44(3):405–20.

[14] Vilos GA. The ABCS of a safer laparoscopic entry. J Minim Invasive Gynecol 2006;13(3):249–51.

[15] Zimberg SE, Sprague ML. Unexpected pathology: severe pelvic adhesions. In: Coomarasamy A, ed. Gynecologic and Obstetric Surgery: Challenges and Management Options. Chichester, West Sussex, Hoboken, NJ: John Wiley & Sons Inc.; 2016:92–93.

[16] Rogers RM Jr, Taylor RH. The Core of a competent surgeon: a working knowledge of surgical anatomy and safe dissection techniques. Obstet Gynecol Clin North Am 2011;38(4):777–88.

[17] Truong M, Kim JH, Scheib S, Patzkowsky K. Advantages of robotics in benign gynecologic surgery. Curr Opin Obstet Gynecol 2016;28(4):304–10.

[18] Liakakos T, Thomakos N, Fine PM, Dervenis C, Young RL. Peritoneal adhesions: etiology, pathophysiology, and clinical significance. Recent advances in prevention and management. Dig Surg 2001;18(4):260–73.

[19] Zimberg SE, Sprague ML. Laparoscopic hysterectomy for large fibroid uterus. In: Coomarasamy A, ed. Gynecologic and Obstetric Surgery: Challenges and Management Options. Chichester, West Sussex, Hoboken, NJ: John Wiley & Sons Inc.; 2016:247–9.

[20] Sinha R, Sundaram M, Lakhotia S, Mahajan C, Manaktala G, Shah P. Total laparoscopic hysterectomy for large uterus. J Gynecol Endosc Surg 2009;1(1):34–9.

[21] Nguyen JH, Tanaka PP. Anesthesia for laparoscopic surgery. In: Wetter PA, ed. Prevention and Management of Laparoendoscopic Surgical Complications, 3rd ed. Miami, FL: Society of Laparoendoscopic Surgeons; 2010.

[22] Srivastava A, Niranjan A. Secrets of safe laparoscopic surgery: anaesthetic and surgical considerations. J Minim Access Surg 2010;6(4):91–4.

[23] Borahay MA, Patel PR, Walsh TM, et al. Intraocular pressure and steep Trendelenburg during minimally invasive gynecologic surgery: is there a risk? J Minim Invasive Gynecol 2013 Nov–Dec;20(6):819–24.

[24] Bogani G, Uccella S, Cromi A, et al. Low vs standard pneumoperitoneum pressure during laparoscopic hysterectomy: prospective randomized trial. J Minim Invasive Gynecol 2014 May–Jun;21(3):466–71.

[25] Gould C, Cull T, Wu YX, Osmundsen B. Blinded measure of Trendelenburg angle in pelvic robotic surgery. J Minim Invasive Gynecol 2012;19(4):465–8.

[26] Borahay MA, Jackson M, Tapısız OL, et al. Assessment of minimally invasive surgical skills of pre-medical students: What can we learn from future learners? J Turk Ger Gynecol Assoc 2014 Jun 1;15(2):69–73.

[27] Öge T, Borahay MA, Achjian T, Kılıç SG. Impact of current video game playing on robotic simulation skills among medical students. J Turk Ger Gynecol Assoc 2015 Mar 1;16(1):1–4.

[28] Borahay MA, Haver MC, Eastham B, Patel PR, Kilic GS. Modular comparison of laparoscopic and robotic simulation platforms in residency training: a randomized trial. J Minim Invasive Gynecol 2013 Nov–Dec;20(6):871–9.

[29] Asoğlu MR, Achjian T, Akbilgiç O, Borahay MA, Kılıç GS. The impact of a simulation-based training lab on outcomes of hysterectomy. J Turk Ger Gynecol Assoc 2016 Jan 12;17(2):60–4.

[30] Shore EM, Grantcharov TP, Husslein H, et al. Validating a standardized laparoscopy curriculum for gynecology residents: a randomized controlled trial. Am J Obstet Gynecol 2016;215(2):204.

[31] Kirby TO, Numnum TM, Kilgore LC, Straughn JM. A prospective evaluation of a simulator-based laparoscopic training program for gynecology residents. J Am Coll Surg. 2008 Feb;206(2):343–8.

[32] Shore EM, Lefebvre GG, Grantcharov TP. Gynecology resident laparoscopy training: present and future. Am J Obstet Gynecol. 2015;2012(3):298–301.

Luz Angela Torres-de la Roche, Lasse Leicher, Rajesh Devassy
and Rudy Leon De Wilde

8 Adhesions after laparoscopic and hysteroscopic surgery, prevention, and treatment

8.1 Introduction

Peritoneal adhesions (PAs) are connective tissue bands between two normally separate anatomical structures within the abdominal or pelvic cavity and are the most common complication after gynecological as well as other abdominal and pelvic surgeries in men and women (Fig 8.1). They lead to clinically and economically significant consequences and negatively influence the quality of health of affected people [1]. Though physicians are aware of PA, critical steps in their pathophysiology remain unidentified and their impact on morbidity is often ignored. Hence, the disease has been dubbed the "ignored iceberg of medicine" [2]. PAs are of considerable importance in women's health, due to the relationship of PA to chronic pelvic pain (CPP), infertility, and repeated readmissions. Despite adhesiolysis being the only treatment option, the clinical benefit of adhesiolysis as part of the management of pain syndromes is still controversial and most patients will not be operated. In this chapter, we will outline the current knowledge of the pathophysiology, the clinical aspects, the importance of surgical technique and the role of the minimal invasive surgery in the diagnosis and treatment of adhesion-related pain and infertility. Finally, we present an outlook on available methods to avoid or reduce the recurrence of PA.

8.2 Pathophysiology

To understand the development of permanent PA, it is necessary to take a closer look at mesothelial repair. It was first noted in 1919 by Hertzler [3] that both small and large peritoneal injuries healed at the same time, and healing differs from healing of injuries to squamous epithelium, where proliferating cells migrate from the edge of the wound inward. Several different theories have since been proposed for mesothelial repair, including:
- Centripetal migration of mesothelial cells
- Macrophage transformation [4]
- Exfoliation of mature or proliferating mesothelial cells from adjacent or opposing surfaces [5]
- Preexisting free-floating serosal reserve cells [4]
- Subserosal mesenchymal precursors [6]
- Bone marrow-derived circulating precursors

https://doi.org/10.1515/9783110535204-008

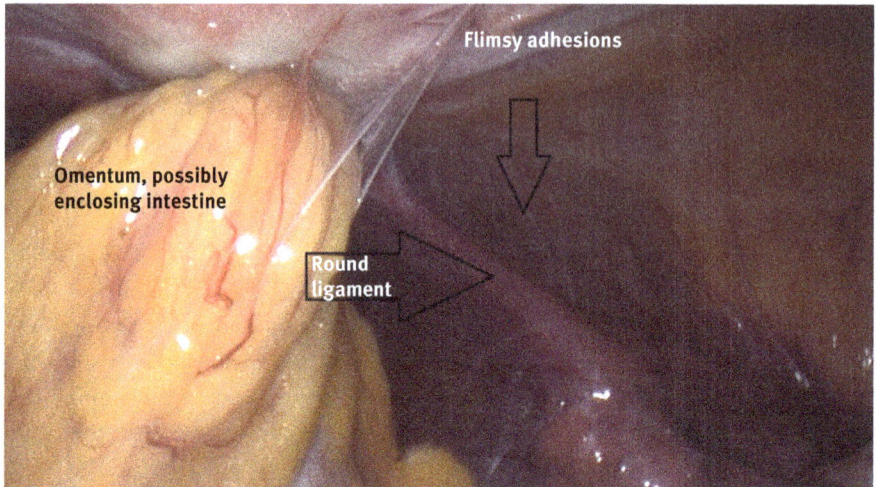

Fig. 8.1: In the foreground, a cohesive adhesion from momentum to abdominal lining is visible. In the background, there is a flimsy adhesion from abdominal wall to the round ligament of the uterus.

Research has failed to find support for most of those theories, and the exact mechanism of mesothelial regeneration is still controversial [7]. However, those studies have given us a better understanding of peritoneal healing: Both the parietal and visceral peritoneum are dynamic membranes involved in homeostasis of the peritoneal cavity and consist of two layers each: a one cell layer thick mesothelium and a submesothelial layer containing fibroblasts, macrophages, and blood vessels. After injury, platelets attach within minutes through the activated coagulation cascade, which also attract mesothelial cells, macrophages, neutrophils, lymphocytes, and fibroblasts. Together, these cells form a fibrin gel matrix, fixating opposing sites to each other. Under normal conditions, the gel matrix is eliminated through a fibrinolytic sequence initiated by plasmin, while mesothelial and fibroblastic cells proliferate over the surface, reestablishing normal peritoneum [8]. The "metabolism" of PA is a time-dependent process. If fibrinolysis is not completed after 3 days, for example as a result of residual blood, damaged mesothelial cells or prolonged inflammation, mature fibroblasts form permanent PA [9], which cannot be fibrinolyzed. However, the properties and capabilities of cells initiating the mesothelial and fibroblastic proliferation have not been characterized as of yet. Multipotent cells have been postulated, with a stem cell or mesenchymal stromal cell population being the most likely candidates.

Contrary to the general assumptions of PA as mostly nonfunctional scar tissue, close examination, and histologic reports show them to consist of mostly vascularized collagen and adipose tissue, with smooth muscle and even myelinated and demyelinated axons.

8.3 Role of mesothelial cells

Mesothelial cells play a crucial role in the development of PA. They are actively involved in local fibrin deposition and clearance in the serosal cavities, having both procoagulant and fibrinolytic activity, and play a role in preventing and removing fibrin deposits after mechanical injury or infection. Their role in the development of PA remains unclear, but recent studies showed evidence for a dedifferentiation process during prolonged healing, called the mesothelial to mesenchymal transition (MMT). MMT is similar to the endothelial to mesenchymal transition that has been observed in fibrosis in peritoneal dialysis patients. In the MMT model, mesothelial cells lose their apico-basal polarity and dedifferentiate toward a fibroblast-like phenotype that allows them to migrate and the capacity to synthesize extracellular matrix components, replacing mesothelial with fibrous tissue [10]. The mechanism explains the way fibroblastic strands develop during prolonged wound healing but does not provide a full understanding of the pathological induction of PA.

8.4 Role of stem cells

The idea of a precursor population, be it of stem cell, mesenchymal stroma cell, or another origin, has been consistently proposed and discussed in theory. However, the lack of convincing data allowed for multiple interpretations, from migrating bone marrow-derived stem cells to hematopoietic-derived mesenchymal stroma cells to subserosal stem cells and more. The discovery of structures from different cell types (muscle, nerve, fat) in mature PA (see pathophysiology) led to a closer characterization of submesothelial cell populations, which showed positive markers for multiple germ layers [11]. This argues the case of a local multipotent precursor population as the key to adhesion formation during prolonged regeneration, although research in this field is ongoing and a causal or lineageal link between precursor cells and PA has not been identified.

8.5 Physician awareness

A 2014 study analyzed 414 gynecological surgeons from the UK, Germany, the Netherlands, and Italy [12]; 70.8% considered PA a source of major morbidity. About half stated that PA represented a major part of their daily work. Two thirds informed their patients about the possibility and risks of adhesion formation. While 60% knew the recommended surgical techniques to reduce PA, only 44% used an antiadhesion agent. Consequently, the PA working group of the European Society for Gynecological Endoscopy (ESGE) recognized PA as the most frequent complication of abdominopelvic surgery with heightened morbidity, mortality, and cost, as the leading cause of bowel obstruction and an important cause of subfertility, pain, etc. [13] and, among others, demanded higher awareness by surgeons, healthcare workers, budget holders, and policy makers and better counseling and information of patients.

8.6 Who is at risk of PA?

Well-known personal risk factors for PA formation include endometriosis, prior pelvic or abdominal surgery, history of pelvic inflammatory disease, history of ectopic pregnancy, inflammatory bowel disease, perforated visceral organ, peritonitis, abscesses, diverticulitis, anastomotic leaks, carcinomatosis, radiation therapy, and long-term peritoneal dialysis [18, 19]. Of those, endometriosis is the most influencing factor on adhesion formation, even of greater influence than the number of previous surgeries. At least 10–28% of women who underwent laparoscopic surgery because of CPP have never had any operation [20, 21].

8.7 Influence of the surgical approach in adhesion formation

When trying to establish surgical techniques to prevent postsurgical adhesion formation, laparoscopic interventions were postulated to be superior to open surgery, because of the smaller injury to the peritoneal lining, the smaller disruption of the moist environment, decreased contact with the peritoneal surface and minimal exposition of the peritoneum. Contrary arguments were the adhesiogenic effect of CO_2 by induction of bulging of the mesothelial membrane cells and local acidosis [14–16] and the incorporation of the complete abdomen, compared to focal peritoneal opening in most open surgeries. Reviewed clinical studies demonstrated laparoscopy producing fewer and less thick PA when compared to laparotomic surgeries for identical diseases [17]. Secondly, laparoscopic procedures achieved fewer reemergencies of PA in adhesiolysis operations when compared to open surgery in animals.

The surgeries with the strongest correlation are endometriosis excision, hysterectomy, ovariectomy, appendectomy, gastrectomy, cholecystectomy, colostomy, abdominoperineal resection, and vascular procedures [19, 22, 24]. The majority of patients (38–55%) will form PA on the ovary, genital tract, and bowel [25].

The incidence of PA is related to the surgery approach, with laparotomy being more adhesiogenic than laparoscopy ($p < 0.000$, 95% confidence interval [CI], 1.02–1.99), regardless of whether clean or dirty [20]. Midline incisions result in more PA than all types of incisions performed for obstetric surgery [20, 26]. In the same way, new minimal invasive techniques via natural orifice transluminal endoscopic surgery or robotics exhibit low PA in animal models, but more studies are required to confirm this in humans [27].

A recent literature review with a consequential proof-of-principal clinical trial showed that the rigorous exercise of all minimally invasive principles, which are (1) atraumatic tissue handling, (2) prevention of hypoxia, reactive oxygen species, desiccation, and local inflammation, together with (3) the use of antiadhesive barriers, resulted in nearly complete prevention of PA, questioning whether the high incidence of PA on a population level could be mostly due to inappropriately or outdated surgical techniques [9].

8.8 Complications and clinical significance

As a result of PA, patients exhibit a range of sequelae, including infertility, CPP, small bowel obstruction, reinterventions, difficulties or inadvertent bowel injury at reoperation or during adhesiolysis, extended reintervention times, and prolonged hospital stays, and it could produce difficulties to apply minimally invasive surgery in further surgeries. In addition, managing these sequelae requires high costs from patients and the health system [23, 28]. Less commonly, PA could produce bladder dysfunction and urethral obstruction and interfere with intraperitoneal therapies [21].

In relation to infertility, PAs are responsible for 20–40% of secondary infertility cases in women [23]. A meta-analysis including 10 studies with 1004 women [24] found that after colorectal surgery for inflammatory bowel disease, only 50% (37–63%) of women achieved a pregnancy up to 158 months after surgery vs. 82% (70–94%) in nonoperated women.

Additionally, PAs increase the risk of intestinal injury during open (19%) and laparoscopic (10–25%) reoperations. In a big case series, enterotomy occurred in 3.7–7.9% of cases when adhesiolysis was performed during gastrointestinal (8.7%) and gynecological (4.8%) surgery. However, in comparison with open surgery, the incidence of intestinal injuries is significantly lower during laparoscopic adhesiolysis (odds ratio [OR], 0.21; CI, 0.05–0.90) [24].

Probably, the most expensive complication of PA is readmissions, but the chance of readmission is equal after laparotomy and laparoscopy. Specifically, in women, previous ovarian surgery and hysterectomy harvest the greatest risk of readmission [29]. It is expected that 5–30% of operated patients will be readmitted within 10 years after an extensive open surgery, greater with bowel obstruction (74% of cases) after lower gastrointestinal tract surgery, urological surgery, or abdominal wall surgery [20, 28, 30, 31]. However, the incidence of intestinal obstruction is lower after laparoscopic procedures (OR, 0.38%; CI, 0.16–0.91). In addition, bowel obstruction cases are responsible for long hospital stays (mean 7.8 days) and 1.9–3.0% of patients will die as a result of this obstruction [24]. The cost of readmission in the United Kingdom is estimated to be circa £24.2–95.2 million at 2 and 5 years after surgery, respectively [23].

8.9 Chronic pain

In CPP, it is often unclear if PAs are the primary or secondary etiology of the pain [19, 30]. PAs were identified as cause of pain in 57% (47%–67%) of patients with a previous surgery and in 40% (34%–47%) of patients after a gastrointestinal surgery for adhesive small bowel obstruction. The highest pain scores are found when the filmy PAs involve movable structures like ovaries or peritoneum, but fixed or dense PAs, independent of their location, have the lowest pain scores [32]. Nevertheless, PAs are not a common cause of chronic pain in men, and there are women without pain who exhibit PA at laparoscopy, even with evidence of nerve fibers within the PA [19]. Pain in patients identifying as colic is mostly due to obstruction and possible ischemia, while chronic pain could stem from the peritoneal lining, the PA itself or traction executed on organs due to PA. To distinguish these entities, multiple surgeries have been conducted on awake patients under local anesthesia, showing that pain was produced by touching the peritoneal lining and PA between movable organs. Touch or traction on dense PAs or PAs that do not limit movement of organs did not produce pain. As chronic pain syndromes often have multiple moderators, such as socioeconomic status and plastic changes in the peripheral and central nervous system, a single causative pathway has not been found. Studies have shown pain score to decrease in up to 70% of chronic pain patients who underwent adhesiolysis, with 29% being pain free [33]. Disappointingly, initial improvements seem to be relatively short-lived, as most studies show pain-free intervals of less than 2 years, which can be explained by an extremely high tendency of PA to recur in up to 97% of cases [34].

8.10 Classification/adhesion risk scores: pre- and intraoperative scores

Efforts have been made in order to establish a classification and standard index to try to predict and to manage PA. They could be classified as PA formed at operative sites, *de novo* at nonoperative sites or formed after the lysis of previous PA, as in the classification proposed by Diamond *et al.* [18].

Based on the macroscopic appearance and their extent to the different regions of the abdomen, Coccolini *et al.* [2] proposed a PA index in 2013, ranging from 0 to 30, according to specific scoring criteria based on a precise description of the intraabdominal condition. This index is a unique system which helps physicians to evaluate patients and compare their conditions after successive surgeries.

However, the mentioned classifications are not useful in distinguishing who is at risk of developing PA. Therefore the Anti-Adhesions in Gynecology Expert Panel (ANGEL) [35] has developed an adhesion risk score (ARS), with the aim to provide a simple tool that will enable gynecologists to routinely identify women at risk of

Tab. 8.1: Ranges and thresholds of low, medium, and high risk of formation of postsurgical PA achievable in women undergoing gynecological surgery.

Level of risk	Preoperative risk score	Perioperative risk score
Low risk	0–12	3–17
Medium risk	13–24	18–28
High risk	25–36	29–31

postsurgical PA. This tool is also useful to facilitate the preoperative assessment and informed consent process as well as to make intraoperative clinical decisions.

The ARS questions 10 preoperative and 10 intraoperative risk factors. The Preoperative Risk Score can range from 0 to 36, identifying the risk prior to surgery, and the Intraoperative Risk Score, ranging from 3 to 31, identifies the risks during surgery.

According to the total pre- and intraoperative scores, surgeons are able to identify women at low, medium, and high risk of postsurgical PA (Tab. 8.1) and adapt the surgical technique with or without using an antiadhesion agent.

8.11 Adhesiolysis

To relieve the patients' symptoms, PA can be removed by open or laparoscopic surgery, but the literature about success rates is variable; cases of chronic recurrent or acute small bowel obstruction (SBO), however, resolve with a conservative treatment in up to 85% of cases [36]. In contrast, other series reported that adhesiolysis is performed in 46% of patients with radiographic and clinical findings of bowel obstruction and CPP secondary to PA [21, 30]. Undeniably, the indications for immediate surgical intervention are failure of conservative management, increasing pain and progressive dilatation of bowel loops, a sign of peritonitis or sepsis [37].

Interestingly, McClain *et al.* (2011) identified that pain resolves quickly when an organ is repaired or resected with the immediate resolution of a partial SBO or after removal of endometriosis foci [38]. In contrast, adhesiolysis alone needs several months to relieve pain, suggesting an involvement of the spinothalamic pathway, like observed in phantom pain after amputation. Specifically after excision of endometriosis, the pain relief and improvement in quality of life persist up to 5 years, and the return of pain (21.5% at 2 years and 40–50% at 5 years) is not always a sign of clinical recurrence [25]. On the other hand, the benefit of adhesiolysis in infertility is clear, particularly when it is related to minimal and mild endometriosis, according to the revised classification of the American Society of Reproductive Medicine (r-ASRM I/II). In the meta-analysis by Jin *et al.* (2014), laparoscopic surgery improves pregnancy rates and live births in comparison with diagnostic laparoscopy [39] (RR, 1.52; 95% CI, 1.26–1.84, $p < 0.01$), with a 1-year cumulative pregnancy rate of

28.7% (CI, 24.7–33.4). Particularly, excision of endometriomas shows better results in pain relief, pain recurrence, fertility, and subsequent spontaneous pregnancy, in comparison with ablation or drainage alone [25].

As regards to the technique of adhesiolysis, laser was initially used because of its theoretical advantages of precision and minimal lateral tissue damage, but further investigations do not confirm its superiority compared with electrocautery or harmonic devices [21]. Meanwhile, laparoscopic adhesiolysis has become popular and safer in virtue of intrinsic advantages of minimal invasive techniques and patient selection criteria. These advantages offer the opportunity to perform it even in some cases of chronic [36] and acute SBO [25, 37] with a success rate of 38–87% and pain recurrence rate up to 26% [34]. Obviously, patients with contraindication for general anesthesia are not candidates for laparoscopic adhesiolysis.

Regardless whether laparoscopic or open adhesiolysis is used, surgeons should be aware of possible complications during surgery, such as injury of intestines (occurrence rate: 5.5%), bladder, uterus, or vascular structures. These could be minimized using subcostal entry, the Hasson technique of "open trocar placement," handling bowel loops gently, and using atraumatic instruments. A laparoconversion should be made when those precautions are not guaranteed or in the presence of fused loops, extremely dense PA, or unclear anatomy. A conversion threshold in 4–32% is reported for cases of acute abdomen secondary to SBO treated by laparoscopy, a morbidity rate between 4% and 75%, and mortality rate of 0.4–25%, but with only 0.5% of recurrent ileus, whereas it presents in 3–5% of cases managed by open surgery [37].

8.12 Prevention of PA

For the purpose of adhesion prevention during gynecological surgery, the European field guideline from the ANGEL group [23] has recommended six basic rules to consider in every single case of adhesiogenic surgeries, that is, adhesiolysis, myomectomy, ovarian, and tubal procedures (Tab. 8.2). As a result, the risk of CPP, infertility, and inadvertent enterotomy in subsequent surgeries could be minimized.

As mentioned, in combination with the principles of good surgical techniques, adhesion reduction agents could be considered for adhesion prophylaxis, taking into consideration their safety, efficacy, manageability, and costs. However, they are not capable of compensating for extensive tissue damage during surgery and cannot completely eliminate the recurrence of PA.

Different pharmacological agents such as steroids, heparin, gonadotropin releasing hormone analogues, nonsteroidal anti-inflammatories, antihistamines, growth factor inhibitors, vitamin E, colloids, and crystalloids alone or in combination have been tested, but none of these agents proved to be effective in adhesion reduction because they do not reach surgical sites, do not stay long enough or do impair normal re-epithelialization [27].

Tab. 8.2: ANGEL's rules of postoperative adhesion prevention in gynecological surgery.

The risk of PA should be systematically discussed with any patient scheduled for open or laparoscopic abdominal surgery prior to obtaining his/her informed consent.

Surgeons need to act to reduce PA in order to fulfill their duty of care toward patients undergoing abdominal surgery.

Surgeons should adopt a routine adhesion reduction strategy at least for patients undergoing high-risk surgery.

Good surgical technique is fundamental to any adhesion reduction strategy.

Surgeons should consider the use of adhesion reduction agents as part of the adhesion reduction strategy.

Good medical practice implies that any serious or frequently occurring risks be discussed before obtaining the patient's informed consent prior to surgery.

In contrast, nonpharmacological agents are available as films, gels, or fluids, most of them having the ability to separate traumatized peritoneal surfaces, acting as barriers and anti-adhesion agents after surgery, being more effective than no treatment in reducing the risk of postsurgical PA [40]. For example, in a retrospective analysis of 48 patients who initially had laparoscopic excision of pelvic endometriosis foci, 97.3% did not have PA at second look [41] when a combination of a highly experienced surgeon, good surgical technique, and application of an antiadhesion agent was used. However, the necessity of an additional major procedure at the time of peritoneal excision was associated with filmy PA (8.7% of cases).

In addition to reducing PA, the Surgical and Clinical PA Research study [42] proved that barrier agents reduce the cumulative costs over 3 years, with a 26–60% reduction of readmission related costs. However, this study was conducted between 1986 and 1996, and many new efficient, safe, and easy-to-use substances have become available; thus, the economic impact could be greater.

There is, however, a lack of comparative studies of superiority between them, and there is no conclusive evidence on the effects of barrier agents used during pelvic surgery on either pain or fertility outcomes in women of reproductive age, although no adverse events directly attributed to the adhesion agents have been reported [40]. For example, the new ADBEE system, a gel composed by a dextrin polymer, has proved to be as safe as a standardized surgical myomectomy [43].

Hence, surgeons should be informed about the risk–benefit profile of each product and use it after high-risk-of-adhesion surgeries such as myomectomy, tubal surgery, ovarian cystectomy, fertility surgery, extensive endometriosis surgery or adhesiolysis [13, 18, 44], irrespective if laparoscopic or open surgery.

Moreover, surgeons should routinely discuss with their patients the personal and procedural risks of PA by means of a written consent form, mainly those with obesity, preexisting PA or medical conditions. Nevertheless, only 44% of German doctors discuss it and 39% of patients felt satisfactorily informed; consequently, most patients are not informed adequately about PA, their complications, and measures to avoid them, leading to successful negligence lawsuits against physicians [45].

Consequently, patient awareness is of utmost importance to avoid legal consequences of complications secondary to PA, which could be realized by means of a leaflet that presents appropriate, patient-orientated information on PA: nature, health risks, long-term consequences, and methods of prevention. Moreover in patients with prior operations, giving the high risk of complications derived of the existing PA and the necessity to perform an adhesiolysis [46].

8.12.1 Intrauterine adhesions

Intrauterine adhesions (IUAs) were first described by Joseph Asherman in 1948 and are also commonly referred as intrauterine synechiae [47, 48]. They develop mainly as a result of trauma during uterine surgery, including D&C, polypectomy, myomectomy or uterine septum removal, uterine artery embolization, or uterine compression sutures for the management of postpartum hemorrhage. IUA could also develop after local infections, prolonged use of an intrauterine device (IUD) or pregnancy. The underlying pathophysiology is mechanical disruption of the endometrial basalis layer that prevents normal endometrial regeneration and leads to subsequent apparition of fibrous connective tissue bands with or without glandular tissue, ranging from filmy to dense [47].

The risk of IUA is related to the type of procedure, being lower for those limited to the endometrium, like polypectomy, and higher for those involving opposing surfaces or entering the myometrial layer. Using electricity for tumor resection or blind removal of gestational tissue also increases the risk of IUA [48]. Due to the resection of extensive areas of endometrium during myomectomy, adhesions develop as soon as 1–2 weeks after surgery and is associated with the number of fibroids resected, 1.5% after a solitary myoma resection and up to 78% after resection of two or more opposing myomata [47].

IUAs are usually suspected and diagnosed 1–3 months after a procedure and could be symptomatic or not. Asymptomatic synechiae are of questionable clinical significance, while partial obliteration of uterine cavity results in abnormal uterine bleeding, chronic dysmenorrhea, female infertility or recurrent miscarriages, referred to as Asherman's syndrome [48]. Hematometra occurs in cases of obliteration of cervical os. Complete uterine cavity obliteration by synechiae leads to secondary amenorrhea. In addition, it is reported that high blood flow impedance of spiral artery in patients with IUA could impair implantation or lead to poor obstetric outcomes [47].

Salpingohysterography (SHG), hysterosonography (HSG) and tridimensional ultrasound (3D-US) imaging are useful for their diagnosis, hysteroscopy being the standard method for final diagnosis and simultaneous treatment [47, 48]. Conventional transvaginal ultrasound fails to demonstrate the IUA extension, with a sensitivity of 52% and specificity of 11% in comparison to hysteroscopy. Transcervical uterine sounding could reveal cervical obstruction and adhesions located near the internal os, but not those laterally or located higher. Compared with hysteroscopy, HSG has a sensitivity of 75–81% and positive predictive value of 43% and false-positive rate of 39%, limiting its use for IUA diagnosis; SHG has a sensitivity of 75% and positive predictive value of 50%. Moreover, both methods fail to demonstrate endometrial fibrosis and extent of adhesions but are reasonable alternatives. New techniques, such as 3D-US and 3D-SHG have higher sensitivity of 87% and 70% and specificity of 45% and 87%, respectively. Magnetic resonance and Doppler sonography are not well studied and are therefore not recommended for routine use [47].

After evaluation of IUA, use of a classification system is recommended, as the severity of the disease is related to prognosis. In 1989, the European Society of Hysteroscopy created a classification based on the extent of IUA at hysteroscopic evaluation [47]. Other classifications have incorporated a combination of clinical symptoms, menstrual characteristics and hysteroscopic and HSG findings, and postoperative pregnancy rates. An international classification system of IUA is still lacking [48].

Because of the absence of malignancy potential of uterine synechiae, expectant management is an option. It is reported that 78% of women resume menstruation and 45% get pregnant within 7 years after diagnosis [48]. Surgical treatment is recommended for symptomatic women or with fertility desire. The aim of therapies is to alleviate the symptomatology and enhance the fertility potential by communicating the uterine tubes, the uterine cavity, and the cervical canal [48].

Adhesiolysis is the treatment of choice to restore the shape and volume of the uterine cavity and cervical canal permeability. With the increasing availability of hysteroscopy, cervical probing and D&C have been abandoned because they do not provide information about the severity of IUA and also carry a higher risk of uterine rupture and further endometrial damage during the procedure. Hysteroscopy has various advantages [47, 48], such as direct vision and magnification, which allow a precise lysis, cutting, and hemostasis and distention through gel or saline solution. However, lateral and severe IUAs increase the potential of uterine perforation and visceral damage during adhesiolysis. Mechanical cutting and adhesion division by means of scissors or needle are preferred to electrosurgical lysis to reduce the risk of endometrial damage and IUA reformation [48]. The 2017 AAGL-ESGE guidelines for the surgical management of IUA are available from Gynecological Surgery (2017) [48].

Unfortunately, *de novo* IUAs occur in 3–24% after lysis of mild IUA and in 30% to 66% of cases after lysis of severe IUA [49, 50]. Different measures have been tested to reduce the incidence of *de novo* IUA after adhesiolysis, including placing a plastic stent, a Foley catheter balloon, an IUD, fresh human amniotic membrane grafts or an antiadhesion barrier, which keep uterine walls apart, as well as hormonal supplementation. However, randomized controlled trials have shown no significant differences in *de novo* adhesion formation or pregnancy outcomes after septoplasty followed by either no treatment, estrogens, a copper IUD, or a copper IUD plus estrogen [47]. In addition, a meta-analysis [48] showed that 14–48% of cases exhibit recurrent IUA after the use of adjuvant measures, such as intrauterine balloon, polyethylene oxide-sodium carboxymethylcellulose gel, hyaluronic acid gel and other antiadhesion barriers. When used in IUA-related infertility, it was found that no significant differences in live-birth rates between antiadhesion therapies and no treatment or placebo (OR, 0.99; 95% CI, 0.46–2.13; p = 0.98). But antiadhesion therapies are associated with fewer IUAs at any second-look hysteroscopy when compared with no treatment or placebo (OR, 0.36; 95% CI, 0.20–0.64; p = 0.0005) [48]. However, there is a lack of evidence in relation with their benefit on subsequent fertility and pregnancy rates.

Prognosis and reproductive outcomes depend on type and severity of IUA. Patients with extensive endometrial destruction are usually unresponsive to treatments, and partial endometrial damage increases the risk for placenta accreata, postpartum hemorrhage, blood transfusion, and postpartum hysterectomy [47]. Normal menstrual pattern is restored in most of cases (81%). After adhesiolysis, full-term pregnancies are achieved by 70–80% of cases with mild to moderate IUA and by 20–40% of those with severe IUA, for an overall live-birth rate between 28% and 32% [47].

Further trials are favoring a second-look hysteroscopy within 2 weeks after surgery for early recognition and mechanical lysis of IUA before they achieve tensile strength [49]. The ongoing OPEN clinical trial is using a new transcervical, intrauterine ultrasound-guided radiofrequency ablation system (The Sonata® System, Gynesonics), which has been designed to minimize or avoid disruption of the endometrial layer. This trial will document the presence or absence of IUA after resection of submucous and/or transmural fibroids.

8.13 Conclusion

As the most common complication of gynecological surgery, the development of PA is not fully understood, but key components, such as mesothelial damage, inflammation, proximity, adhesiogenicity of different organs and time dependency, have been identified. Prevention is the single most important pillar in surgical practice, regardless of open or laparoscopic approach. The use of generally advocated surgical techniques in combination with barrier agents and the creation of a peritoneal-friendly environment can greatly decrease the incidence of PA. Compared to open approaches, minimally invasive surgery is less adhesiogenic and associated with higher pregnancy rates, lower pain scores, and fewer adhesion-related sequelae. Moreover, laparoscopic adhesiolysis improves adhesion-related infertility and pain syndromes. Unfortunately, PAs virtually always reappear. Therefore, future research should focus on the treatment of existing PAs and the understanding of their pathophysiology, to develop more effective antiadhesion substances.

Compared to PA, IUAs have limited clinical implications. Most of the typical sequelae (amenorrhea, dysmenorrhea, uterine cavity deformity) can very well be treated. Infertility, however, shows lower response rates to treatment and is inversely correlated to the severity of the disease, which can be attributed to the irreversible change of endometrial tissue to epithelial and connective tissue in the initial stage of the disease. As mechanical barriers and antiadhesive gels are available but comparative studies on antiadhesive barriers and gels up to now are underpowered and of low quality, focus should be directed toward multicenter comparative analysis and the development of a classification of IUA as well as therapeutic options for their prevention.

References

[1] Wallwiener M, Brölmann H, Koninckx PR, et al. Adhesions after abdominal, pelvic and intra-uterine surgery and their prevention. Gynecol Surg 2012;9(4):465–6.
[2] Coccolini F, Ansaloni L, Manfredi R, et al. Peritoneal adhesion index (PAI): proposal of a score for the "ignored iceberg" of medicine and surgery. World J Emerg Surg 2013;8(1):6.
[3] Hertzler AE. The Formation of fibrous tissue. In The peritoneum. Hertzler AE, ed. C. V. Mosby Company, St. Louis. USA, 1919: 238–272.
[4] Ryan GB, Grobéty J, Majno G. Mesothelial injury and recovery. Am J Pathol 1973;71(1):93–112.
[5] Whitaker D, Papadimitriou J. Mesothelial healing: morphological and kinetic investigations. J Pathol 1985;145(2):159–75.
[6] Raftery AT. Regeneration of peritoneum: a fibrinolytic study. J Anat 1979;129(Pt 3):659–64.
[7] Mutsaers SE. Mesothelial cells: their structure, function and role in serosal repair. Respirology 2002;7(3):171–91.
[8] Maciver AH, McCall M, James Shapiro AM. Intra-abdominal adhesions: cellular mechanisms and strategies for prevention. Int J Surg 2011;9(8):589–94.
[9] Koninckx PR, Gomel V, Ussia A, Adamyan L. Role of the peritoneal cavity in the prevention of postoperative adhesions, pain, and fatigue. Fertil Steril 2016;106(5):998–1010.
[10] Sandoval P, Jiménez-Heffernan JA, Guerra-Azcona G, et al. Mesothelial-to-mesenchymal transition in the pathogenesis of post-surgical peritoneal adhesions. J Pathol 2016;239(1):48–59.
[11] Foroutan T, Hosseini A, Pourfathol AA, Soleimani M, Alimoghada K, Mosaffa N. Peritoneal mesothelial progenitor or stem cell. J Biol Sci 2010;10(5):460–4.
[12] Wallwiener M, Koninckx PR, Hackethal A, et al. A European survey on awareness of post-surgical adhesions among gynaecological surgeons. Gynecol Surg 2014;11:105–12.
[13] De Wilde RL, Bakkum EA, Brölmann H, et al. Consensus recommendations on adhesions (version 2014) for the ESGE Adhesions Research Working Group (European Society for Gynecological Endoscopy): an expert opinion. Arch Gynecol Obstet 2014;290(3):581–2.
[14] Molinas CR, Mynbaev O, Pauwels A, Novak P, Koninckx PR. Peritoneal mesothelial hypoxia during pneumoperitoneum is a cofactor in adhesion formation in a laparoscopic mouse model. Fertil Steril 2001;76(3):560–7.
[15] Molinas CR, Binda MM, Manavella GD, Koninckx PR. Adhesion formation after laparoscopic surgery: what do we know about the role of the peritoneal environment? Facts Views Vis Obgyn 2010;2(3):149–60.

[16] Hazebroek EJ, Schreve MA, Visser P, De Bruin RWF, Marquet RL, Bonjer HJ. Impact of temperature and humidity of carbon dioxide pneumoperitoneum on body temperature and peritoneal morphology. J Laparoendosc Adv Surg Tech A 2002;12(5):355–64.

[17] Schemmer P, Mehrabi A, Büchler MW, Gutt CN, Oniu T. Fewer adhesions induced by laparoscopic surgery? Surg Endosc 2004;18(6):898–906.

[18] Diamond MP, Wexner SD, diZereg GS, et al. Adhesion prevention and reduction: current status and future recommendations of a multinational interdisciplinary consensus conference. Surg Innov 2010;17(3):183–8.

[19] Styer AK. Prevalence and incidence in primary care of chronic pelvic pain in women: evidence from a national general practice database. Br J Obstet Gynecol. 1999;106:11149–55.

[20] Shehata F, Zarei A, Shalom-Paz E, Tulandi T. Predictors of intra-abdominal adhesions. Gynecol Surg 2011;8(4):405–8.

[21] Kavic SM, Kavic SM. Adhesions and adhesiolysis: the role of laparoscopy. JSLS 2002;6(2):99–109.

[22] Gao X, Li, Luo, et al. Novel thermosensitive hydrogel for preventing formation of abdominal adhesions. Int J Nanomedicine 2013;2453.

[23] De Wilde RL, Brölmann H, Koninckx PR, et al. Prevention of adhesions in gynaecological surgery: the 2012 European field guideline. Gynecol Surg 2012;9(4):365–8.

[24] ten Broek RPG, Kok-Krant N, Bakkum EA, Bleichrodt RP, van Goor H. Different surgical techniques to reduce post-operative adhesion formation: a systematic review and meta-analysis. Hum Reprod Update 2012;19(1):12–25.

[25] Laborda E, Clarke A, Carpenter T. The threshold for laparoscopy for pelvic pain. Obstet Gynaecol 2010;12(1):7–12.

[26] Awonuga AO, Fletcher NM, Saed GM, Diamond MP. Postoperative adhesion development following cesarean and open intra-abdominal gynecological operations: a review. Reprod Sci 2011;18(12):1166–85.

[27] Brüggmann D, Tchartchian G, Wallwiener M, Münstedt K, Tinneberg H-R, Hackethal A. Intra-abdominal adhesions: definition, origin, significance in surgical practice, and treatment options. Dtsch Arztebl Int 2010;107(44):769–75.

[28] Qin F, Ma Y, Li X, et al. Efficacy and mechanism of tanshinone IIA liquid nanoparticles in preventing experimental postoperative peritoneal adhesions in vivo and in vitro. Int J Nanomedicine 2015;10:3699–716.

[29] Ellis H, Moran BJ, Thompson JN, et al. Adhesion-related hospital readmissions after abdominal and pelvic surgery: a retrospective cohort study. Lancet 1999;353(9163):1476–80.

[30] Warren JW, Morozov V, Howard FM. Could chronic pelvic pain be a functional somatic syndrome? Am J Obstet Gynecol 2011;205(3):199.e1–5.

[31] ten Broek RPG, Bakkum EA, Mvan CJ, van Goor H. Epidemiology and Prevention of Postsurgical Adhesions Revisited. Ann Surg 2016;263(1):12–9.

[32] Demco L. Pain mapping of adhesions. J Am Assoc Gynecol Laparosc 2004;11(2):181–3.

[33] Leidig P, Krakamp B. Laparoscopic lysis of adhesions—a simple method of diagnosis and therapy of abdominal pain caused by adhesions]. Leber Magen Darm 1992;22(1):27–8.

[34] van der Wal JBC, Halm JA, Jeekel J. Chronic abdominal pain: the role of adhesions and benefit of laparoscopic adhesiolysis. Gynecol Surg 2006;3(3):168–74.

[35] Lundorff P, Brölmann H, Koninckx PR, et al. Predicting formation of adhesions after gynaecological surgery: development of a risk score. Arch Gynecol Obstet 2015;292(4):931–8.

[36] Reissman P, Spira RM. Laparoscopy for adhesions. Semin Laparosc Surg 2003;10(4):185–90.

[37] Majewski WD. Long-term outcome, adhesions, and quality of life after laparoscopic and open surgical therapies for acute abdomen: follow-up of a prospective trial. Surg Endosc 2005;19(1):81–90.

[38] McClain GD, Redan JA, McCarus SD, Caceres A, Kim J. Diagnostic laparoscopy and adhesiolysis: does it help with complex abdominal and pelvic pain syndrome (CAPPS) in general surgery? JSLS 2011;15(1):1–5.

[39] Jin X, Beguerie JR. Laparoscopic surgery for subfertility related to endometriosis: a meta-analysis. Taiwan J Obstet Gynecol 2014;53(3):303–8.

[40] Ahmad G, O'Flynn H, Hindocha A, Watson A. Barrier agents for adhesion prevention after gynaecological surgery. Cochrane Database of Systematic Reviews 2015, Issue 4. Art. No.: CD000475. DOI: 10.1002/14651858.CD000475.pub3

[41] Oboh A, Trehan AK. Pelvic adhesion formation at second-look surgery after laparoscopic partial and total peritoneal excision for women with endometriosis. Gynecol Surg 2007;4(4):261–5.

[42] Parker MC, Wilson MS, Menzies D, et al. The SCAR-3 study: 5-year adhesion-related readmission risk following lower abdominal surgical procedures. Colorectal Dis 2005;7(6):551–8.

[43] Cezar C, Korell M, Tchartchian G, et al. How to avoid risks for patients in minimal-access trials: Avoiding complications in clinical first-in-human studies by example of the ADBEE study. Best Pract Res Clin Obstet Gynaecol 2016;35:84–96.

[44] Rimbach S, Korell M, Tinneberg H-R, De Wilde R-L. Adhäsionen und ihre Prävention in der gynäkologischen Chirurgie: Standortbestimmung und aktueller Konsensus basierend auf den Ergebnissen von vier Workshops. Geburtshilfe Frauenheilkd 2004;64(9):891–9.

[45] Hirschelmann A, Wallwiener CW, Wallwiener M, et al. Is patient education about adhesions a requirement in abdominopelvic surgery? Geburtshilfe Frauenheilkd 2012;72(4):299–304.

[46] Herrmann A, De Wilde RL. Adhesions are the major cause of complications in operative gynecology. Best Pract Res Clin Obstet Gynaecol 2016;35:71–83.

[47] Berman JM. Intrauterine adhesions. Semin Reprod Med 2008;26(4):349–55.

[48] AAGL Elevating Gynecologic Surgery. AAGL practice report: practice guidelines on intrauterine adhesions developed in collaboration with the European Society of Gynaecological Endoscopy (ESGE). Gynecol Surg 2017;14(1):6.

[49] Yang J-H, Chen C-D, Chen S-U, Yang Y-S, Chen M-J. The influence of the location and extent of intrauterine adhesions on recurrence after hysteroscopic adhesiolysis. BJOG 2016;123(4):618–23.

[50] Pabuçcu R, Atay V, Orhon E, Urman B, Ergün A. Hysteroscopic treatment of intrauterine adhesions is safe and effective in the restoration of normal menstruation and fertility. Fertil Steril 1997;68(6):1141–3.

Gokhan Sami Kilic and Burak Zeybek

9 Laparoscopy/robotically assisted simple hysterectomy procedure

9.1 Introduction

One in three women in the USA will have a hysterectomy before she turns 60 [1]. Since the Food and Drug Administration's (FDA's) statement in 2014 warning against power morcellation, the rate of any type of laparoscopic hysterectomy for benign indications decreased from 57.3% to 55.4% [2, 3]. As a consequence, postoperative morbidity rose in parallel with this change in practice [2, 4–6]. The data have been accumulating since the FDA's warning that the risk and benefit ratio favors a minimally invasive approach versus open hysterectomy [2, 4–6].

In this chapter, we describe the step-by-step approach to robotically assisted/laparoscopic simple hysterectomy and provide updated useful knowledge about laparoscopic and robotically assisted hysterectomy practice for all professionals, especially general gynecologists, urogynecologists, and gynecologic oncologists.

9.2 Positioning the patient/uterine manipulator

After anesthesia, the patient is placed in the dorsal lithotomy position, and both of her arms are tucked in by passing a sheet under the patient, wrapping it around the arms, and then passing it back underneath the patient once again for traction to prevent the patient from sliding. The legs are placed in Allen stirrups (Allen Medical System, Acton, MA, USA). The skin is prepped below the breast line, down to the bilateral knees, and laterally to the posterior axillary line.

To gain maximum exposure to the deep pelvic area, a 25-degree Trendelenburg is optimal. The robotically assisted Si model (DaVinci, Intuitive, Silicon Valley, Sunnyvale, CA, USA) must be in the Trendelenburg position at the beginning of the surgery following the trocar placement. However, the robotically assisted Xi or laparoscopy can be adjusted to the Trendelenburg position, as required, at any time during the surgery.

Surgical team members should synchronize their duties before the docking process to decrease the operating time. For instance, while the uterine manipulator is placed by the surgeon, the scrub, circulating nurses, and assistant surgeon should be focusing the camera, light sources, and energy sources, as well as setting the gas tubes up.

Worldwide, the most commonly used uterine manipulators for hysterectomy are the Advincula Delineator (Cooper-Surgical, Trumbull, CT, USA), V-Care

https://doi.org/10.1515/9783110535204-009

(V-CARE Standard, CONMED Corporation, Utica, NY, USA), and Rumi II (Rumi Koh-Efficient, Cooper-Surgical, Trumbull, CT, USA). They all give the opportunity to manipulate the uterus and delineate the vaginal cuff properly. Using the appropriate cup size is of paramount importance for effective use of the manipulator (or to get its full benefits during the surgery). A cup size that is too small for the cervix would compromise the delineation component. On the other hand, a cup size that is too large would increase the risk of ureteral injury. The Advincula Delineator and V-Care provide an additional advantage during the bladder flap creation. The handle of these two manipulators can be rotated 180 degrees to create a very prominent cervico-vesical delineation.

The balloon at the tip of the uterine manipulator will be insufflated with 7 mL of air in a normally sized uterus. Insufflation will facilitate manipulating the uterus as well as pulling and removing the uterus transvaginally after the uterus is fully detached. It is the authors' opinion that fixing the uterine manipulator with anchor sutures on the cervix is not practical most of the time, especially for in-bag morcellations in larger uteruses or when rotating the manipulator 180 degrees during bladder flap creation.

9.3 Trocar placement/instrumentation

Depending on the size of the uterus, surgeries additional to hysterectomy and the surgeon's comfort level, total trocar numbers may vary from one to five. If a robotically assisted Si or laparoscopy technique is being used either in midline or at the Palmer point (located 2 cm below the left arcus costarium in the midaxial line), a 5-mm optic trocar under direct visualization will be introduced. Entering with the 5-mm laparoscopic scope in the beginning reduces the potential injury size to the surrounding organs. If a robotically assisted Xi is used, a 12-mm optic trocar under direct visualization will be the initial trocar choice at the Palmer point. Laparoscopic entry proceeds by using either a visual cannula Endoscopic Threaded Imaging Port (EndoTIP, Karl Storz GmbH & Co., Tuttlingen, Germany) or optical trocar VISIPORT (Covidien Surgical, Mansfield, MA, USA). First, the uterus should be pushed cephalad to its maximum level using the uterine manipulator. If a midline entrance is chosen, trocar entry should be 10 cm above the fundus of the uterus to give enough space for the camera to view the whole surgical field. Usually, the 8-mm robotic working trocars are placed lateral to the rectus abdominis muscle at the umbilical level. The Si model gives the flexibility to place robotic trocars in a W formation, which maintains a distance of 10 cm between each trocar (Fig. 9.1). The Xi model requires all the robotic trocars to be on the same line (Fig. 9.2). Unfortunately, finding a place for all four trocars in very thin patients can be problematic. However, the Xi model tolerates up to an 8-cm proximity in between the trocars. In our practice, a laparoscopic

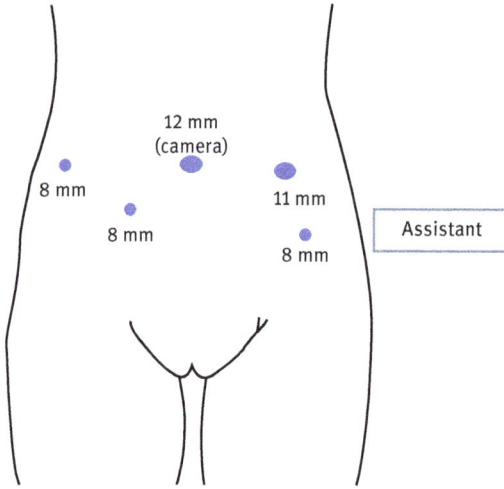

Fig. 9.1: Robotically assisted trocar placement for the Si model.

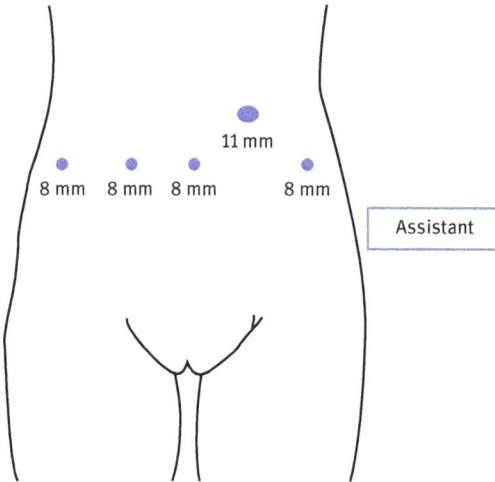

Fig. 9.2: Robotically assisted trocar placement for the Xi model.

12-mm trocar is placed on the left upper quadrant and a 5-mm trocar is placed on the left lower quadrant. If needed, another 5-mm assistant trocar will be placed at the umbilical level on the patient's right side (Fig. 9.3).

Robotically assisted cases can easily be performed with lower abdominal pressure, such as 11–12 mmHg. Maintaining pneumoperitoneum during the colpotomy might be challenging in patients with copious vaginal space. To overcome this effect,

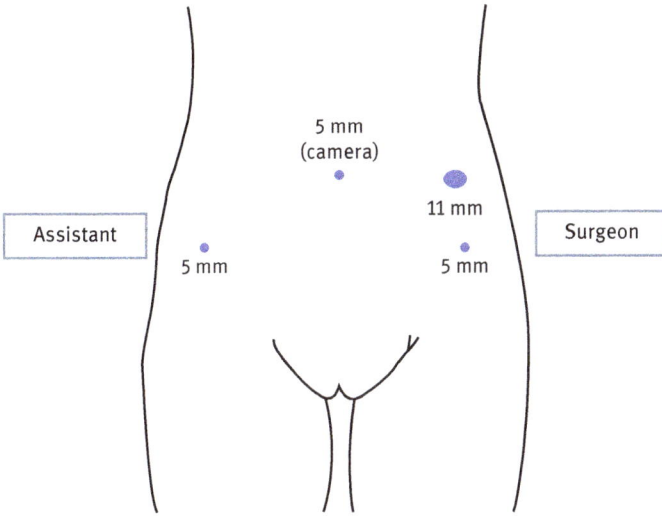

Fig. 9.3: Laparoscopic trocar placement.

either two separate insufflators running simultaneously or high flow insufflation will be helpful. Laparoscopic, robotic Xi, and robotic Si with side docking all provide a comfortable space between the patient's legs for uterine manipulation.

In robotically assisted cases, EndoWrist® Monopolar Curved Scissors are commonly used on the right, with a bipolar grasper on the left. On the third robotic arm, the preferred forceps are usually a ProGrasp or Cardiere grasper. As needed, a traumatic grasper or suction irrigator may be used via the assistant trocar. The assistant trocar is also used to transport sutures, morcellation bags or Ray-Tec® (4 × 4) X-ray Detectable Sponges. Harmonic Ace® (Ethicon Endo-Surgery, Inc., Cincinnati, OH, USA) and Enseal® (Ethicon Endo-Surgery, Inc., Cincinnati, OH, USA) are available for robotic use. Energy sources vary in laparoscopic use. None of them have significant advantages or disadvantages over the others, so it is the surgeon's discretion to choose.

For robotically assisted single-site procedures, port placement is performed using a standard Hasson's technique: A 2.0–2.5-cm midline intraumbilical incision is made and special da Vinci single-site port equipment is used for the Si model. The single-site port has five lumens: four to hold cannulas and one for the insufflation adapter (Fig. 9.4).

The da Vinci SP system is also available and fully designed for single-port procedures that include three multijointed, wristed instruments and a fully wristed 3D HD camera. The instruments and the camera all emerge through a single cannula and are properly triangulated around the target anatomy to avoid instrument collisions.

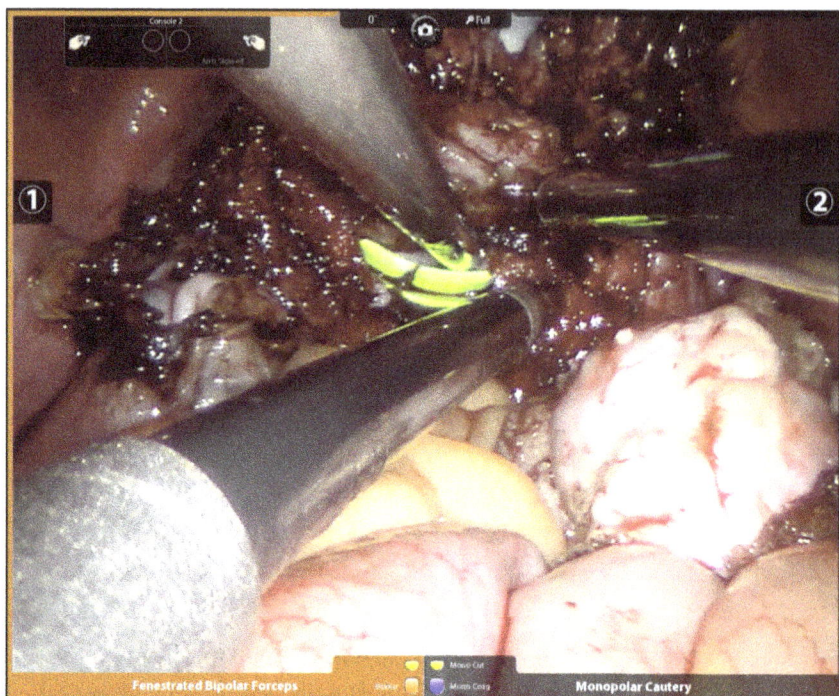

Fig. 9.4: Robotic endoscopic single-site surgery.

9.4 Step-by-step approach to simple hysterectomy

Pelvic space and the upper abdominal area will be explored initially during laparoscopy. For ergonomic reasons, hysterectomy starts with transection of the round ligament on the patient's left side using a three-step approach:

Step 1—Using the plasma kinetic (PK)/bipolar cutting forceps, grasp, and coagulate the round ligament close to the uterus (Fig. 9.5).

Step 2—Grasp and coagulate the ligament 1 cm distal to the first bite (Fig. 9.6).

Step 3—Without letting the PK/bipolar go, use monopolar scissors to cut between the two previous bites to the tip of the PK/bipolar, simultaneously using sharp and cutting modes of the monopolar power (Fig. 9.7).

This three-step rule naturally does not apply to other energy sources.

After completing the round ligament transaction, the PK/bipolar instrument is used to dissect the broad ligament parallel to the uterus anteriorly. Care is taken to avoid getting too close to the uterus to avoid injuring the ascending branch of the uterine vessels and to prevent unintended bleeding. When the dissection reaches the utero-vesical junction, it should turn at approximately a 90-degree angle toward the cervix (Fig. 9.8). The broad ligament dissection continues until reaching the

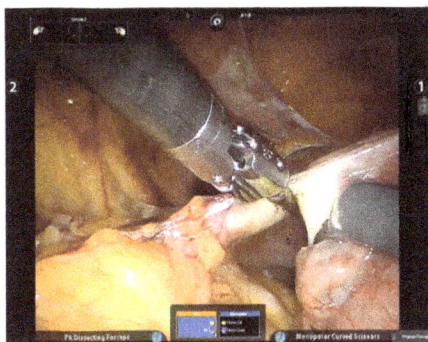

Fig. 9.5: Step 1, coagulating the left round ligament.

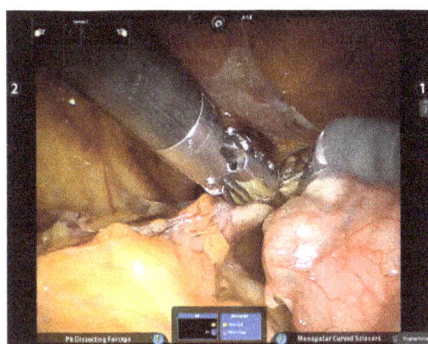

Fig. 9.6: Step 2, second line of coagulation, placed 1 cm away from the first bite.

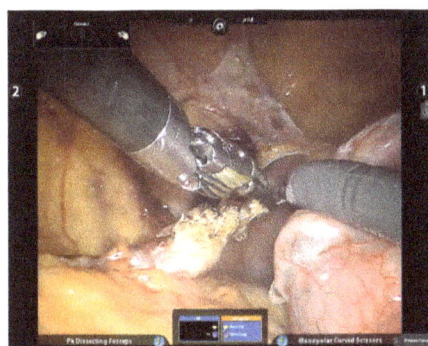

Fig. 9.7: Step 3, transecting the round ligament with monopolar scissors.

contralateral round ligament (Fig. 9.9). The right-side broad ligament is coagulated and transected using same three-step technique. The only difference from the left side is that the first-step coagulation is performed laterally to the uterus to prevent the two robotic arms from crossing each other. Then attention is turned to completing the bladder flap using monopolar scissors. The cutting power should be dropped to 20 W to prevent bladder coagulation injuries later.

Using the uterine manipulator, the uterus is anteverted completely. After transsectioning the round ligament, the broad ligament dissection is extended posteriorly. The posterior broad ligament dissection is usually performed parallel to the

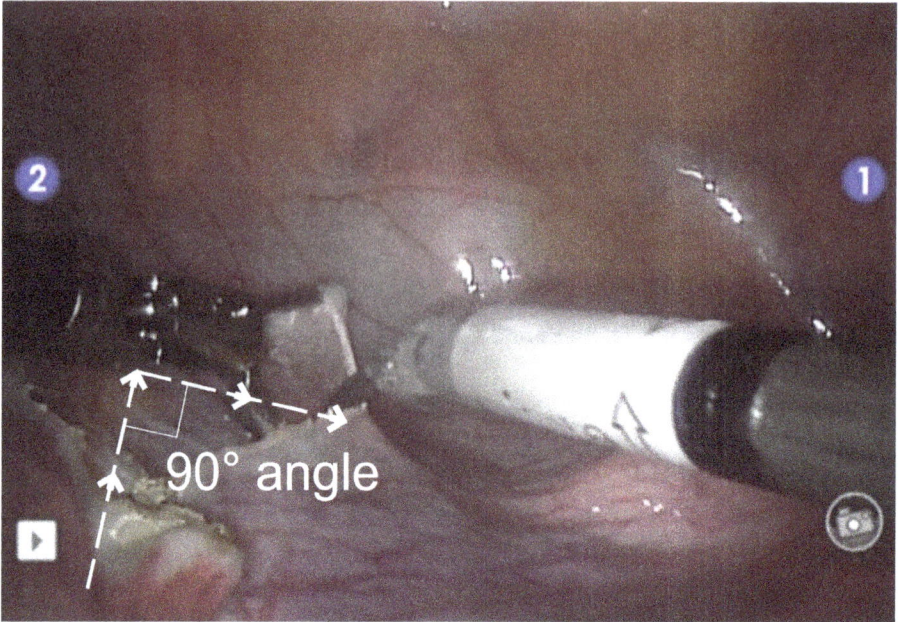

Fig. 9.8: Broad ligament dissection turning at an approximately 90° angle at the utero-vesical junction.

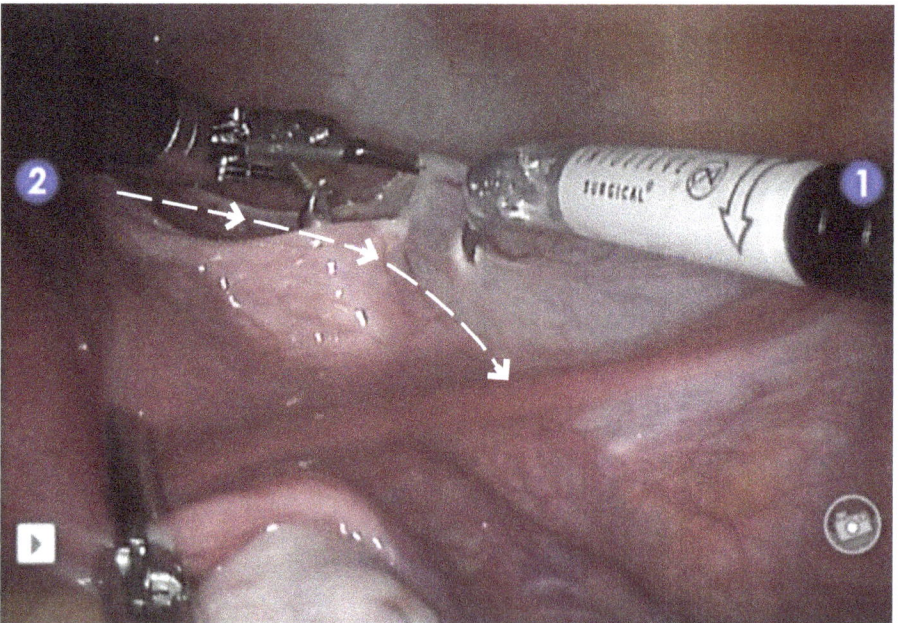

Fig. 9.9: Broad ligament dissection to contralateral round ligament.

infundibulopelvic (IP) ligament since this approach makes identification and dissection of the ureter easier if necessary. The IP or utero-ovarian ligaments are coagulated and transected with the same three-step technique. The posterior peritoneum is dropped to the lower uterine segment.

Special care should be given to skeletonization of both uterine vessels (Fig. 9.10). PK/bipolar is used to coagulate, not to transect, the ascending branch of the uterine vessels to prevent back bleeding. Uterine vessels should be coagulated after pushing the uterus maximally cephaled with the uterine manipulator to decrease the risk of ureteral injuries (Fig. 9.11).

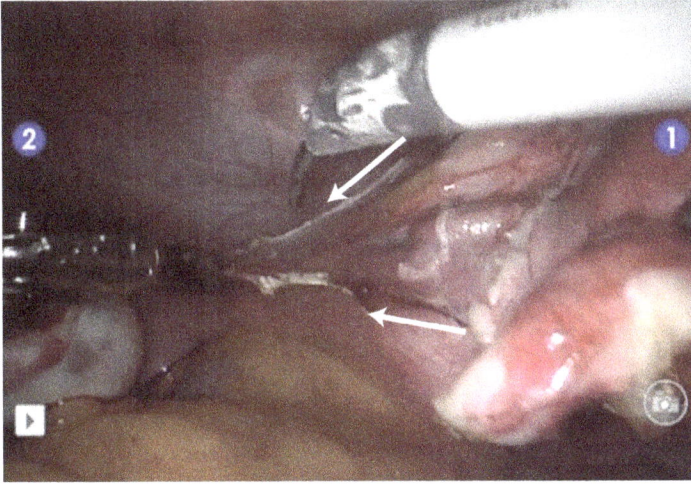

Fig. 9.10: Skeletonization of the uterine vessels.

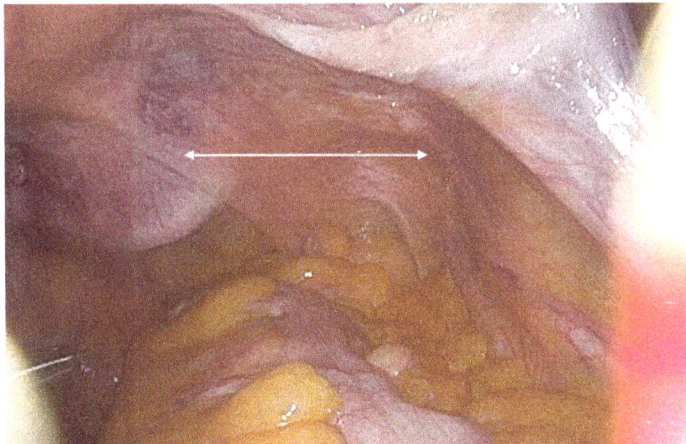

Fig. 9.11: Uterine manipulator pushed cephalad to increase the distance of ureters from surgi-cal field.

Uterine vessels should first be transected inside the ring provided by uterine manipulator. After transecting the uterine vessels, the vessel stumps are clamped away from the uterine lower segment toward the uterine manipulator ring, continuing until vessel bundles peel off outside the uterine manipulator ring (Fig. 9.12).

At this point, the vaginal cuff will be delineated by the uterine manipulator ring, and it is safe to start the colpotomy since all the major vessels are transected and moved away from the incision area. The cut mode power on the monopolar scissors is increased to 40 W before cutting the vaginal cuff, using single blade of the scissors to gain more precise cutting. If using a Rumi manipulator, the vaginal occluder balloon is filled with 60 cc normal saline. It is helpful to activate two separate insufflators through the trocars to maintain pneumoperitoneum. The vaginal cuff is cut with monopolar scissors layer by layer using brush-stroke-type movements, which will help maintain the pneumoperitoneum until the last moment (Fig. 9.13). After completing the colpotomy, the specimen is removed vaginally, using morcellation as needed.

The vagina is occluded using laparotomy sponges covered by a sterile glove depending on the size of the vagina. Aggressive homeostasis using the energy modality should be avoided to preserve vascularization and facilitate cuff healing. For cuff closure, different combinations of instruments are available. Two needle holders provide an advantage in handling the suture needle. One needle holder and one grasper provide an advantage in holding the vaginal cuff during suturing. Either

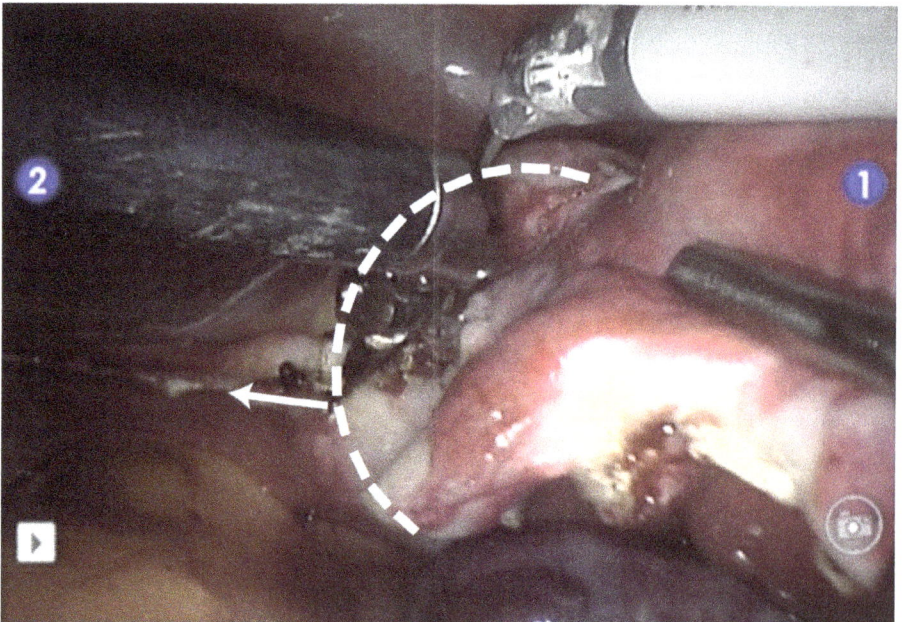

Fig. 9.12: Lateralization of the uterine vessels' stumps on patient's left side (peel off).

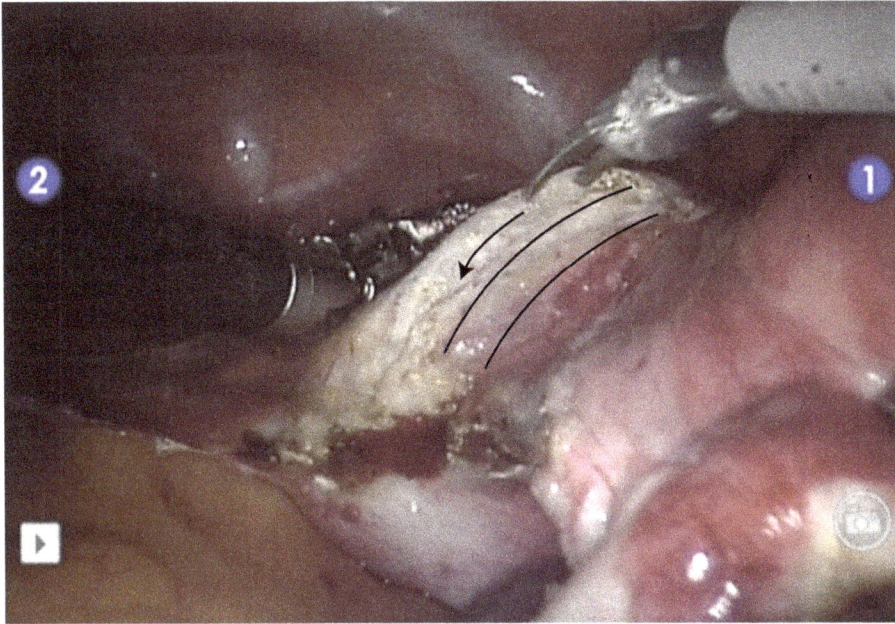

Fig. 9.13: Layer-by-layer excision of the vaginal cuff with monopolar scissors.

option provides opportunity and trade-offs; the final choice will depend on the surgeon's discretion. Commonly used suture material is barbed bidirectional suture 2-0 or 0 absorbable polyglyconate (V-Loc TM 180 Absorbable Polyglyconate Knotless Wound Closure Device, Covidien Ilc, Mansfield, MA). Special care should be given closing the vaginal cuff angles. Angles should close in a triangle fashion to avoid uterine vessel injury yet properly close the cuff angles (Fig. 9.14).

If no assistant arm is used during the surgery, the CT-1 needle can be introduced into the abdominal cavity by bending it slightly to fit into the 8-mm robotic trocar.

Previous meta-analyses show that cuff dehiscence is slightly higher in minimally invasive surgery (MIS) cases compared to open and vaginal hysterectomies: 0.6%, 1.2%, and 4% for open, laparoscopic, and robotic, respectively [7]. Therefore, longer-acting suture material is a reasonable choice for cuff closing in robotic surgery.

During the undocking process, special care should be given to avoid letting the robotic arms touch the patient. The robotic camera is exchanged for a 5-mm laparoscopic camera, caps are placed on the robotic trocars to serve as 5-mm laparoscopic access ports and the laparoscopic camera is introduced into one of these 8-mm robotic trocars. Intraabdominal pressure is dropped to 5 mmHg to assure homeostasis, and the Trendelenburg position is reversed to the horizontal level after the pressure reaches 15 mmHg again.

The fascia for all 10-mm and larger trocar incisions is closed. The author prefers using an endoclose technique (Carter-Thompson CloseSure System, CooperSurgical,

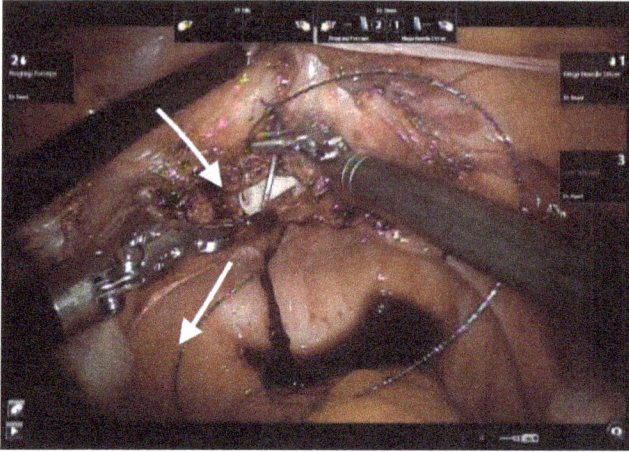

Fig. 9.14: Cuff angle closure.

Trumbull, CT) under direct visualization. Robotic trocar incisions between the skin and the fascia are closed using 2/0 vicryl UR-6 needle (Polyglactin 910 Synthetic Absorbable Suture, Ethicon, Inc., Somerville, NJ). The skin can be closed with the surgeon's preferred method.

Robotic or laparoendoscopic single-site surgery (LESS) is also an option for simple hysterectomy. Although a single-site laparoscopic approach is used for different medical fields, the requirements of the learning curve and technical considerations, including external clashes, poor visualization of critical structures, and surgeon fatigue, continue to be major disadvantages of single-site surgery. To overcome some of these difficulties, novel articulated instrumentation, such as flexible scopes, angle instruments, and novel robotic technologies (platforms), have been developed and/or applied. The advantage of robotically assisted over laparoscopic on LESS cases would be the orientation of the surgeon. In laparoscopy, the surgeon's hands are crossed, which has the potential to cause disorientation, while in robotically assisted cases, the surgeon can set up the arms based on his or her preference, e.g., to adjust the right robotic hand to the surgeon's left hand and vice versa.

References

[1] Hysterectomy. MedlinePlus, US National Library of Medicine. https://medlineplus.gov/hysterectomy.html. Updated 2012. Accessed October 22, 2012.
[2] Multinu F, Casarin J, Hanson KT, et al. Practice patterns and complications of benign hysterectomy following the FDA statement warning against the use of power morcellation. JAMA Surg 2018;153:e180141.

[3] US Food and Drug Administration. UPDATED Laparoscopic Uterine Power Morcellation in Hysterectomy and Myomectomy: FDA Safety Communication. 2014. https://www.burgsimpson. com/wp-content/uploads/2016/08/FDA_Safety_Communication_11-24-2014.pdf. Published on November 24, 2014. Accessed February 6, 2018.

[4] Wright JD, Chen L, Burke WM, et al. Trends in use and outcomes of women undergoing hysterectomy with electric power morcellation. JAMA 2016;316:877–8.

[5] Ottarsdottir H, Cohen SL, Cox M, Vitonis A, Einarsson JI. Trends in mode of hysterectomy after the U.S. food and drug administration power morcellation advisory. Obstet Gynecol 2017;129:1014–21.

[6] Barron KI, Richard T, Robinson PS, Lamvu G. Association of the U.S. Food and Drug Administration morcellation warning with rates of minimally invasive hysterectomy and myomectomy. Obstet Gynecol 2015;126:1174–80.

[7] Sarlos D, Kots L, Stevanovic N, von Felten S, Schar G. Robotic compared with conventional laparoscopic hysterectomy: a randomized controlled trial. Obstet Gynecol 2012;120:604–11.

Chetna Arora and Arnold P. Advincula

10 Abdominal approaches to uterine myomas (laparoscopic myomectomy) and morcellation

10.1 Introduction

During the reproductive years, uterine myomas are the most common benign tumor encountered in women and are the single most frequent indication for hysterectomy [1]. As a result, they represent a significant morbidity to many women and a major public health problem. The majority of the symptoms related to myomas are associated with their mass effect on surrounding structures, heavy menstrual bleeding, pelvic pain, recurrent pregnancy loss and even infertility. Interestingly, many women are asymptomatic [2, 3].

Several medical and nonsurgical therapies exist for the treatment of uterine myomas. For those women who are asymptomatic, expectant management is advised as the risk of malignancy is low and the majority of myomas decrease in size during menopause [4]. If symptomatic and treatment is desired, management should be tailored to each patient. Therapy should be dependent on the size and location of the myomas, the patient's age, the symptom profile and the desire to maintain fertility.

If medical treatment is preferred, there are many options currently available that can be customized to the patient's symptom profile. Medical treatment includes the use of hormonal therapy, nonsteroidal anti-inflammatory drugs, tranexamic acid, gonadotropin-releasing hormone agonists and selective receptor modulators. Often, if the symptoms are largely due to heavy menstrual bleeding, dysmenorrhea, or even pelvic pain, these therapies can allow for significant improvement [2, 5].

Alternatively, if the myomas are implicated in infertility or cause bulk symptoms such as pelvic pressure, urinary/bowel changes, or recurrent pregnancy loss, or they have failed medical management, interventional/surgical therapy may be considered. These options include uterine artery embolization, magnetic resonance-guided high-intensity focused ultrasound, ultrasound-guided radiofrequency ablation, myomectomy, and definitive treatment with a hysterectomy [5, 6].

In this chapter, we will discuss the surgical abdominal approach to uterine myomas via a laparoscopic myomectomy as well as the history and current techniques of morcellation and tissue extraction.

10.2 Laparoscopic myomectomy

The various surgical approaches to a myomectomy include conventional laparoscopy, robotic-assisted laparoscopy, operative hysteroscopy and the traditional abdominal incision (either via midline or Pfannenstiel). Operative hysteroscopy is the intervention of choice for all submucosal myomas under 3 cm with >50% intracavitary

https://doi.org/10.1515/9783110535204-010

component (The International Federation of Gynecology and Obstetrics (FIGO) 0 or 1 classification) [7]. Each route is chosen based on myoma burden (of both size and number), myoma location, patient preference, patient comorbidities, and surgeon skill. For those women in which fertility is desired or simply uterine preservation in the setting of symptoms, myomectomy is the leading intervention [8]. In this chapter, we will focus on the conventional (nonrobotic) laparoscopic route.

There are many benefits to a conventional laparoscopic approach compared to the alternative routes. These include less blood loss, decreased postoperative pain, shorter recovery time, shorter hospitalization time, and decreased perioperative complications [9]. The laparoscopic approach should be considered first-line for patients unless the presence of an intramural myoma exceeds 10–12 cm or there are multiple myomas (consensus is approximately four or more) that require several incisions based on varying locations within the uterus [10, 11]. While this is a recommendation, successful laparoscopic approaches to myomas >20 cm have been published, proving that experienced surgeons can safely perform this type of procedure despite the aforementioned recommendations [12–14].

The first step to a laparoscopic myomectomy is abdominal entry. This should be governed by previous surgical history, clinical examination of myoma burden, preoperative imaging, and surgeon preference to optimize access. For patients with a surgically naïve abdomen and small myoma(s), entry via the umbilicus is appropriate. In the event access is constrained due to suspected or known adhesions or uterine size >20 weeks, Palmer's point (left upper quadrant entry) should be employed. Finally, port placement should be individualized to the patient's pathology and abdominal topography (Fig. 10.1). Three or more incisions are required to accommodate the camera as well as at least two operative instruments. The sizes of these ports vary from 5 mm to 10 mm depending on the desired equipment and surgeon preference. Single-site laparoscopy has also been performed but does require specialized and flexible laparoscopic equipment [9, 15].

Another crucial step when performing a laparoscopic myomectomy is the use of a uterine manipulator. Myomas can be difficult to remove if located on the posterior or lateral aspects of the uterus and can be even more challenging when large enough to abut surrounding structures, such as the rectum or the pelvic side wall. The benefits of uterine manipulators are multifold. Not only do they allow for better visualization and exposure in addition to traction-countertraction, but they also push the uterus and the associated pathology away from vital structures such as the ureters, major pelvic vasculature, and bowel [16–18].

With the uterus now optimally visualized with a global view via the uterine manipulator and the individualized ports placed, the myomas are identified and subsequently enucleated. Firstly, not only is there the inherent benefit of laparoscopy over laparotomy via entry, but also blood loss can be further minimized before complete removal if the myomas are first injected with vasopressin into the pseudocapsule [19–21]. Other alternative or synergistic ways of mitigating blood loss also include the use of vascular clamps, clips, or ties (both permanent and temporary)

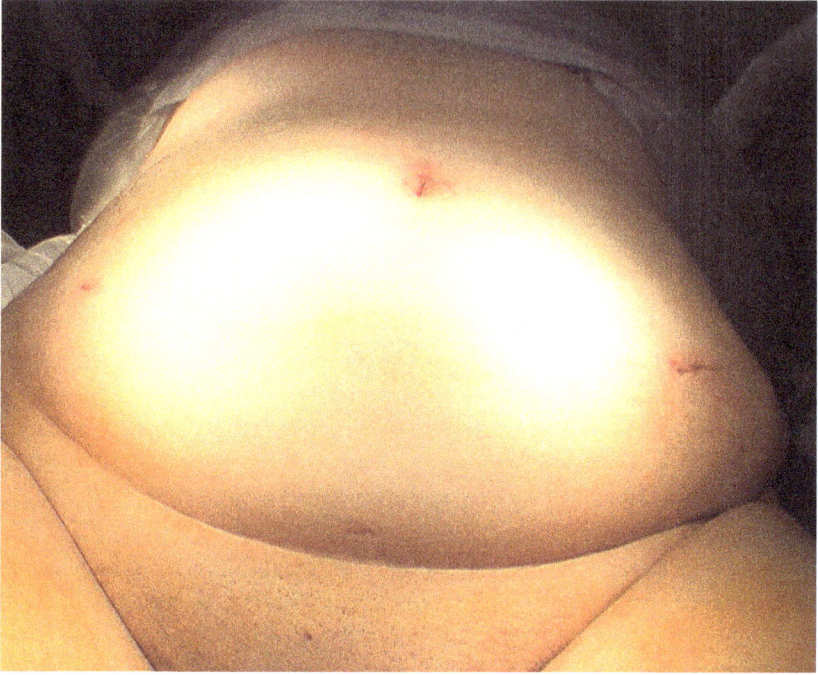

Fig. 10.1: Sample configuration of incision sites during 4-port laparoscopy.

of bilateral uterine arteries, intravaginal prostaglandins, oxytocin infusions, intravenous tranexamic acid, loop ligation of the myoma pseudocapsule once the majority of a large myoma has been enucleated and peri-cervical tourniquets, as well as the use of gelatin thrombin matrices or cell salvage systems. Many of these methods have been extrapolated from their uses in abdominal myomectomies and applied with success laparoscopically [15, 19]. Once adequate hemostatic approaches have been utilized, the surgeon must carefully dissect out an intramural myoma by first incising the serosa and myometrium to the level of the pseudocapsule. Transverse incisions allow the surgeon to ergonomically close the wound, but vigilance when near the uterine arteries is indicated. With careful attention to follow the tissue planes of the pseudocapsule, the myoma can be circumferentially enucleated and dissected from its fibrous attachments to the surrounding myometrium. The devices used to perform the enucleation are largely surgeon preference, but it can be accomplished with a variety of instruments such as an ultrasonically activated scalpel or electrosurgical instruments such as scissors, bipolar forceps, and monopolar needles. An effort should be made to minimize the number of incisions to not only minimize further blood loss as the majority of bleeding ensues from the surrounding myometrium but also minimize serosal injury, limit the chances of disruption of the endometrium and maintain the integrity of the uterine body and cornuas [15] (Fig. 10.2).

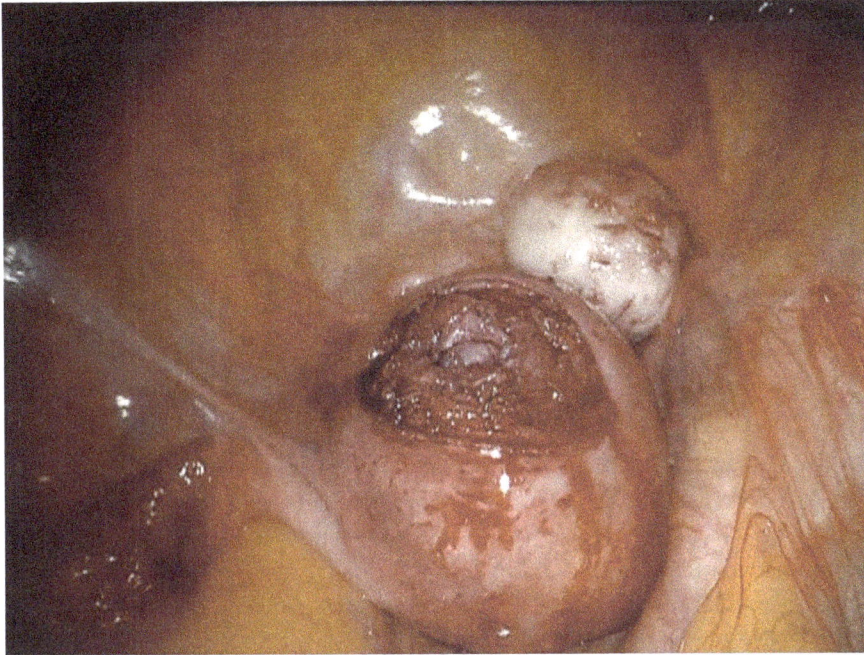

Fig. 10.2: Excised myoma placed in anterior cul de sac after antero-fundal hysterotomy with subsequent enucleation.

With the myoma placed aside within the pelvis or upper abdomen, the uterine incisions are then closed. Tissue extraction and morcellation will be discussed in the following section. Closure of the uterine incisions is modeled after the traditional abdominal myomectomy closure technique. With the intent to close the defect from the inside-out, often, a three-layer closure is employed if the endometrium is not disturbed [22]. Identification of a breach in the endometrium can be readily identified by injecting methylene blue into the uterine manipulator, which distends the uterine cavity. In the event there is evidence of endometrial disruption with release of methylene blue within the abdomen, an extra layer of suture closure may be required. Hemostasis is largely achieved by rapid re-approximation with suture, but diathermy may be required. Minimal use of energy is advised to maintain the viability of the surrounding myometrium and decrease the possible risk of future obstetrical complications, such as uterine rupture [23, 24]. Closure of the incisions can be performed with either barbed or nonbarbed suture. If barbed suture is employed, unidirectional or bidirectional sutures are available on a delayed absorbable monofilament. The suture itself contains small barbs that are arranged in a helical array to securely grasp the tissue and maintain tension. Bidirectional sutures have two needles (the surgeon starts at the middle and sutures in both directions to the ends of the incision), whereas unidirectional sutures have a single needle with a loop at the end (allowing for the suture to be anchored) [25]. As a result of the barbed suture's design, it also eliminates the need for surgical knots, thus leading to a significantly shorter operating time as seen by Alessandri *et al.* (9.6–13.4 vs 15.7–19.1 minutes; $p < 0.001$) and lower estimated blood loss ($\Delta Hb = 0.5–0.7$ versus 0.7–1.1; $p = 0.004$) [25, 26]. Once the myometrium has been sutured closed, attention can then be directed to the serosa. A finer suture can be used to imbricate this layer in a baseball stitch to decrease suture exposure thus minimizing possible foreign body reactions and adhesions [23].

10.3 Morcellation/tissue extraction

Removal of the myomas is the concluding and crucial step in the achievement of a minimally invasive approach to myomectomy. While laparoscopic surgery has been proven to be associated with fewer perioperative complications, lower mortality, faster recovery, better cosmesis, and improved quality of life, tissue extraction of large pathology can be a challenge [9, 27, 28]. Further challenges arose with the strong warning issued by the Food and Drug Administration (FDA) in spring of 2014 contraindicating the use of power morcellation for presumed uterine myomas. This advisory was published after a grassroots movement to ban morcellation was launched by a patient with an undiagnosed leiomyosarcoma who underwent a hysterectomy with morcellation of her uterus and subsequent worsening of her prognosis by occult dissemination [29]. Following this safety communication, there was an 11% absolute increase in the use of abdominal myomectomy. While the spreading of malignancy is a large concern, even benign, problematic pathology such as endometriosis or leiomyomatosis can occur due to iatrogenic dispersal as well. Complications with the use of the uncontained power morcellator have been published and include damage to surrounding structures from the motorized blade, in addition to the scattering of benign or malignant cells [30–32]. While these recommendations from the FDA are strong, both the American College of Obstetricians and Gynecologists and American Association of Gynecologic Laparoscopists have made statements to support the continued use of the power morcellator in select patients with consideration for preoperative endometrial cavity evaluation either by means of direct sampling or imaging American College of Obstetricians and Gynecologists (ACOG) [29]. Given these limitations, alternative techniques for tissue extraction have been reengineered to allow for continued safe and minimally invasive gynecologic surgery to be performed for myoma management.

An alternative to uncontained power morcellation is in-bag manual morcellation. While this option does have an improved safety profile, there is a drawback of potentially increased operative time [33]. Multiple routes for tissue extraction have been performed with success. The removal of specimens can be via a posterior colpotomy, thereby avoiding intracorporeal morcellation altogether, through extension of an incision to create a mini-laparotomy, thus facilitating removal with minimal to no morcellation or with reduction of the specimen to smaller fragments in order to be removed via the trocar sites. All three techniques are viable options without significant differences in perioperative complications [34, 35].

At our institution, we have developed a trainee-friendly and reproducible technique to simply extract even the largest myomas from the trocar sites safely and efficiently. This published technique is called extracorporeal C-incision tissue extraction, or the ExCITE technique. It models the same cutting principles of a power morcellator, but it is manual and contained within an endoscopic specimen bag [36].

The ExCITE technique is broken into five key steps.
1. Specimen retrieval and containment
2. Self-retaining retractor placement
3. Creation of the C-incision
4. Tissue extraction
5. Fascial closure

In step 1 of the ExCITE technique, the myoma(s) are placed within an endoscopic specimen retrieval bag. The incision at the level of the umbilicus (or the largest incision used during trocar placement) is extended approximately 2.5 to 3.5 cm. The bag edges are then exteriorized and held in place.

Step 2 of the technique involves the placement of a self-retaining retractor within the bag. This placement not only allows for a wider exposure during tissue extraction but also holds the endoscopic specimen bag open and in place (Fig. 10.3). Both the inner and outer rings should be fully deployed. Because an air-tight seal is created at the extraction site, pneumo-peritoneum can be maintained if desired, thereby elevating the contained specimen from critical structures such as the bowel.

Step 3 is the creation of the C-incision. First, grasp the specimen with a type of penetrating clamp (Lahey or single-tooth tenaculum unless the specimen is calcified or friable). Using a #11 scalpel blade, a reverse C-incision is created with the clamp providing upward traction in the nondominant hand and the scalpel starting the incision from the nondominant side toward the dominant side. By making the incisions wide, a specimen strip will be created that can be efficiently removed. A reciprocating sawing motion is preferred over single sweeping motions.

Step 4 is tissue extraction. With the basics of surgical traction-countertraction in mind, the strip of specimen being created is re-grasped near the base with the penetrating clamp, allowing for the maintenance of tension. As the reciprocating sawing motions are continued, the tissue should progressively lengthen into one completely intact strip—similar to what one would see with a power morcellator (Fig. 10.4).

Step 5 is the standard fascial closure. The specimen bag, with the self-retaining retractor within it, is removed without contaminating the abdomen with either microscopic cells or gross tissue fragments.

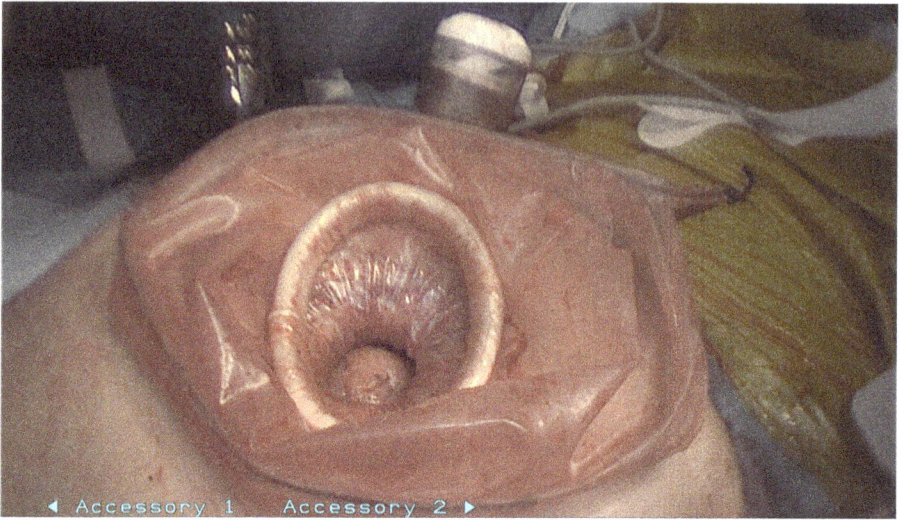

Fig. 10.3: Self-retaining retractor placed within specimen retrieval bag at the level of the umbilicus.

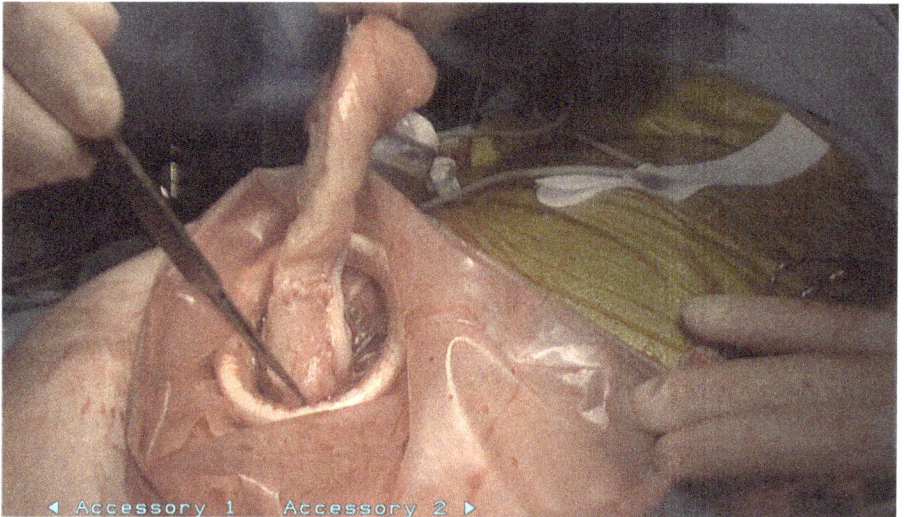

Fig. 10.4: Elongation of myoma strip during manual cold-knife tissue extraction.

10.4 Conclusion

Laparoscopic myomectomy should be considered as the first-line management of symptomatic uterine fibroids not amenable to conservative interventions, especially in patients desiring future fertility. This procedure is associated with proven success, even with large or multiple fibroids, especially when performed by experts in the field of minimally invasive gynecologic surgery. Regardless of the limitations enacted by the FDA's stance on the power morcellator, many viable—and expeditious—tissue extraction alternatives allow surgeons to continue to provide this route of surgery to the appropriate patients.

References

[1] Stewart EA, Laughlin-Tommaso SK, Catherino WH, Lalitkumar S, Gupta D, Vollenhoven B. Uterine fibroids. Nat Rev Disease Primers 2016;2:16043.
[2] Haney AF. Clinical decision making regarding leiomyomata: what we need in the next millennium. Environ Health Perspect 2000;108(Suppl 5):835–9.
[3] Stewart EA. Clinical practice. Uterine fibroids. N Engl J Med 2015;372:1646–55.
[4] Schwartz PE, Kelly MG. Malignant transformation of myomas: myth or reality? Obstet Gynecol Clin North Am 2006;33:183–98, xii.
[5] De La Cruz MS, Buchanan EM. Uterine fibroids: diagnosis and treatment. Am Fam Phys 2017;95:100–7.
[6] Silberzweig JE, Powell DK, Matsumoto AH, Spies JB. Management of uterine fibroids: a focus on uterine-sparing interventional techniques. Radiology 2016;280:675–92.
[7] Munro MG, Critchley HO, Broder MS, Fraser IS. FIGO classification system (PALM-COEIN) for causes of abnormal uterine bleeding in nongravid women of reproductive age. International journal of gynaecology and obstetrics: the official organ of the International Federation of Gynaecology and Obstetrics 2011;113:3–13.
[8] Flake GP, Andersen J, Dixon D. Etiology and pathogenesis of uterine leiomyomas: a review. Environ Health Perspect 2003;111:1037–54.
[9] Stoica RA, Bistriceanu I, Sima R, Iordache N. Laparoscopic myomectomy. J Med Life 2014;7:522–4.
[10] Donnez J, Dolmans MM. Uterine fibroid management: from the present to the future. Hum Reprod Update 2016;22:665–86.
[11] Holub Z. [Laparoscopic myomectomy: indications and limits]. Ceska Gynekologie 2007;72:64–8.
[12] Sinha R, Hegde A, Mahajan C, Dubey N, Sundaram M. Laparoscopic myomectomy: do size, number, and location of the myomas form limiting factors for laparoscopic myomectomy? J Minim Invasive Gynecol 2008;15:292–300.
[13] Aksoy H, Aydin T, Ozdamar O, Karadag OI, Aksoy U. Successful use of laparoscopic myomectomy to remove a giant uterine myoma: a case report. J Med Case Rep 2015;9:286.
[14] Damiani A, Melgrati L, Marziali M, Sesti F, Piccione E. Laparoscopic myomectomy for very large myomas using an isobaric (gasless) technique. JSLS 2005;9:434–8.
[15] Gingold JA, Gueye NA, Falcone T. Minimally invasive approaches to myoma management. J Minim Invasive Gynecol 2017;25(2):237–250.
[16] van den Haak L, Alleblas C, Nieboer TE, Rhemrev JP, Jansen FW. Efficacy and safety of uterine manipulators in laparoscopic surgery: a review. Arch Gynecol Obstet 2015;292:1003–11.
[17] Janssen PF, Brolmann HA, Huirne JA. Causes and prevention of laparoscopic ureter injuries: an analysis of 31 cases during laparoscopic hysterectomy in the Netherlands. Surg Endosc 2013;27:946–56.
[18] Agdi M, Tulandi T. The benefits of intrauterine balloon: an intrauterine manipulator and balloon proved useful in myomectomy. Am J Obstet Gynecol 2008;199:581.e1.

[19] Hickman LC, Kotlyar A, Shue S, Falcone T. Hemostatic techniques for myomectomy: an evidence-based approach. J Minim Invasive Gynecol 2016;23:497–504.

[20] Lin XN, Zhang SY, Fang SH, Wang MZ, Lou HY. [Assessment of different homeostatic methods used in laparoscopic intramural myomectomy]. Zhonghua yi xue za zhi 2008;88:905–8.

[21] Cohen SL, Wang KC, Gargiulo AR, et al. Vasopressin administration during laparoscopic myomectomy: a randomized controlled trial. J Minim Invasive Gynecol 2015;22:S39.

[22] Guarnaccia MM, Rein MS. Traditional surgical approaches to uterine fibroids: abdominal myomectomy and hysterectomy. Clin Obstet Gynecol 2001;44:385–400.

[23] Kim HS, Oh SY, Choi SJ, et al. Uterine rupture in pregnancies following myomectomy: a multicenter case series. Obstet Gynecol Sci 2016;59:454–62.

[24] Pistofidis G, Makrakis E, Balinakos P, Dimitriou E, Bardis N, Anaf V. Report of 7 uterine rupture cases after laparoscopic myomectomy: update of the literature. J Minim Invasive Gynecol 2012;19:762–7.

[25] Tulandi T, Einarsson JI. The use of barbed suture for laparoscopic hysterectomy and myomectomy: a systematic review and meta-analysis. J Minim Invasive Gynecol 2014;21:210–6.

[26] Alessandri F, Remorgida V, Venturini PL, Ferrero S. Unidirectional barbed suture versus continuous suture with intracorporeal knots in laparoscopic myomectomy: a randomized study. J Minim Invasive Gynecol 2010;17:725–9.

[27] Wright KN, Jonsdottir GM, Jorgensen S, Shah N, Einarsson JI. Costs and outcomes of abdominal, vaginal, laparoscopic and robotic hysterectomies. JSLS 2012;16:519–24.

[28] Stentz NC, Cooney LG, Sammel M, Shah DK. Changes in myomectomy practice after the U.S. Food and Drug Administration safety communication on power morcellation. Obstet Gynecol 2017;129:1007–13.

[29] AAGL practice report: morcellation during uterine tissue extraction. J Minim Invasive Gynecol 2014;21:517–30.

[30] Milad MP, Milad EA. Laparoscopic morcellator-related complications. J Minim Invasive Gynecol 2014;21:486–91.

[31] Milad MP, Sokol E. Laparoscopic morcellator-related injuries. J Am Assoc Gynecol Laparosc 2003;10:383–5.

[32] Wright JD, Tergas AI, Cui R, et al. Use of electric power morcellation and prevalence of underlying cancer in women who undergo myomectomy. JAMA Oncol 2015;1:69–77.

[33] Frasca C, Degli Esposti E, Arena A, et al. Can in-bag manual morcellation represent an alternative to uncontained power morcellation in laparoscopic myomectomy? A randomized controlled trial. Gynecol Obstet Investig 2017;83(1):52–56.

[34] Meurs E, Brito LG, Ajao MO, et al. Comparison of morcellation techniques at the time of laparoscopic hysterectomy and myomectomy. J Minim Invasive Gynecol 2017;24:843–9.

[35] Ghezzi F, Casarin J, De Francesco G, et al. Transvaginal contained tissue extraction after laparoscopic myomectomy: a cohort study. BJOG 2017;125(3):367–373.

[36] Truong MD, Advincula AP. The extracorporeal C-incision tissue extraction (ExCITE) Technique. OBG Manag 2014;26(11):56.

Arnaud Wattiez

11 Surgical treatment of endometriosis

11.1 Introduction

Endometriosis is a chronic gynecologic condition in which endometrial glands and stroma are present outside the uterus. These implants are predominantly found in the pelvis but may be present anywhere in the body. Lesions range from superficial deposits scattered throughout the pelvic and abdominal cavity, to deep and invasive endometriosis with adhesions (Fig. 11.1).

Endometriosis is a progressive, debilitating disease that affects 10–15% of women during their reproductive years. Treatment decisions should be individualized and consider clinical presentation (e.g., pain, infertility, mass), symptom severity, disease extent and location, reproductive desires, patient's age, medication side effects, surgical complication rates, and cost.

Currently, laparoscopy is the recognized route of surgery for endometriosis.

11.2 Preoperative assessment

Diagnostic preoperative examination must include in all patients a thorough history taking and physical examination. The imaging techniques have a fundamental role in the diagnosis of endometriosis [1]. Ovarian and deep (vagina, uterosacral, ureter, and bowel) endometriosis can be recognized using transvaginal ultrasound and/or magnetic resonance imaging (MRI). Although transvaginal ultrasound is the first choice of imaging modality when investigating women with pelvic pain, MRI has a role for the wider field of visions. Transvaginal ultrasound is superior to MRI with reported high sensitivity and specificity of 97% and 80%, respectively.

MRI can be very useful in patients in whom ultrasound findings are ambivalent and in carefully selected high-risk population. It is especially beneficial in identifying endometriomas, adhesions, superficial peritoneal implants, and extraperitoneal lesions, particularly those in the rectovaginal space and uterosacral ligaments as well as in solid endometriotic nodules.

If deep infiltrative endometriosis is suspected based on symptomatology (such as dyspareunia, dysuria, dyschezia, and hematochezia) and/or physical examination (e.g., uterosacral ligament tenderness with dense nodules and nonmobile uterus), the preoperative evaluation can include tests targeted to the specific organ, such as bladder, ureter, and kidney, lower gastrointestinal (GI) tract such as rectum and sigmoid, but also the caecum and the appendix [2]. In addition, ultrasound and MRI can provide more details for the higher lesions. Colonoscopy is of limited value [3].

https://doi.org/10.1515/9783110535204-011

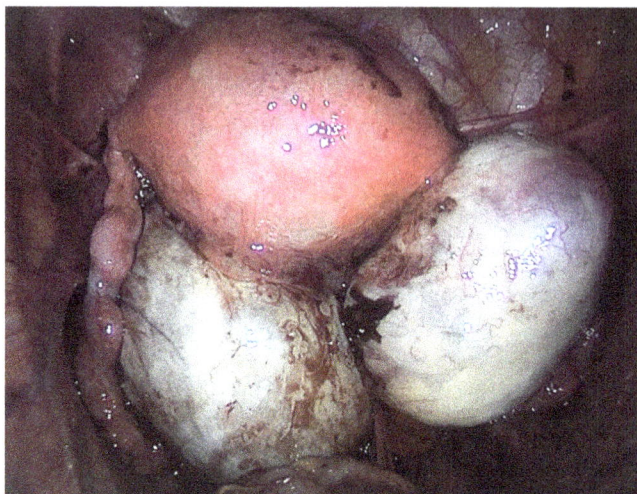

Fig. 11.1: Severe pelvic endometriosis with bilateral endometriomas, adherence of the ovaries to each other and the posterior uterine wall, and adhesions between the large bowel and ovaries.

Unfortunately, blood serum levels of antiendometrial antibodies and placental proteins PP14 and CA125 marker do not have sufficient sensitivity or specificity to be routinely used for diagnostic evaluation [2].

Preoperative informed consent and counseling should be targeted toward the aim of the intended surgery, covering its risks and benefits. There is no evidence for preoperative medical suppressive therapy.

A low-residue diet is prescribed 5 days before surgery, which eases the displacement of the bowel during surgery, allowing for adequate exposure. Rectal enema is used in cases of deeply infiltrating endometriosis (DIE) the night before surgery. A systematic antibiotic prophylaxis is recommended in all cases of DIE by a preoperative shot half an hour prior the incision.

11.3 Surgical technique

Surgical treatment involves both the assessment of the location and the extent of endometriotic lesions followed by the surgical treatment. However, total removal of all endometriotic cells from all sites is not clinically possible.

The surgical technique can be divided into general and specific steps. The general strategy involves basic steps and ergonomic principles that have to be performed in all cases [4].

The woman is placed in the lithotomy position with both arms located alongside the body and the coccyx at the edge of the table. The legs must be semiflexed, and their position must give the third surgeon optimal access to use vaginal and rectal instruments. Strict caution must be paid to positioning, avoiding both vascular and nerve compression. Vaginal and rectal examination under anesthesia must be systematically carried out to evaluate the endometriotic lesion before surgery begins.

A 10-mm, 0-degree laparoscope is introduced at umbilicus level, and three 5-mm accessory trocars are placed, respectively, in the iliac fossa and in the suprapubic midline. The midline trocar is located at the level of the lateral ones, or higher, to obtain a more ergonomic set-up. In cases of a big uterus due to adenomyosis or associated other pathology such as fibroids, the midline trocars can be placed at the level of the umbilicus and 10 mm trocar supra-umbilical for the laparoscope.

A systematic inspection of the abdominal and pelvic cavity must be carried out to map the endometriotic lesions and adapt the surgical strategy. More specifically, the diaphragm and the appendix should always be assessed.

At the end of this inspection, the surgeon compares the laparoscopic findings to the preoperative diagnosis and the objectives and the consent of the patient and can decide to proceed if the pre- and intraoperative assessments match or to abort the surgery if the intraoperative findings exceed the preoperative assessment. If the decision to proceed is taken, it comes with the obligation to do a complete surgery.

Adequate exposure is then achieved by several steps:

– First, the woman is placed in a Trendelenburg position, and a uterine manipulator is used. Bowel should be moved out of the pelvis if they are free of adhesions. Adhesiolysis is then carried out to reestablish normal anatomy. During this process, the physiological attachment of the sigmoid colon is freed to allow access to the left adnexa and the left ureter.
– If endometriotic cysts are present, the ovaries are freed, and usually, during this process, they are opened, drained, and suspended to the anterior abdominal wall using a suspension method.
– When dealing with more complex cases, other organs can be suspended. The rule is that if an organ should be reclined permanently, it should be done by a suspension method and not by an instrument.

These maneuvers are helpful because they improve the exposure of the surgical field and free the assistant's hand to help the surgeon.

Suspension of both ovaries and sigmoid colon is usually conducted in DIE surgery using straight needles or special devices such as T-Lift.

Ureteral identification is mandatory and may require their dissection. Of note, the left ureter crosses the common iliac artery and the right ureter crosses the external iliac artery. Hydrodissection and use of liquids is not recommended because the subsequent edema will hide the anatomical plane and make the dissection more difficult and the use of electrosurgery less efficient.

Once the normal anatomy is restored, the lesions are reevaluated and the specific strategy is then implemented. The specific strategy depends on the location and importance of the lesions, the goal being to be as complete as possible.

11.4 Ovarian endometriosis

Laparoscopic surgery is the gold standard approach for the management of endometriomas. The main indications are a symptomatic endometriosis or a cyst larger than 4–5 cm. Several techniques have been described to treat endometriomas. In most of these techniques, the procedure consists of opening and draining the cyst, followed by either excision (stripping technique), fulguration, or vaporization of the cystic wall (ablative technique). Drainage alone is not recommended because of the high recurrence rate. Excisional surgery is usually preferred as it provides better outcomes than ablative treatment in terms of spontaneous pregnancy rate, recurrence, and pain symptoms [5]. However, the balance between different techniques should be tailored according to the patient needs, i.e., fertility preservation or pain symptoms.

The ovary is freed from the posterior leaf of the broad ligament by traction. This procedure induces cyst rupture in almost all cases; if not, the cyst is intentionally emptied with immediate aspiration of the chocolate like material to prevent pelvic contamination. The cystic cavity is repeatedly irrigated with suction irrigation and inspected by cystoscopy [4]. If dealing with DIE, we proceed with the ovarian suspension to the abdominal wall, leaving cystectomy to the end of the surgery. The recommended way of cystectomy is to evert the cyst, incise its base, and carry out a reverse cystectomy for both halves of the cyst (Fig. 11.2). Two grasping forceps are used to exert traction and countertraction in the incision margins. The cyst's capsule is then detached from the ovarian parenchyma by stripping. The correct plane of dissection is chosen when the capsule appears white or slightly yellow without red streaks; this will allow bloodless dissection without any hemorrhage and will reduce the inadvertent removal of ovarian parenchyma. Precise hemostasis of the ovarian bed is obtained by dripping saline and bipolar coagulation electrode. Blind coagulation must be

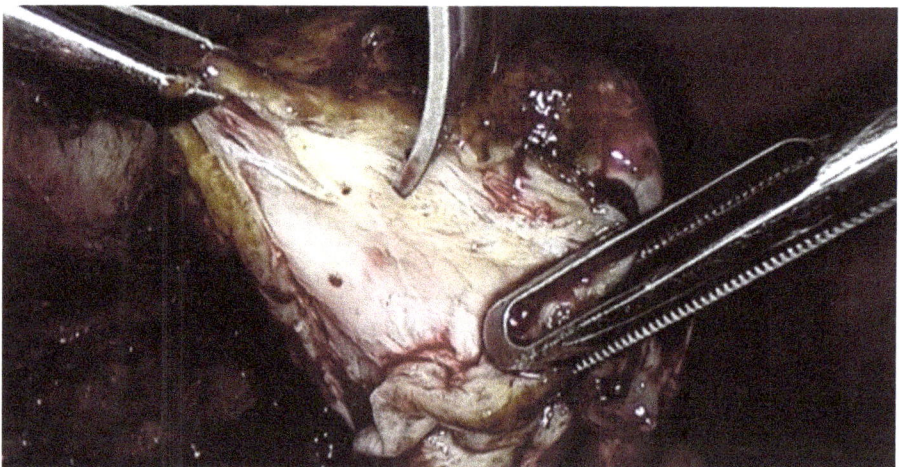

Fig. 11.2: After drainage, the ovary with endometrioma is everted and an incision is made to its base. The plane between the cyst capsule and ovarian cortex can be clearly seen.

avoided. Generally, the ovary is left open without any need for suturing. Antiadhesion barriers are placed at the end of the procedure to decrease the risk of postoperative adhesions.

It must be remembered that endometriomas are frequently associated with advanced-stage endometriosis, so it must be considered as a marker of more extensive pelvic and intestinal disease. In many cases, endometriomas are fixed to the ipsilateral uterosacral ligament by dense adhesions, and this may involve and displace the ureter medially which often necessitate careful ureterolysis.

11.5 Deep infiltrating endometriosis of Douglas's pouch

Deep infiltrating endometriosis is defined by the presence of endometriosis lesions penetrating more than 5 mm under the peritoneal surface with variable distribution. Technical difficulties are expected usually in surgeries for DIE. The surgeon should balance his or her skills against the anticipated difficulty and duration of surgery. This highlights the need for a team with an assistant experienced in deep endometriosis surgeries, when endometriosis nodule is more than 3 cm.

Lesions of DIE can be classified either as anterior, when they invade the detrusor muscle, or as posterior, when they are located at the pouch of Douglas. At this level, the most frequent sites affected by the disease are the uterosacral ligaments, the posterior vaginal wall, and the anterior rectosigmoid.

After lysis of sigmoid adhesions and drainage and stripping of endometriomas, ureters and large vessels are localized and the ureter is then exposed down to the ureteric canal following its course in the pelvis until healthy tissue is reached (Fig. 11.3). If uterosacral ligaments are involved, the anatomical landmarks for uterosacral ligament excision (ureters, uterine arteries, hypogastric nerves, and the rectosigmoid) should be identified. In isolated lesions, dissection should begin with a peritoneal window, medial to the ureter, to dissect the nodule until the ascending uterine artery and torus uterinus. Special attention should be paid not to get too close to the rectum.

On the contrary, in cases of extensive adhesive disease, the dissection should not extend below the deep uterine vein, avoiding harm to the inferior hypogastric plexus that contains branches from the inferior hypogastric nerve and from the splanchnic autonomic nerves responsible for urinary and bowel function.

The left ureter and the left inferior hypogastric nerve are left lateral and the Okabayashi part of the pararectal space is dissected caudally and medially to the course of hypogastric nerve. Dissection should continue lateral to the rectum and then to the rectovaginal nodule until the disease is passed caudally, with attention to the middle rectal artery. The dissection is made in the same manner on the right side, pushing the right ureter and the right nerve laterally. Once healthy connective tissue is reached downward in the posterior vaginal wall, it is possible to begin the dissection of the anterior rectal wall. Dissection should be tailored to the needs, and extensive dissection should be avoided.

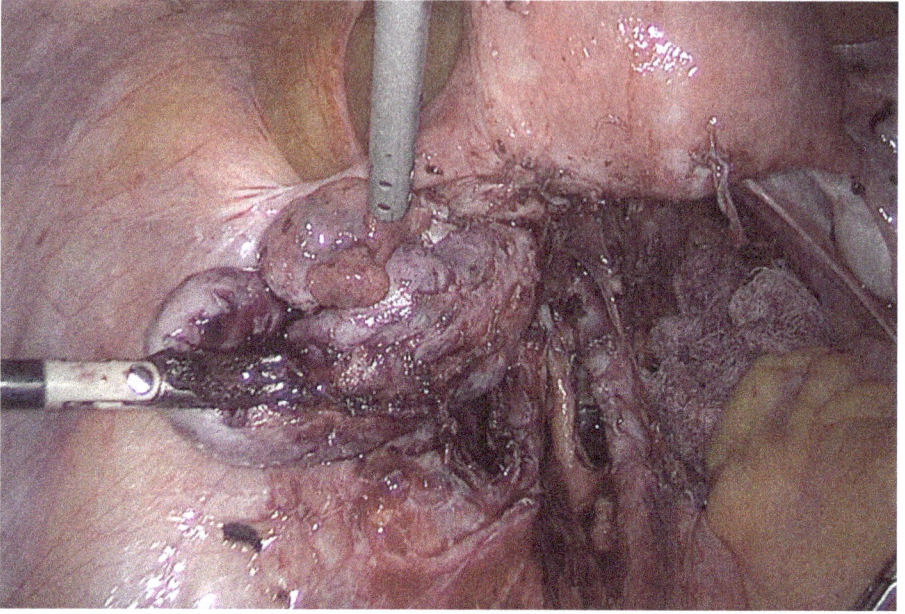

Fig. 11.3: After adhesiolysis, the left ureter is exposed down to the ureteric canal.

Once this step is achieved, the fibrotic/endometriotic tissue is shaved from the rectum. It is essential to divide the nodule as close as possible to the rectal wall, leaving as much endometriosis tissue attached to the uterus and the vaginal wall. The shaving is continued downward along the posterior cervical and vaginal wall and as caudal as the rectovaginal space is entered caudal to the lesion. At that point, the lesion is totally dissected and all necessary anatomical landmarks under vision. Finally, once the rectum has been detached, the nodule can be dissected from the posterior vaginal wall.

The lesions are reassessed, and further decisions are taken in order to tailor the surgery to the needs. Decisions have to be taken concerning the uterosacral ligaments, the vagina, the rectum, and the sigmoid.

The uterosacral ligaments are resected at the site of insertion of the cervix. In bilateral uterosacral involvement, the surgeon should decide whether a radical or conservative approach should be taken according to the neural risk. Bilateral excision of nodules at the uterosacral ligaments has a high risk of hypogastric nerve damage, exposing the woman to postsurgical bladder voiding problems. Although transient in most women, in some cases, it might last for weeks, requiring self-catheterization. Nerve-sparing surgery has been advocated to limit voiding dysfunctions. Nevertheless, extensive fibrosis and secondary inflammatory reaction make the nerve dissection difficult, even in expert hands. This highlights the need for good anatomical knowledge, and the feasibility of nerve-sparing procedures in severe DIE needs to be questioned. In our opinion, it may be better to limit the extent of surgery than to leave the woman with permanent voiding dysfunction.

In most of the cases, the vagina is involved. When the implants are visible vaginally, the situation is clear and a vaginal resection should be performed. If the vagina is infiltrated and the implants are not seen vaginally, the indications for vaginal opening and resection are not clear. Some authors advocate a systematic resection of the vagina, arguing the decrease of recurrence [6]. In that case, the vagina is opened as the surgeon follows the nodule between normal and diseased tissue. Once the vagina is opened, the gas leak and the vision are impaired. A number of solutions can be implemented to solve this problem: packing the vagina with swabs, using a manipulator with an antileak system or removing the manipulator, packing the vagina, and suspending the uterus. The nodule can be extracted through the vaginal opening. The vagina is closed longitudinally using a monofilament (absorbable) number 0 interrupted suture material and intracorporeal knot tying.

11.6 Bowel endometriosis

Two techniques can be proposed: a radical technique, with the aim of a complete resection of the lesions to prevent recurrence, and a more conservative technique that could decrease the rate of functional disorders. Consultation with a general or colorectal surgeon should be take place before or during surgery.

Bilateral opening of the pararectal fossas and the lateralization of the ureters are mandatory before detaching the bowel from the rectovaginal septum (Fig. 11.4). To do so, the assistant pulls the rectum cephalad by means of a flat atraumatic forceps, and the posterior part of the uterus and the vagina are detached from the bowel,

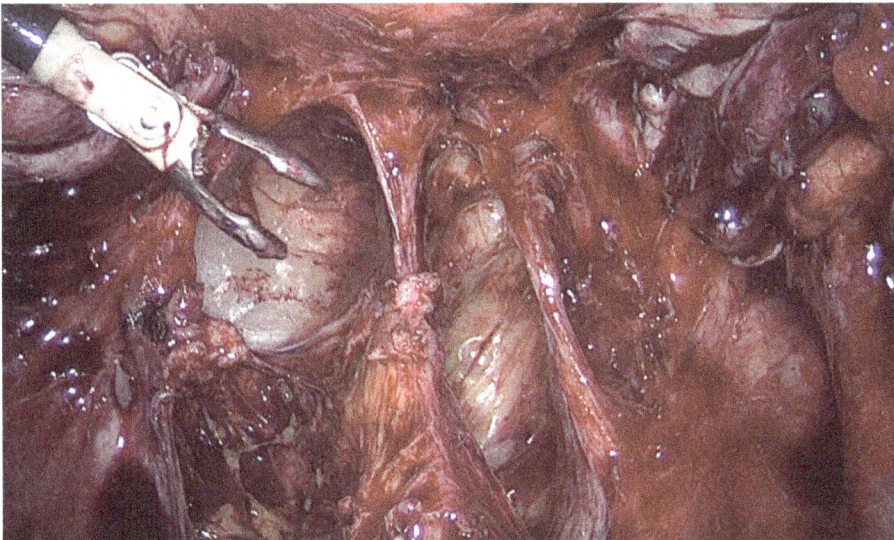

Fig. 11.4: Pararectal spaces have been opened before detaching the bowel from the rectovaginal septum.

progressively turning the lesion around with scissors. Aggressive coagulation of the bowel wall, especially when thin, is avoided. The surgeon should leave as much of the disease as possible on the posterior vaginal wall. The nodule is then detached from the vagina, with attention not to open the vagina if the disease does not infiltrate the mucosa. Once the bowel has been detached, a rectal probe is used to check if stenosis is present and to control the circumference of bowel involvement.

Occasionally, adhesiolysis is sufficient and no more surgery on the bowel is required. Shaving techniques consist of resection of superficial lesions of the serosa or of the muscular layer. Muscularis defect will be closed with a single layer running transversal suture. A full thickness defect is sutured in two layers. When the lesion is deeper than the mucosa and not larger than 3 cm, a discoid resection can be carried out using a circular stapler (discoid resection) or a linear stapler (wedge resection).

For segmental bowel resection, the mesentery is dissected close to the digestive tract above the fascia proprietary of the rectum to preserve vascular lymphatic vessels as well as surrounding sympathetic and parasympathetic nerves. A linear endoscopic stapler is used to resect the bowel at the edge of the nodule. It is proven that an intracorporeal anastomosis provides a faster recovery of bowel function, decreases postoperative narcotic use, length of stay, and morbidity. Conventionally, a 4-cm Pfannenstiel's incision is made to resect the rectum and place an Alexis retractor, and an end-to-end or side-to-end anastomosis is carried out intracorporeally with GI stapler transanally. Less invasive approaches, such as transanal and transvaginal natural orifice specimen extraction, have been developed in colorectal surgery.

The integrity of the anastomosis is systematically controlled with air and methylene blue tests. Vascularization of the anastomosis, and absence of tension or twists are checked. The two doughnut rings of tissue are also checked.

Although there is no evidence demonstrating its efficacy, an omental flap can be placed to separate the anastomosis from the vagina if they are at the same level. When the resection is ultralow (less than 6 cm from the anal verge), a protective ileostomy might be considered according to the technical complexity and length of the operation. Postoperative care must be done with caution to detect early leaks of the anastomosis.

The anterior compartment endometriosis is less frequent but is addressed with the same strategy compared to the posterior compartment. The bladder can be involved as well as the ureter. Even if the ureter is more frequently involved with posterior lesion, we will discuss the ureteric problem as part of the urinary tract endometriosis.

11.7 Bladder endometriosis

Bladder endometriosis is defined as the presence of endometrial glands and stroma in the detrusor muscle. Symptoms can be dysuria, hematuria, or recurrent urinary tract infections, but in 50% of the cases, the symptoms are not characteristic.

Cystoscopy should eventually be carried out at the beginning of the procedure to check the localization of the nodule and to assess the distance of the nodule to the ureteric ostia. Ureteral double-J stents should be placed if partial cystectomy is planned, when the lesion is located at the bladder trigone or when the lesion is close to the ureteral orifices. Multiple surgical alternatives are available according to the degree of bladder-wall involvement. Shaving could be considered when superficial endometriosis is found on the bladder peritoneum. The bladder should be opened in case of full thickness resection, and care is taken not to damage the intramural part of the ureter. The bladder should be opened as high as possible, permitting identification of the exact location of the ureter. The bladder wall is closed in a single- or double-layer interrupted suture using intracorporeal knots. Its integrity is checked using methylene blue test, and ureteral stents should be left in place for 6–8 weeks. An indwelling catheter should be left in place for 10–15 days and should be removed after confirmation of the absence of contrast medium leak by cystography.

11.8 Ureteral endometriosis

Ureteral endometriosis is usually classified into extrinsic, which includes the infiltration of the surrounding connective tissue and adventitia, and intrinsic, where muscularis mucosa or uro-epithelium is involved. Ureteral involvement should always be suspected in the presence of retrocervical nodules larger than 2 cm as it could lead to the silent death of the kidney, and the urinary tract should always be assessed in case of rectovaginal nodules. Changes in the ureteric course from its lateral to medial, particularly at the lower third, are expected in cases of DIE due to the presence of periureteral fibrosis that causes retraction and distortion. Special attention should be paid not to harm the ureteral adventitia to avoid ureteral devascularization (Fig. 11.5). In most cases, ureterolysis is the only treatment required, and if severe devascularization is observed, it is recommended that a double-J stent is inserted to decrease the risk of ureteral fistula. Preoperative stenting is necessary in cases of ureteral stenosis.

End-to-end anastomosis is required in the case of intrinsic ureteral endometriosis or persistent stenosis after relieving extrinsic compression. The double-J stent should be left in place for 6–8 weeks.

Ureteral reimplantation is recommended when the lesion is located at the ureterovesical junction. A Psoas hitch suspension can be carried out in cases where the ureter's length is insufficient, to ensure a tension-free anastomosis. A double-J stent and an indwelling catheter should be left in place for 7–10 days. Before removing the bladder catheter, it is recommended that a cystography is carried out to test the integrity of the anastomosis.

11.9 Postoperative care

Depending on the difficulties encountered during laparascopy, patients are usually discharged home 24 to 48 hours postoperatively. Clamping of Foley's catheter and

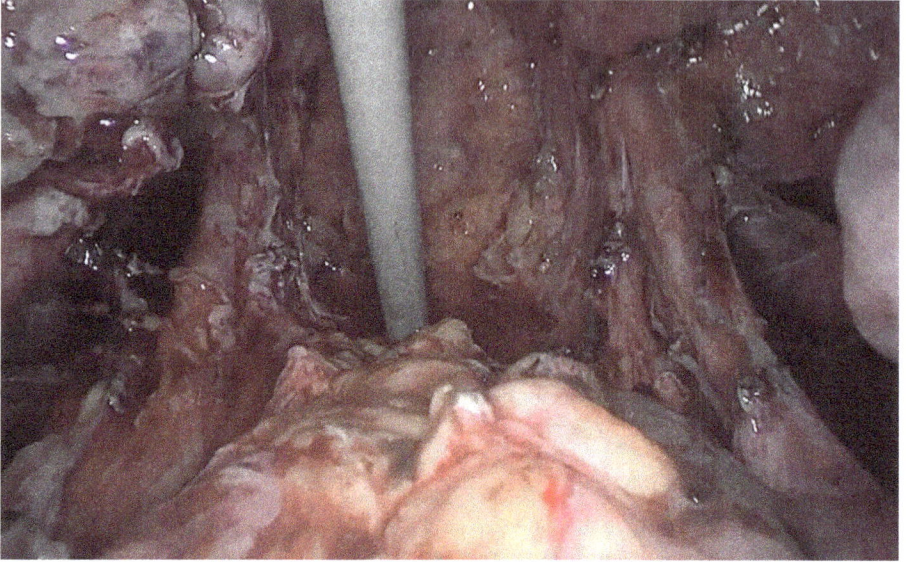

Fig. 11.5: Appearance of the ureters after bilateral ureterolysis, note well preserved adventitia.

testing for bladder sensation before removal are advised in cases of DIE. Mild analgesics usually will be sufficient to control the pain. Use of mechanical or pharmacological venous thromboembolism prophylaxis depends upon the procedure and the patient's risk factors.

Postoperative medical therapy (such as gonadotropin releasing hormone analogues and oral contraceptive pills) may be prescribed to prevent recurrence, reduce pelvic pain, and facilitate subsequent induction of ovulation in fertility treatment.

References

[1] Nisenblat V, Bossuyt PM, Farquhar C, Johnson N, Hull ML. Imaging modalities for the noninvasive diagnosis of endometriosis. Cochrane Database Syst Rev 2016;2:CD009591.

[2] Dunselman GA, Vermeulen N, Becker C, et al. ESHRE guideline: management of women with endometriosis. Hum Reprod 2014;29(3):400–12.

[3] Koninckx PR, Ussia A, Adamyan L, Wattiez A, Donnez J. Deep endometriosis: definition, diagnosis, and treatment. Fertil Steril 2012;98(3):564–71.

[4] Wattiez A, Puga M, Albornoz J, Faller E. Surgical strategy in endometriosis. Best Pract Res Clin Obstet Gynaecol 2013;27(3):381–92.

[5] Hart R, Hickey M, Maouris P, Buckett W, Garry R. Excisional surgery versus ablative surgery for ovarian endometriomata: a Cochrane review. Hum Reprod 2005;20(11):3000–7.

[6] Matsuzaki S, Houlle C, Botchorishvili R, Pouly JL, Mage G, Canis M. Excision of the posterior vaginal fornix is necessary to ensure complete resection of rectovaginal endometriotic nodules of more than 2 cm in size. Fertil Steril 2009;91(4 Suppl):1314–5.

Liselotte Mettler and Ibrahim Alkatout

12 Management of benign adnexal masses

12.1 Introduction

Adnexal masses are common and are one of the leading cause of surgery in gynecological practice. The vast majority of adnexal masses is functional and/or asymptomatic and can be managed conservatively. A recent international multicenter prospective study showed that, among women with adnexal masses thought to be benign at initial diagnosis, risk of complications was found to be low (0.4% for ovarian torsion and 0.2% for cyst rupture). In the same study, spontaneous resolution occurred in 20% and risk of malignant or borderline ovarian tumors was 0.4% and 0.3%, respectively [1]. The diagnosis of adnexal masses has been covered in Chapter 2. In this chapter, we exclude tubal disease as well as ovarian endometriomas and focus on surgical management of benign adnexal masses.

12.2 Indications for surgery for adnexal masses

There are no universally accepted indications for surgery for benign adnexal masses. Adnexal torsion, cyst rupture, concern of borderline or malignant tumor, and persistent/significant pain are probably the commonly agreed reasons. Some clinicians or centers use a certain size as an indication for surgery, but there is no overall consensus if this is a valid indication and what the cutoff should be.

In premenopausal women, when there is no concern of malignancy and surgical treatment is indicated due to cyst accidents (see adnexal torsion below) or pain symptoms, conservative surgery, i.e., cystectomy with preservation of the ovary and fallopian tube, is usually the treatment of choice. In the presence of recurrent or very large cysts—especially in older women—an adnexectomy may be chosen, even when there is no concern of malignancy. If there is concern of malignancy, rupture of the cyst and spillage of the contents may potentially be harmful to the survival of the patient; hence, cystectomy by laparoscopy is not the proper technique in this scenario. Removal of the adnexa is the optimal approach in postmenopausal women when surgery is indicated.

Functional ovarian cysts resolve without surgery, with or without the use of hormonal contraceptives [2]. Hence, when functional cysts are diagnosed, expectant management for one to two cycles would be appropriate, even if they are symptomatic.

Optimal management of incidentally detected asymptomatic benign ovarian cysts is not known, as the natural course of these is still unknown [3]. However, as mentioned above, spontaneous resolution occurs in a significant proportion of masses, and risks of torsion or rupture are uncommon [1].

https://doi.org/10.1515/9783110535204-012

12.2.1 Dermoid cysts

Dermoid cysts (mature cystic teratomas) are the most common ovarian neoplastic lesions found in adolescents and approximately 70% of benign ovarian tumors in women under 30 years of age [4, 5]. They contain tissues deriving from the three embryonic layers (ectoderm, mesoderm, and endoderm) and are frequently filled with fatty, thick, sebaceous material with bone, hair, and cartilage.

When surgery is indicated, a minimally invasive approach by laparoscopy offers many benefits. However, when very large, bilateral dermoids or cysts with suspicious areas are present, some surgeons prefer laparotomy. Spillage of the cyst contents during laparoscopy may lead to adhesion formation and chemical peritonitis, but in the hand of an expert surgeon, laparoscopic approach with preservation of the ovary in young women is the method of choice.

12.2.2 Serous and mucinous cystadenoma

Serous cystadenoma is common in women aged between 30 and 40 years. Their diameter is usually less than 15 cm. They may have smooth internal surface or papillary projection in the internal wall. Mucinous cystadenomas are commonly unilateral and may reach 30–50 cm or even more in diameter.

12.3 Surgical approach

As with the other surgical procedures, better surgical skills lead to better results and fewer complications of surgery. The surgeon should be experienced and should understand the disease that is being treated. Whether the plan is organ conservation or removal, it should be discussed with the patient before the operation. Route and type of surgery, complications, risk of oophorectomy (when cystectomy is planned), and possibility of conversion to laparotomy should be discussed and documented via an informed consent. Those patients in whom severe adhesions might be detected should have preoperative bowel preparation. All patients should receive preoperative prophylactic antibiotics and wear antithrombotic stocking and/or sequential compression devices.

The surgery is performed under general anesthesia with tracheal intubation. Foley catheter should be placed to empty the bladder and reduce the risk of bladder injury. Abdominal skin should be prepared from xiphoid process to mons pubis as for an abdominal laparotomy preparation. If the patient has a uterus, uterine manipulator may be helpful to facilitate the adnexal dissection. In the cases of previous hysterectomy, introduction of a vaginal sponge-on-stick is helpful.

In a standard laparoscopic technique, after induction of general anesthesia, pneumoperitoneum is attained using a Veress needle. Then, a 10-mm laparoscope is introduced through a 1-cm umbilical incision, and on direct view, two to three accessory 5–12-mm trocars are placed through lower abdominal incisions for introduction of accessory instruments. After initial diagnostic evaluation of the pelvis and abdomen by rotating the scope around, any sign of adhesion or malignancy should be evaluated. Adhesiolysis is performed when indicated to reestablish the normal anatomy. The ovaries should be assessed for the presence of nodules, abnormal vascularity, and external vegetations. If ascites is present, or in the presence of suspicious peritoneal lesions, samples or peritoneal washings should be obtained for cytology. Suspicion of malignancy should be proved by biopsy and frozen sectioning. In this situation, management should be continued with the involvement of a gynecological oncologist.

12.3.1 Cystectomy

If spillage is expected, it may be sensible to aspirate the cyst contents before a cystectomy is started. This can be achieved by inserting the closest laparoscopic port into the cyst and inserting the suction device directly into the cyst while the port is in the cyst cavity. This will minimize the spillage of cyst contents. After aspiration, the port insertion site can be extended to start cystectomy.

When intact cyst removal is anticipated, an incision is made on the antimesenteric surface of the cyst to reveal the plane between the cyst wall and ovarian cortex. The plane is developed further by use of appropriate instruments, careful traction and countertraction without tearing the ovarian cortex may be applied, and the cyst is enucleated from its bed inside the ovarian tissue. At the ovarian hilus, the dissection is often more difficult, but nevertheless, dissection should continue until the cyst capsule is completely removed from the ovary. Hemostasis is achieved by bipolar coagulation, suturing, or hemostatic sealant agents.

A specimen retrieval bag is usually utilized to remove the cyst from the peritoneal cavity. If the cyst is removed intact, its contents are first aspirated in the bag before retrieving the specimen. Smaller cysts may be removed through a 10- or even 5-mm port if the cyst contents have been aspirated.

A thorough peritoneal irrigation and aspiration should be undertaken to eliminate any spilled cyst content or blood. This is particularly important after spillage of a dermoid cyst. Antiadhesion agents may be used to reduce risk of adhesion formation.

12.3.2 Oophorectomy

The indications for laparoscopic oophorectomy usually include large cysts and benign ovarian cysts in peri- or postmenopausal women. A Properly placed uterine manipulator is important to get a good exposure of the ovaries and tubes. Three techniques have been described for managing the infundibulopelvic ligament: bipolar electrodessication, suture ligation with pretied loop, and stapling. Ultrasound energy devices may also be used. A bipolar coagulation forceps is used to coagulate the ovarian pedicle. After total desiccation of the tissue, 5-mm scissors or a CO_2 laser is used to cut. Before starting the procedure, it is important to observe the course of the ureter as it crosses the external iliac artery near the bifurcation of the common iliac artery at the pelvic brim.

Specimen retrieval is usually in a specimen retrieval bag through a 10-mm port site.

12.4 Adnexal torsion and treatment by laparoscopy

Adnexal torsion is an uncommon condition that predominantly occurs in the reproductive age group, although it has also been reported in premenarcheal girls. Unilateral torsion associated with an adnexal mass is seen more commonly, although cases of torsion of normal adnexa have been reported. Adnexal torsion involving previously normal adnexa in premenarchal girls may constitute up to 15–50% of adnexal torsion cases [6, 7]. It can be difficult to diagnose because although adnexal torsion may present in the form of acute pelvic pain, the symptoms can sometimes be misleading. When the lesions are asymptomatic, the diagnosis may be made only during the surgical procedure. Doppler evaluation in cases of ovarian torsion can be a useful tool, but it was found to be normal in 60% of these cases. The absence of Doppler flow was predictive of surgically confirmed cases of ovarian torsion, demonstrating the low sensitivity but high specificity of Doppler studies in the diagnosis of torsion [8, 9].

In our unit, we managed 33 patients with adnexal torsion over an 11-year period between December 1999 and September 2010.

The mean age of the patients was 34.9 years (range 14–68 years). Four patients (12%) were in the premenarcheal age group, 23 patients (70%) were in the reproductive age group, and 6 patients (18%) were postmenopausal. Of 23 patients in the reproductive age group (17%), 4 were pregnant at the time of the operative intervention. One of them had a singleton pregnancy of 10 weeks' gestation and two patients had triplets (in vitro fertilization (IVF)/Intracytoplasmic Sperm Injection (ICSI) cycle) of 7 and 14 weeks' gestation, respectively. Both of them had multiple ovarian cysts because of ovarian hyperstimulation syndrome. One patient had a cornual interstitial ectopic pregnancy of 6 weeks' gestation as well as a dermoid cyst on the same side.

All 33 patients had a unilateral torsion. The torsion was more common on the right side (61%, $n = 20$) than on the left side (39%, $n = 13$). Fourteen patients (43%) had only an ovarian torsion, 10 patients (30%) had only a tubal torsion, and 9 patients (27%) had a torsion of the entire adnexa.

The diameter of the cyst ranged from 3 to 15 cm, with a median size of 8 cm.

The categorization of the operations ranged from a conservative procedure, such as laparoscopic detorsion, to an aggressive procedure, such as adnexectomy. There was no conversion to laparotomy. In 17 cases (52%), the adnexae were preserved by performing detorsion. In two cases (6%), detorsion alone was performed; in 13 cases (40%), detorsion and cyst enucleation were performed; and in a further two cases (6%), detorsion and cyst aspiration were performed.

The histopathological reports revealed functional or developmental adnexal cyst in 15 cases (45%), dermoid cyst in four cases (12%), endometrioma in two cases (6%), serous cystadenoma in three cases (9%), ovarian fibroma in only one case (3%), hydrosalpinx in three cases (9%), and normal adnexa in one case (3%) [10, 11].

12.5 Tubectomy and ovariectomy/adnexectomy during hysterectomy beyond the reproductive age

Concomitant tubectomy, ovariectomy, or adnexectomy may be considered in women undergoing hysterectomy. As oophorectomy is associated with decreased long-term health outcomes, ovarian conservation should be considered in premenopausal women having pelvic surgery. Salpingo-oophorectomy should be considered for "ovarian/tubal" cancer prophylaxis in women with endometriosis, in the presence of a suspicious adnexal mass, or after numerous previous surgical interventions on the adnexae.

Tubectomy or salpingectomy during hysterectomy (Opportunistic Salpingectomy), however, is considered today as good standard of care for adnexal cancer prevention.

12.5.1 Tubectomy during hysterectomy

Prophylactic bilateral salpingectomy (PBS) without ovariectomy has been proposed as a new preventive approach to reduce the risk of sporadic neoplasia in women at average risk of ovarian cancer [12] without exposing these patients to the adverse effects of iatrogenic premature menopause.

A 2011 position paper by the Society of Gynecologic Oncology of Canada [12] encouraged physicians to discuss the risks and benefits of PBS at the time of hysterectomy or tubal ligation with women at average risk for ovarian cancer, and this recommendation has been confirmed in 2015 by the American College of Obstetricians and Gynecologists.

The advantage of PBS has been estimated also in term of cost-effectiveness. A recent analysis on PBS (elective salpingectomy at hysterectomy or instead of tubal ligation) showed that salpingectomy with hysterectomy for benign conditions will reduce ovarian cancer risk at acceptable cost and is a cost-effective alternative to tubal ligation for sterilization.

The new proposed theory shifts the early events of carcinogenesis to the Fallopian tube instead of the ovary [13], suggesting that types II tumors derive from the epithelium of the Fallopian tube, whereas clear cell and endometrioid tumors derive from

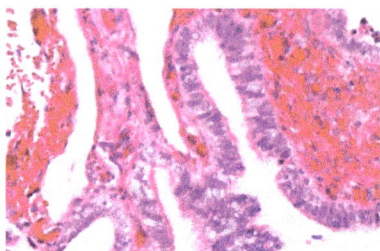

Fig. 12.1: Histologic view of a serous tubal intraepithelial cancer.

endometrial tissue that migrate to the ovary by retrograde menstruation. These observations have been mainly collected from women carrying BRCA1/2 mutations and undergoing prophylactic salpingo-oophorectomy, in which most of the incidentally diagnosed *in situ* carcinomas or intraepithelial precursors of cancers (serous tubal intraepithelial cancer) were detected not in the ovary but in the fimbrial end of the Fallopian tube [14–16] (Fig. 12.1).

12.6 Summary

1. Benign ovarian cysts can usually be managed by cystectomy, and appropriate surgical technique should be used in the hands of an experienced surgeon. Oophorectomy may be required in a minority of women with benign adnexal masses.
2. Adnexal torsion: Conservative treatment should be considered in women within the reproductive age, still desiring fertility. Only beyond the reproductive age, adnexectomy should be considered, and really only in cases with extreme pathology on the adnexa. Laparoscopy is the primary therapeutic option in patients with adnexal torsion.
3. Tubectomy, ovariectomy, and adnexectomy: Tubectomy and ovariectomy at the time of hysterectomies are being reconsidered. While ovariectomy decreases definitely the long-term health outcome of women, ovarian conservation is advised in premenopausal women. Bilateral tubectomy should be performed during hysterectomy (Opportunistic Salpingectomy) at any age, carefully and not compromising the vascular supply of the ovaries.

References

[1] Froyman W, Landolfo C, De Cock B, et al. Risk of complications in patients with conservatively managed ovarian tumours (IOTA5): a 2-year interim analysis of a multicentre, prospective, cohort study. Lancet Oncol 2019 Mar;20(3):448–58.

[2] MacKenna A, Fabres C, Alam V, Morales V. Clinical management of functional ovarian cysts: a prospective and randomized study. Hum Reprod 2000 Dec;15(12):2567–9.

[3] Valentin L. Use of morphology to characterise and manage common adnexal masses. Best Pract Res Clin Obstet Gynaecol 2004 Feb;18(1):71–89.

[4] Templeman CL, Fallat ME, Lam AM, Perlman SE, Hertweck SP, O'Connor DM. Managing mature cystic teratomas of the ovary. Obstet Gynecol Surv 2000 Dec;55(12):738–45.

[5] O'Neill KE, Cooper AR. The approach to ovarian dermoids in adolescents and young women. J Pediatr Adolesc Gynecol 2011 Jun;24(3):176–80.

[6] Balci O, Icen MS, Mahmoud AS, Capar M, Colakoglu MC. Management and outcomes of adnexal torsion: a 5-year experience. Arch Gynecol Obstet 2010 Sep;284(3):643–6.

[7] Pansky M, Abargil A, Dreazen E, Golan A, Bukovsky I, Herman A. Conservative management of adnexal torsion in premenarchal girls. J Am Assoc Gynecol Laparosc 2000 Feb;7(1):121–4.

[8] Pena JE, Ufberg D, Cooney N, Denis AL. Usefulness of Doppler sonography in the diagnosis of ovarian torsion. Fertil Steril 2000 May;73(5):1047–50.

[9] Erdemoglu M, Kuyumcuoglu U, Guzel AI. Clinical experience of adnexal torsion: evaluation of 143 cases. J Exp Ther Oncol 2011;9(3):171–4.

[10] Fleischer AC, Brader KR. Sonographic depiction of ovarian vascularity and flow: current improvements and future applications. J Ultrasound Med 2001 Mar;20(3):241–50.

[11] Argenta PA, Yeagley TJ, Ott G, Sondheimer SJ. Torsion of the uterine adnexa. Pathologic correlations and current management trends. J Reprod Med 2000 Oct;45(10):831–6.

[12] Harris AL. Salpingectomy and ovarian cancer prevention. Nurs Womens Health 2015 Dec–2016 Jan;19(6):543–9.

[13] Kurman RJ, Shih Ie M. Molecular pathogenesis and extraovarian origin of epithelial ovarian cancer—shifting the paradigm. Hum Pathol 2011 Jul;42(7):918–31.

[14] Crum CP, Drapkin R, Kindelberger D, Medeiros F, Miron A, Lee Y. Lessons from BRCA: the tubal fimbria emerges as an origin for pelvic serous cancer. Clin Med Res 2007 Mar;5(1):35–44.

[15] Manchanda R, Abdelraheim A, Johnson M, Rosenthal AN, Benjamin E, Brunell C, et al. Outcome of risk-reducing salpingo-oophorectomy in BRCA carriers and women of unknown mutation status. BJOG 2011 Jun;118(7):814–24.

[16] Powell CB, Chen LM, McLennan J, et al. Risk-reducing salpingo-oophorectomy (RRSO) in BRCA mutation carriers: experience with a consecutive series of 111 patients using a standardized surgical-pathological protocol. Int J Gynecol Cancer 2011 Jul;21(5):846–51.

Ertan Sarıdoğan and Kuhan Rajah

13 Surgery for fallopian tube disorders

Fallopian tubes have an essential role in reproduction as an active participant in the transport of gametes and embryos. Disorders of fallopian tubes may affect this function, resulting in infertility and ectopic pregnancy. Tubal function may be disrupted by a number of conditions, including salpingitis and pelvic peritonitis, endometriosis, and postoperative pelvic adhesions. In this chapter, we will cover the minimally invasive procedures that are performed to manage disorders of the fallopian tubes. In addition, tubal re-anastomosis following tubal ligation for contraceptive purposes will be discussed.

13.1 Ectopic pregnancy

Approximately 1.1% of pregnancies develop within the fallopian tubes [1]. Risk factors include previous sexually transmitted infections, endometriosis, infertility, smoking, and previous tubal surgery.

The United Kingdom National Institute for Health and Care Excellence (NICE) recommends that women who have been diagnosed with a tubal ectopic pregnancy should undergo surgical management when there is significant pain, the serum human chorionic gonadotropin (hCG) level is 5000 iu/l or greater or when the adnexal mass is 35 mm or larger and contains a live embryo. Women who are haemodynamically unstable, have evidence of significant intraabdominal bleeding on ultrasound, are unable to comply with follow-up with medical or expectant management, or have a heterotopic pregnancy with a viable intrauterine pregnancy should also undergo surgical management [1, 2].

The laparoscopic route is preferable to the open approach for the management of ectopic pregnancy due to several advantages, including lower blood loss, shorter hospital stay, less postoperative pain, and being less expensive [3–5].

The two surgical approaches available are a salpingectomy, which is the partial or complete removal of the Fallopian tube, or salpingotomy, which is removal of the ectopic pregnancy through an incision on the Fallopian tube while conserving the rest of the tube. The European Surgery in Ectopic Pregnancy Study, a large multicenter randomized control trial, found that salpingotomy does not improve future fertility outcomes compared to salpingectomy in the presence of a healthy contralateral tube. The cumulative ongoing pregnancy rate following spontaneous conception within a 3-year time period was 60.7% following salpingotomy and 56.2% following salpingectomy (p = 0.678) [6]. The Royal College of Obstetricians and Gynaecologists therefore recommends that a salpingectomy be performed if the contralateral tube is healthy but that a salpingotomy should be considered if there are known fertility-reducing factors, including previous ectopic pregnancy and contralateral

https://doi.org/10.1515/9783110535204-013

tubal damage. Women also need to be counseled regarding the risk of persistent trophoblastic disease, which is reported to be between 3.9% and 11% [2]. NICE recommends that women undergoing a salpingotomy have a serum hCG level taken 7 days after surgery and then weekly until a negative result is obtained [1]. The management of persistent trophoblastic disease includes further surgery to perform a salpingectomy or systemic methotrexate.

In a salpingotomy, diluted synthetic vasopressin (20 IU diluted with 20–100 ml of isotonic sodium chloride) is injected into the mesosalpinx just below the ectopic pregnancy to minimize blood loss. A 1–2-cm incision is then made over the ectopic pregnancy on the antimesenteric side of the fallopian tube using electrosurgery or cold scissors. The pregnancy tissue typically protrudes out of the tube at this point. The tissue can be released from the tube through hydrodissection using pressurized irrigation and gentle dissection with a suction irrigator. The alternative is to remove the tissue with forceps, but this is may lead to the tissue breaking up into smaller pieces. The fallopian tube is irrigated thoroughly and any bleeding is controlled through applying pressure or the use of bipolar diathermy. Suture ligation of the vessels in the mesosalpinx may be attempted if bleeding persists [7]. The incision on the fallopian tube is left to heal by secondary intention, as there is no benefit from primary closure [8, 9].

A salpingectomy can be performed through a few different methods. Conventional bipolar energy to seal the vessels in the mesosalpinx and then scissors to excise the specimen is one approach. The salpingectomy can be started either from the fimbrial end or from excising the proximal isthmic portion from the uterus. It is important to elevate the tube and cut the mesosalpinx close to the tube to minimize damage to the ovarian vasculature. A second approach is to use an advanced energy device, either an advanced bipolar, ultrasonic, or hybrid device, to perform the salpingectomy. The third approach is to use a pretied surgical loop such as ENDOLOOP®. The tube is brought through the loop, the loop is tightened, and the tube is then excised with scissors. The surgical method of choice will be dependent on the experience of the surgeon, complexity of surgery, and available resources.

13.2 Tubal surgery for infertility

Tubal damage is thought to be responsible in approximately 14% of women with infertility [10], and 10–30% of women with tubal factor infertility have hydrosalpinges [11]. While surgery to repair damaged fallopian tubes to improve the chances of spontaneous pregnancy has been largely replaced by assisted reproductive technology (ART), tubal surgery still has a place in a subgroup of women. It has a role in women with mild to moderate tubal damage that is mostly associated with flimsy pelvic adhesions with relatively well-preserved tubal anatomy and in those who underwent tubal sterilization in the past. ART is usually the preferred method in cases of severe tubal damage when the size of hydrosalpinx is greater than 3 cm, the tubal wall is thickened, mucosal folds are lost and flattened, intraluminal adhesions are present, extensive and dense peritubal adhesions are present, and there is bipolar (both distal and proximal) tubal damage.

Tubal surgery was initially developed by a small number of pioneers who applied the principles of microsurgery before the era of ART. Microsurgical principles include magnification, minimal tissue handling, use of starch-free gloves and fine and nonreactive suture material, judicious use of diathermy, frequent irrigation, and aspiration to avoid tissue drying and avoiding the use of dry towels or sponges. Advances in endoscopic surgery have made it possible to apply these same microsurgical principles to laparoscopic surgery, eliminating the need for open surgery. Minimally invasive procedures to improve tubal-related infertility include adhesiolysis, fimbrioplasty, neosalpingostomy, and tubal reanastomosis.

13.2.1 Adhesiolysis

Tubo-ovarian adhesions may develop as a result of pelvic inflammatory disease (PID), previous pelvic surgery such as myomectomy or adnexal surgery, and endometriosis. Adhesions secondary to endometriosis tend to be dense and vascular, while PID adhesions are more likely to be flimsy and avascular. Postoperative adhesions, on other hand, may include both types. Adhesiolysis for flimsy adhesions is known to give better spontaneous pregnancy outcomes when the fallopian tubes, including tubal mucosa, are relatively normal. The condition of the fimbrial end and tubal mucosa should be assessed when the fimbrial end is accessible. This may, however, be possible only after adhesiolysis if the fimbrial end is covered with adhesions. Tubal mucosa can easily be assessed by inserting a small endoscope with saline (distal salpingoscopy) through one of the secondary ports. The loss of mucosal folds and intratubal adhesions are indicative of poor prognosis.

The aim of adhesiolysis is to free up pelvic organs and restore pelvic anatomy. It is preferable to excise adhesions instead of just dividing them as removing the adhesion tissue will reduce the chances of reformation postoperatively (Fig. 13.1). The application of antiadhesive agents over the areas where adhesions have been excised or divided is recommended to reduce recurrence rates. Laparoscopic adhesiolysis tends to give good reproductive outcomes, with intrauterine pregnancy rates of 44–62% and ectopic pregnancy rates of 4–8%. High pregnancy rates are achieved when adhesions are the only cause of infertility [12].

13.2.2 Fimbrioplasty

Fimbrioplasty is used when the fimbriated end of the fallopian tube is not entirely blocked but is damaged due to adhesions. The damage may be in the form of

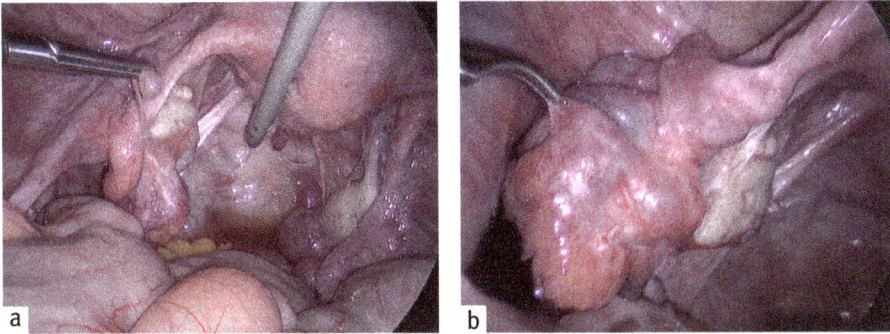

Fig. 13.1: (a) Flimsy left perituboovarian adhesions covering the ovary and fimbrial end. A hydrosalpinx can be seen on the right. (b) The left Fallopian tube after excision of left adnexal adhesions.

agglutination when there are adhesions across the fimbriae, blunting when there is side to side adherence of fimbriae giving a "mitten" appearance and when there is phimosis or narrowing of the fimbriated end [13].

Fimbrioplasty involves excising or dividing adhesions covering the fimbriae, separating fimbriae that are adherent to each other, and widening the phimotic end of the fallopian tube, which may require cruciate incisions using fine-needle diathermy. Blunt dissection and widening of the fimbriated end can be achieved by inserting a fine tip curved or right angle tip grasping forceps. The quality of mucosa should then be assessed as described above. The fimbriated end should be everted by suturing the edges onto the serosa using fine monofilament nonabsorbable material to reduce risk of recurrence and closure (Fig. 13.2).

Intrauterine pregnancy rates of 17–51% and ectopic pregnancy rates of 4–23% have been reported following fimbrioplasty [12].

13.2.3 Neosalpingostomy

Neosalpingostomy is performed when the fimbriated end is completely blocked. Methylene blue dye is administered via a uterine manipulator to distend the fallopian tube and identify the location of the occlusion. Three or four cruciate incisions are then made using fine-needle diathermy to open the fimbriated end of the fallopian tube. Care should be taken to minimize diathermy damage to the fimbriated end at this stage by using a fine needle with high power pure cutting that will minimize lateral spread of diathermy and exercising targeted coagulation for hemostasis. The fimbriated ends are then everted using fine monofilament nonabsorbable sutures, as described above. Some surgeons use laser vaporization or gentle bipolar coagulation of the serosa of the tubal infundibulum to evert the fimbriated end, but this may carry the risk of further damage to the fallopian tube.

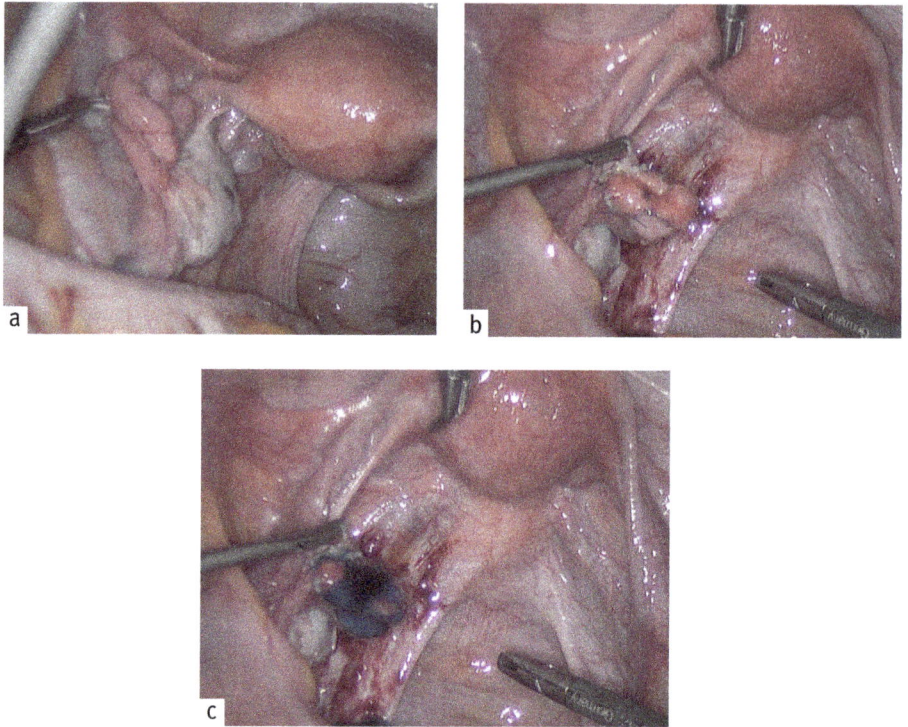

Fig. 13.2: (a) Phimosis of the left fimbrial end and a small left hydrosalpinx. (b) The left fimbrial end has been opened and everted with sutures. (c) Tubal patency after fimbrioplasty.

A systematic review and meta-analysis of salpingostomy for hydrosalpinx at laparoscopy and laparotomy showed clinical pregnancy rates of 25.5% at 24 months with ectopic pregnancy rates of 10% [14].

13.2.4 Tubal reanastomosis

Tubal reanastomosis is performed in the presence of proximal tubal pathology such as previous tubal sterilization and salpingitis isthmica nodosa. Regret or change in personal circumstances after tubal sterilization are the two most common reasons for tubal reanastomosis, and the procedure has particularly high success rates in this group of women with previously proven fertility and no other contributing factor. A number of prognostic factors have been evaluated after reversal of sterilization, including the age of the woman, method of sterilization, time interval between sterilization and reversal, and length of the remaining fallopian tube. The age of the woman was found to be the most significant prognostic indicator, with better pregnancy rates in younger women. There are no direct comparisons with in vitro fertilization (IVF), but it is quite likely that sterilization reversal is more favorable in younger women, while IVF may be preferable in older women [15].

Laparoscopic tubal reanastomosis should ideally be performed using specially designed 3-mm laparoscopic microsurgical instruments. A very high-quality image is required to see the details of tubal layers, small-diameter tubal lumen, and fine suture material that is used for this technique. In conventional laparoscopy, three or four ancillary ports are used in addition to the camera port. The location of the ports depends on the suturing technique of the surgeon, with one of the ports being a 5-mm port to allow insertion of the suture material into the abdominal cavity. Robotic surgery would fulfill the image quality requirements and provide additional flexibility for suturing with the fine suture material, but larger ports are required.

After the initial assessment of pelvis and upper abdomen, the fallopian tubes are assessed closely for their length and appearance of the fimbriated end. Adhesions are excised or divided if present. Diluted synthetic vasopressin may be injected into the mesosalpinx to reduce bleeding. Fibrotic or scarred tissue, together with the serosa at the tip of proximal and distal ends that will be anastomosed, is excised using needle diathermy. Following this, the distal end of the proximal tube and the proximal end of the distal tube are cut at right angles either using cold scissors or specially designed "guillotine" device. The ends that will be anastomosed are then examined closely and ideally the diameter of the lumens should be very similar. Methylene blue dye is then administered via the uterine manipulator to confirm the patency of the proximal end. Distal part patency can also be checked using a specially designed device to instill methylene blue.

The ends are then anastomosed using fine polyprolene sutures. Initially, a single suture is placed to approximate the mesosalpinx at the anastomosis site. Following this, 7/0 or 8/0 interrupted sutures are placed at 6, 12, 3, and 9 o'clock positions (in this order) to bring the muscularis and mucosa together. Two or three interrupted serosal sutures are applied to complete the anastomosis. Tubal patency is then checked with methylene blue dye administered through the uterine manipulator.

13.2.5 Hydrosalpinx and ART

Damaged fallopian tubes, particularly hydrosalpinges, have a detrimental impact on ART outcome. Surgical treatment of hydrosalpinges is known to improve the pregnancy rates of ART. Surgery may be in the form of salpingectomy or proximal tubal occlusion (PTO), as a number of randomized controlled trials have shown that both procedures improve clinical pregnancy rates [16]. Salpingectomy may reduce ovarian reserve more than PTO can, as measured by anti-Müllerian hormone level and antral follicle count, as well as being associated with longer ovarian stimulation and higher gonadotrophin requirements. Pregnancy rates, however, appear to be similar after both approaches [17]. The reduction in ovarian reserve is likely to be related to the disruption of blood supply to the ovaries, and for this reason, any technique to perform PTO or salpingectomy should aim to avoid disruption of ovarian vasculature.

PTO may be performed by either bipolar diathermy of the proximal isthmus or by applying clips or rings that are used for tubal sterilization, such as Filshie clips. This may be combined with fenestration of the distal end of the tube to drain the hydrosalpinx fluid.

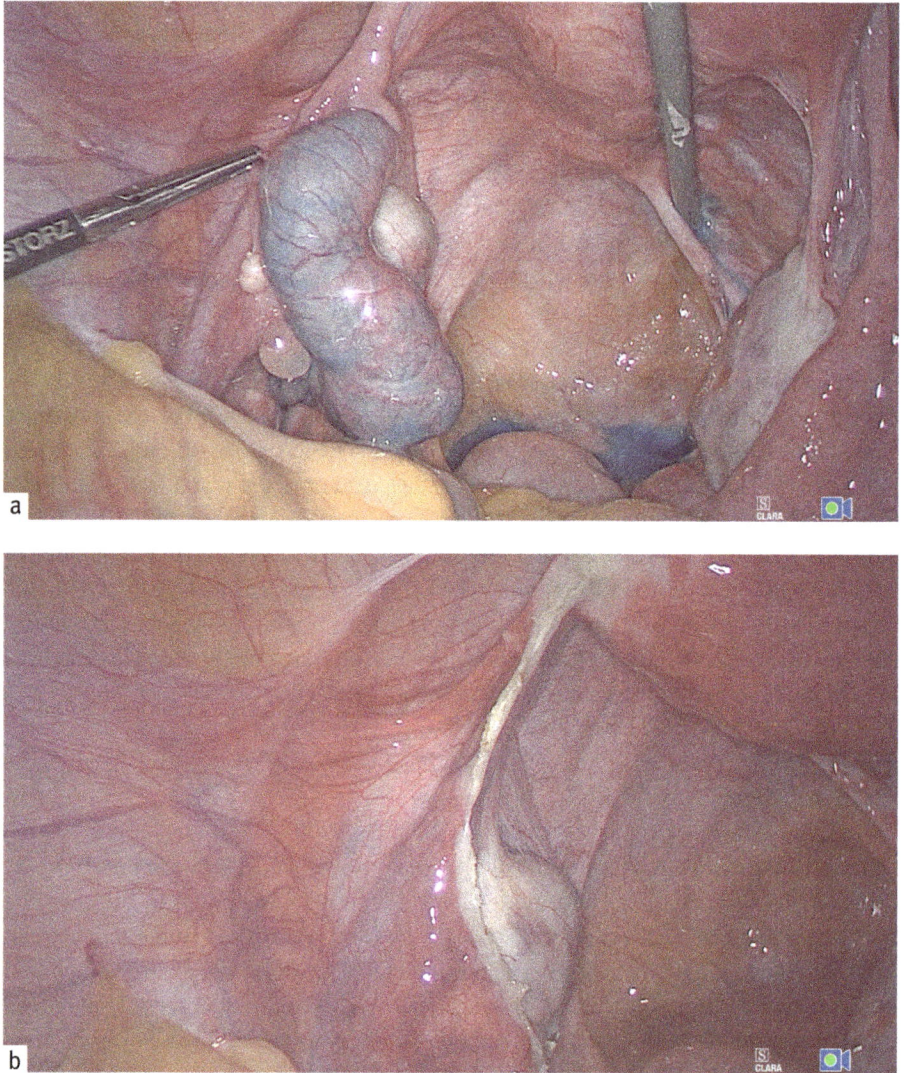

Fig. 13.3: (a) Left hydrosalpinx. (b) Left tubal mesentery and intact blood vessels can be seen after salpingectomy.

Salpingectomy may be performed by one of the techniques described above, keeping in mind to avoid the mesosalpingeal collateral vessels between the uterine and ovarian arteries (Fig. 13.3). If the tube and ovary are densely adherent to each other, as in cases of severe endometriosis, PTO may be preferable over salpingectomy.

13.2.6 Hysteroscopic tubal cannulation for proximal tubal obstruction

Proximal tubal obstruction may be secondary to the presence of mucus, debris, or fibrosis. Unblocking the obstruction may be particularly successful in cases of mucus or debris, when the rest of the tubes are normal. Tubal cannulation may be performed under fluoroscopic guidance as an outpatient procedure. It is a relatively simple and inexpensive procedure but does not allow the assessment of the rest of the tube, presence of peritubal adhesions, or other pelvic pathology such as endometriosis. An alternative approach is to perform hysteroscopic tubal cannulation in combination with laparoscopy. While the latter method usually requires general anesthesia and is more expensive, it enables the clinicians to assess the fallopian tube and other pelvic organs more reliably. A recent meta-analysis showed results that were comparable to IVF, with a cumulative pregnancy rate of 26% after fluoroscopic tubal cannulation and 31% after laparoscopy guided hysteroscopic tubal cannulation [18].

Hysteroscopic tubal cannulation technique involves utilization of a hysteroscope with an operating channel which can accommodate 5Fr instruments. Concomitant laparoscopy is performed, usually using a second camera stack, to assess the pelvis and simultaneously confirm successful cannulation and tubal patency. A 5Fr ureteric catheter with guidewire or specially designed tubal cannulation catheters can be used to cannulate the fallopian tube after identifying the tubal ostium. Once the catheter is successfully inserted into the proximal part of the tube, the guidewire is withdrawn and methylene blue dye is administered to confirm tubal patency. Tubal patency rates of approximately 70% are achieved with this approach.

13.3 Conclusion

While the use of surgical procedures to improve fertility has decreased with the advances of ART, tubal surgery still has a role in a selected group of patients. Tubal surgery is particularly more successful in younger women with mild to moderate tubal damage and in those who have previously undergone tubal sterilization. It may also have a place to increase the chances of spontaneous conception in women with reduced ovarian reserve and consequently lower chances of success with ART.

References

[1] National Institute for Health and Care Excellence. Ectopic Pregnancy and Miscarriage: Diagnosis and Initial Management in Early Pregnancy of Ectopic Pregnancy and Miscarriage. London: National Institute for Health and Care Excellence; 2012.

[2] Elson CJ, Salim R, Potdar N, Chetty M, Ross JA, Kirk EJ on behalf of the Royal College of Obstetricians and Gynaecologists. Diagnosis and management of ectopic pregnancy. BJOG 2016;123:e15–5.

[3] Vermesh M, Silva PD, Rosen GF, Stein AL, Fossum GT, Sauer MV. Management of unruptured ectopic gestation by linear salpingostomy: a prospective, randomized clinical trial of laparoscopy versus laparotomy. Obstet Gynecol 1989;73:400–4.

[4] Lundorff P, Thorburn J, Hahlin M, Kallfelt B, Lindblom B. Laparoscopic surgery in ectopic pregnancy. A randomized trial versus laparotomy. Acta Obstet Gynecol Scand 1991;70:343–8.

[5] Gray DT, Thorburn J, Lundorff P, Strandell A, Lindblom B. A cost-effectiveness study of a randomised trial of laparoscopy versus laparotomy for ectopic pregnancy. Lancet 1995;345:1139–43.

[6] Mol F, van Mello NM, Strandell A, et al.; European Surgery in Ectopic Pregnancy (ESEP) study group. Salpingotomy versus salpingectomy in women with tubal pregnancy (ESEP study): an open-label, multicentre, randomized controlled trial. Lancet 2014;383:1483–9.

[7] Ectopic pregnancy: surgical treatment. UpToDate, 2017. Available at: https://www.uptodate.com/contents/ectopic-pregnancy-surgical-treatment. Accessed March 18, 2019.

[8] Tulandi T, Guralnick M. Treatment of tubal ectopic pregnancy by salpingotomy with or without tubal suturing and salpingectomy. Fertil Steril 1991;55:53.

[9] Fujishita A, Masuzaki H, Khan KN, et al. Laparoscopic salpingotomy for tubal pregnancy: comparison of linear salpingotomy with and without suturing. Hum Reprod 2004;19:1195.

[10] Hull MG, Glazener CM, Kelly NJ, et al. Population study of causes, treatment and outcome of infertility. Br Med J (Clin Res Ed) 1985 Dec 14;291(6510):1693–7.

[11] Mansour R, Aboulghar M, Serour GI. Controversies in the surgical management of hydrosalpinx. Curr Opin Obstet Gynecol 200 Aug;12(4):297–391.

[12] Posaci C, Camus M, Osmanagaoglu K, Devroey P. Tubal surgery in the era of assisted reproductive technology: clinical options. Hum Reprod. 1999 Sep;14 (Suppl 1):120–36.

[13] Abuzeid MI, Mitwally MF, Ahmed AI, et al. The prevalence of fimbrial pathology in patients with early stages of endometriosis. J Minim Invasive Gynecol 2007 Jan–Feb;14(1):49–53.

[14] Chu J, Harb HM, Gallos ID, et al. Salpingostomy in the treatment of hydrosalpinx: a systematic review and meta-analysis. Hum Reprod 2015 Aug;30(8):1882–95.

[15] van Seeters JAH, Chua SJ, Mol BWJ, Koks CAM. Tubal anastomosis after previous sterilization: a systematic review. Hum Reprod Update 2017 May 1;23(3):358–70.

[16] Johnson NP, van Voorst S, Sowter MC, Strandell A, Mol BW. Surgical treatment for tubal disease in women due to undergo in vitro fertilization. Cochrane Database Syst Rev 2010;(1):CD002125.

[17] Vignarajan CP, Malhotra N, Singh N. Ovarian reserve and assisted reproductive technique outcomes after laparoscopic proximal tubal occlusion or salpingectomy in women with hydrosalpinx undergoing in vitro fertilization: a randomized controlled trial. J Minim Invasive Gynecol 2018 Oct 24. pii:S1553-4650(18)31318-9.

[18] De Silva PM, Chu J, Gallos ID, Vidyasagar AT, Robinson L, Coomarasamy A. Fallopian tube catheterization in the treatment of proximal tubal obstruction: a systematic review and meta-analysis. Hum Reprod 2017 Apr 1;32(4):836–52.

Olivier Donnez

14 Cesarean section scar defects and their management

14.1 Introduction

Over the recent decades, the number of cesarean sections (CSs) has continued to rise worldwide. In the United States, the proportion of CSs performed in 2007 was over 30% [1–4], while rates in China have climbed as high as 35–58% in 2010 and even 80% in private practice in Brazil, resulting in increasing obstetric sequelae, such as placenta accreta, scar dehiscence, and ectopic scar pregnancy due to incomplete healing of the CS incision. Described for the first time as an "isthmocele" by Morris in 1995 [5], a defect on the anterior wall of the uterine isthmus located at the site of previous CS is also known as a "cesarean scar defect" (Fig. 14.1) or niche [6, 7]. CS scar defects are increasingly more frequently described, and the reported incidence is as high as 61% after one CS, reaching 100% after three or more [8]. As reported by Vervoort *et al.* [9], a number of hypotheses may explain cesarean scar defect development: (1) a very low incision through the cervical tissue, (2) inadequate suturing or incomplete closure of the uterine wall due to a single-layer endometrial-saving closure technique or use of locking sutures, and (3) surgical interventions that encourage adhesion formation (namely, nonclosure of the peritoneum, inadequate hemostasis, visible sutures, etc.).

14.2 Symptoms

Although these defects could be asymptomatic, they may be associated with complications in later pregnancies, such as uterine rupture, abnormally adherent placenta, or scar rupture [10, 11].

 Gynecological sequelae, such as abnormal bleeding, chronic pelvic pain, dysmenorrhea, dyspareunia, and infertility, have also been increasingly reported in the last decade in case of CS scar defects [12]. The collection of menstrual blood in the uterine defect, with intermittent passage through the cervix, may explain the occurrence of vaginal bleeding or spotting. Retention of blood inside the uterine scar defect can originate from endometriotic lesions [13] but also from typical hypervascularization [14] or the inability of the myometrium covering the defect to exhibit sufficient contractility to expel blood from endometrial shedding during menstruation. This might be due to the significant decrease in muscular density we observed

https://doi.org/10.1515/9783110535204-014

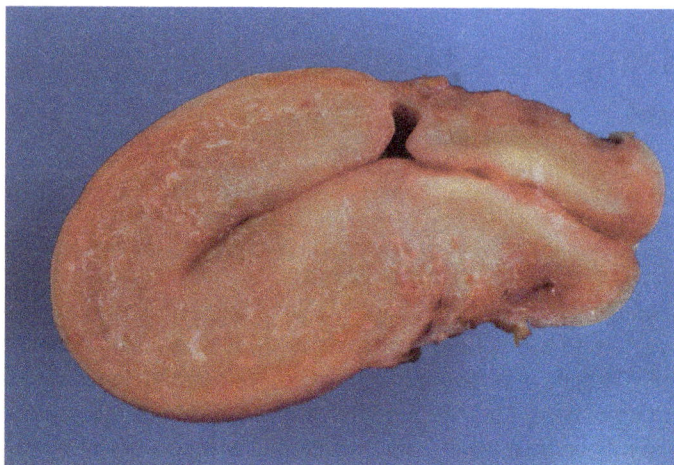

Fig. 14.1: Sagittal view of a frozen section from a hysterectomy specimen. A deep anterior defect covered with a thin layer of myometrium (white circle) can be observed at the level of the presumed site of CS. From Donnez O. Laparoscopic repair of cesarean scar defects. Fertil Steril 2016.

in the myometrium covering the defect compared with adjacent myometrium [13]. According to the literature [15–17], subsequent fertility may be impaired, with the risk of infertility estimated to be between 4% and 19%. Accumulation of mucus or blood in the defect, leading to the presence of intrauterine fluid, could prevent transport of sperm or embryo implantation [15–19]. This toxic environment could be responsible for the decrease in fertility, even though the association between a cesarean scar defect and infertility has never been proven. Nevertheless, some mechanisms may be speculated to play a role. Bloody fluid or bleeding from the cesarean scar flows into the vagina and also the uterine cavity, which could result in infertility via a process similar to hydrosalpinx [20]. The cytotoxicity of iron is well known, and an excess of iron after degradation of hemoglobin in the uterine cavity [21, 22] may be embryotoxic and/or impair embryo implantation via disturbed endometrial receptivity, as in case of endometriosis [22] or disrupted expression of the cytokine cascade [23].

Although the risks associated with cesarean scar defects remain unclear, there is obviously an association between large defects detected in nonpregnant women and dehiscence or uterine rupture in subsequent pregnancy (odds ratio [OR], 11.8; 95% confidence interval [CI], 0.7–746) [24]. The risk of uterine rupture or dehiscence was reported to be even higher in another study in women with large defects (OR, 26.05; 95% CI, 2.36–287.61) [25].

14.3 Diagnosis

Anomalies in a cesarean scar can be visualized by hysterosalpingography, transvaginal sonography (TVS), saline infusion sonohysterography, hysteroscopy, and magnetic resonance imaging (MRI) and are characterized by a defect within the myometrium, reflecting a breach at the site of a previous CS [26]. The most useful discriminating measurement is the thickness of the remaining myometrium [8, 24].

14.3.1 Ultrasound

Ultrasound (TVS) is an accurate method used to diagnose and measure a caesarean scar defect, with or without saline or gel [7, 27], with high detection rates.

14.3.2 Hysteroscopy

Cesarean scar defects can also be diagnosed during hysteroscopy. A cavity is then observed at the level of the isthmus. The presence of hypervascularized areas and dendritic vessels with hemorrhage (Fig. 14.2a), observed by some authors [14, 23] at hysteroscopy, could suggest that the bleeding originates from the scarred area.

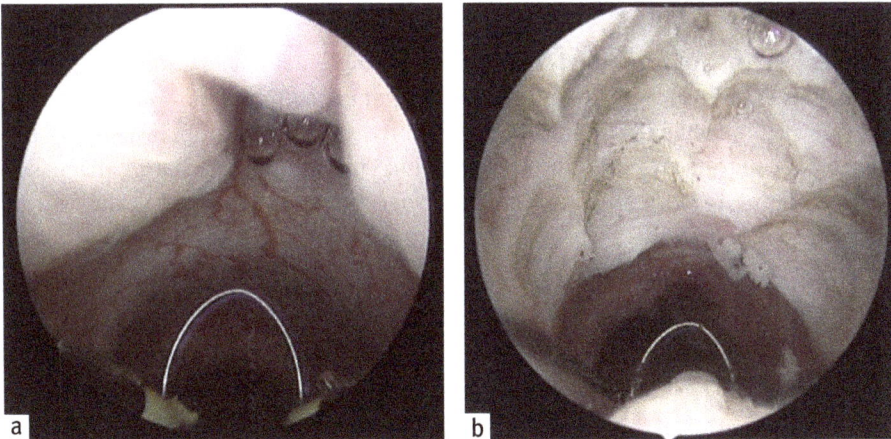

Fig. 14.2: (a) Hysteroscopic view of the endocervical canal showed an anterior pseudocavity at the level of the dehiscence and the defect running along the whole breadth of the anterior uterine wall. Dendritic blood vessels are seen in the defect (white arrows). (b) Hysteroscopic view of the endocervical canal after complete resection of the pseudocavity.

However, there is no additional information regarding residual myometrial thickness regarding diagnosis made by hysteroscopy.

14.3.3 Magnetic resonance imaging

MRI gives the precise mapping of defects. Residual myometrium can be easily measured, and on T1-weighted images with saturation of fatty tissue, hypersignal spots are frequently detected in the defect due to the presence of residual menstrual blood. This was observed in 89% of the patients from our series [13]. In the other cases, the signal was present, but less intense, revealing the presence of mucus. Microscopic residual myometrium has recently been correlated to ultrasound and MRI measurements [13].

MRI and ultrasound are thus appropriate tools to determine the thickness of residual myometrium. The advantages of MRI are reproducibility of measurements and a clearer view of the defect before surgery. However, its use may be disputed, as preoperative residual thickness values were found to be similar by both MRI and ultrasound [13]. Further studies are needed to identify the most accurate means of imaging, taking into account the cost-effectiveness of both methods.

14.4 Treatment

Of course, in case of incidental diagnosis in asymptomatic women, surgery is not recommended. Nevertheless, as stated by Nezhat *et al.* [28], asymptomatic women who wish to conceive in the future may also require surgical repair owing to the high risk of uterine rupture, and the pros and cons should at least be discussed with the patient. More studies are clearly needed to shed further light on this specific issue.

14.4.1 Medical treatment

The use of progestogen or oral contraceptive may be useful but with various efficacy in terms of bleeding and pain [29, 30], as some authors report failure of medical treatment [5, 31, 32]. Regarding these results, medical treatment can be proposed to symptomatic women without desire of further pregnancy and information should be given regarding surgical correction in case of failure.

14.4.2 Surgical treatment

14.4.2.1 Hysteroscopic resection

Hysteroscopic resection of cesarean scar defects was first described in 1996 [33]. Hysteroscopic treatment includes resection of the fibrotic tissue covering the scar to facilitate further evacuation of blood during menstruations. This is the most commonly reported technique [32, 34–37]. Initial reports recommended complete resection of the defect cavity [38] (Fig. 14.2b), while a recent study evaluated the possibility of resecting only the distal edge of the defect [39]. Postmenstrual spotting and spotting-related discomfort can be reduced by hysteroscopic resection in women with a defect with residual myometrium of ≥3 mm. Standard practice would have involved performing hysteroscopic resection of the defect in all patients who no longer wished to conceive [28]. However, in our series, hysteroscopic resection was not offered due to the risk of bladder injury and uterine perforation in patients with myometrial thickness of less than 3 mm [14].

Most series on hysteroscopic management do not provide any information [19, 32, 34–37] on residual myometrial thickness before and after surgery, although myometrial thickness before and after hysteroscopy was reported to be similar in a series of 24 women treated by hysteroscopy (4.4 mm vs. 5.3 mm) [40].

According to several reports on hysteroscopic resection, intermenstrual bleeding can be improved in 59–100% of cases, with pregnancy rates climbing to 77.8% to 100% of cases [32, 35, 38].

Gubbini *et al.* [34, 38] published their prospective series of 37 patients who delivered by CS after hysteroscopic resection at the level of the cesarean scar defect. Unfortunately, as the investigators failed to provide information on residual myometrial thickness before and after surgery, no conclusions could be drawn on the efficacy of the technique in terms of preventing uterine dehiscence or rupture.

Hysteroscopic treatment most likely corrects the scar defect but does not strengthen the uterine wall, while laparoscopic/vaginal repair of the defect may potentially reinforce myometrial endurance.

14.4.2.2 Laparoscopic repair

The first laparoscopic repair of a uteroperitoneal fistula caused by CS was performed by the group of Nezhat [41]. Laparoscopic repair of large defects was subsequently described by Donnez *et al.* in 2008 [42], showing an increased risk of uterine rupture, and the first series of 13 patients was reported several years later [14].

Using CO_2 laser (Lumenis-Sharplan), the scar was opened up from one end to the other (Fig. 14.3a). The fibrotic tissue was then excised from the edges of the defect to

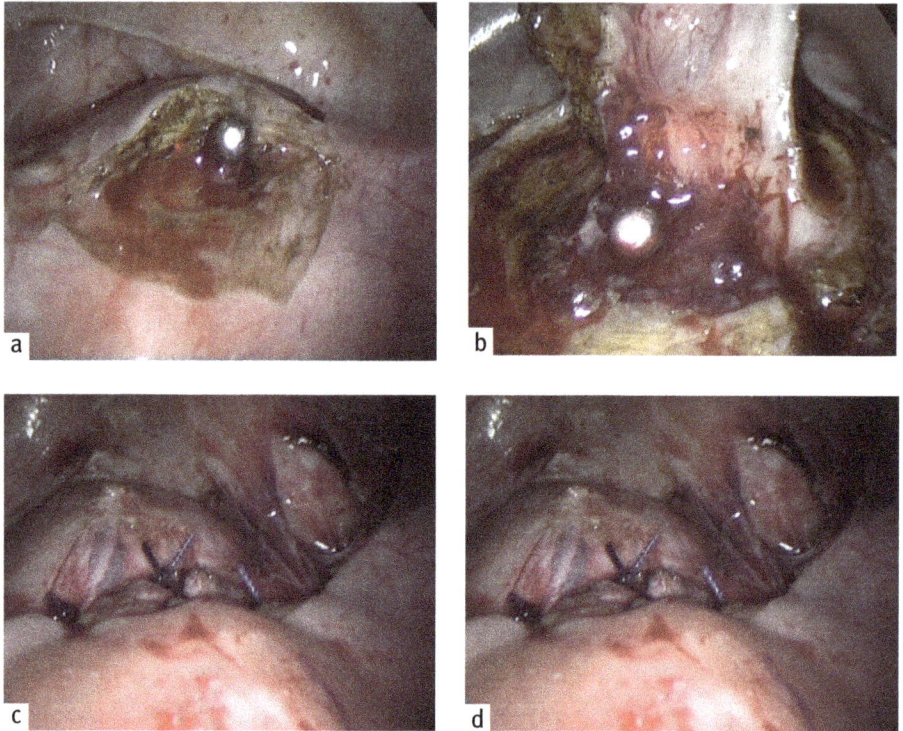

Fig. 14.3: (a) Laparoscopic view of the cesarean scar with a probe inserted into the endocervix. The residual myometrium covering the scar is very thin. (b) Laparoscopic view of the cesarean section scar defect cavity. (c) Laparoscopic view of the first layer of suture. (d) Laparoscopic view of the second layer of suture.

access healthy myometrium and facilitate further healing (Fig. 14.3b). Before closing the defect, a Hegar probe was inserted into the cervix to preserve the continuity of the cervical canal with the uterine cavity. For the first layer, three separate sutures were placed to close the scar using 2-0 Vicryl SH (Johnson & Johnson) (Fig. 14.3c). A second layer of separate stitches was applied to achieve double-layer closure (Fig. 14.3d). The peritoneum was then closed using Monocryl 0 MH+ (Johnson & Johnson) running suture. Vervoort *et al.* [9] suggested that retroflexion of the uterus may impair wound healing after CS and encourage formation of cesarean scar defects. For this reason, the round ligaments were shortened bilaterally in case of a retroflexed uterus. At the end of surgery, hysteroscopy was performed to visualize the repair of the cervical canal, which showed complete correction of the defect and normal patency of the cervix. All the patients were discharged from hospital within 24 hours of surgery. After a period of 3 months and subsequent pelvic MRI, the women were told they could attempt pregnancy.

Residual myometrial thickness increased from 1.4 ± 0.76 mm to 9.6 ± 1.8 mm, proving adequate reinforcement of the myometrium. This surgical technique is able to restore the thickness of the anterior uterine wall. These results are comparable to those obtained by Tanimura *et al.* [23] but superior to those achieved by Chang *et al.* [32] and Vervoort *et al.* [43]. However, despite residual myometrial thickness being considered the best discriminating factor, this important information was missing from the last series of Zhang *et al.* [44] and Li *et al.* [45]. Vervoort *et al.* reported 5.3 mm of residual myometrial thickness, but in their series, 22% and 34% of the patients respectively presented spotting and dysmenorrhea after surgery, with 12% residual myometrium still under 3 mm. The technique we use is associated with high success rates in terms of symptoms, as 91% of our patients were asymptomatic after laparoscopic repair. Only two women underwent hysteroscopic resection to treat residual intermenstrual bleeding, despite a good anatomical result, and one of them was able to achieve pregnancy. It is important to note one serious failure occurring in a patient with three previous CSs. The myometrium was unable to heal correctly, which could have been due to excessive fibrotic tissue surrounding the scar or the inability of the surgeon to distinguish healthy tissue after three CS.

14.4.2.3 Hysterectomy

Hysterectomy is the radical surgical treatment for cesarean scar defects. This option must be discussed in case of <3 mm residual myometrium and clear absence of pregnancy desire.

14.5 Conclusions

Cesarean scar defect is a relatively new entity. The anterior uterine wall should be evaluated in case of symptomatic patient (chronic pelvic pain, dysmenorrhea, intermenstrual bleeding, infertility) in women with history of CS. Based on the data available in the literature, the choice of therapy will depend on the severity of the symptoms, the size of the defect, the residual myometrial thickness, and the wish to conceive or preserve uterus. An algorithm can be proposed (Fig. 14.4). Progestogen or oral contraceptive may be proposed to symptomatic patient without desire of further pregnancy. In symptomatic women with residual myometrial thickness of less than 13 mm who wish to conceive, laparoscopic repair should be proposed, as it was demonstrated that it significantly strengthens the myometrial wall and uterine antefixation can be easily performed during laparoscopy. In case of symptoms like dysmenorrhea, bleeding, or pelvic pain, hysteroscopic resection may be carried out if the residual thickness is more than 3 mm but the postoperative residual myometrial thickness still needs evaluation.

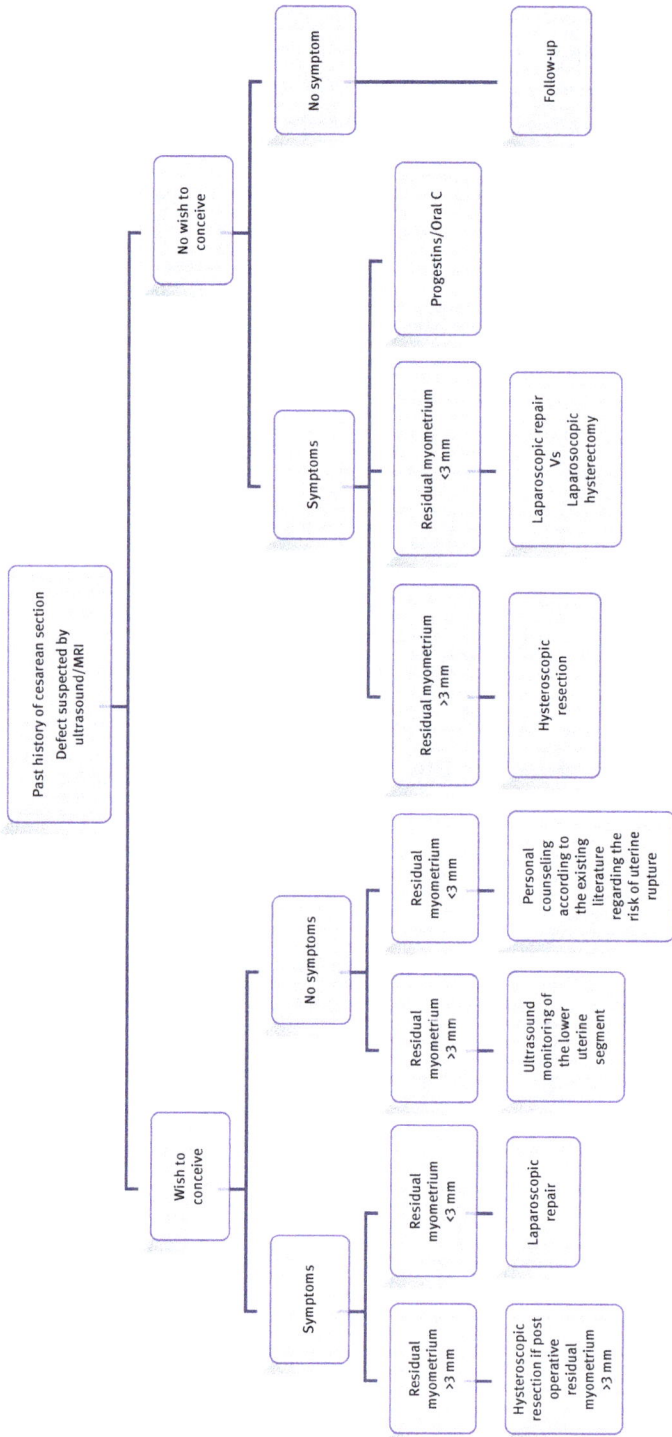

Fig. 14.4: Algorithm of treatment of cesarean scar defect.

References

[1] Souza JP, Gülmezoglu A, Lumbiganon P, et al., the WHO Global Survey on Maternal and Perinatal Health Research Group. Cesarean section without medical indications is associated with an increased risk of adverse short-term maternal outcomes: the 2004–2008 WHO Global Survey on Maternal and Perinatal Health. BMC Med 2010;10:71.

[2] Hamilton BE, Martin JA, Osterman MJ, Curtin SC, Matthews TJ. Births: final data for 2014. Natl Vital Stat Rep 2015;64:1–64.

[3] Martin JA, Hamilton BE, Ventura SJ, et al. Births: final data for 2009. Natl Vital Stat Rep 2011;60:1–70.

[4] Menacker F, Hamilton BE. Recent trends in cesarean delivery in the United States. NCHS Data Brief 2010;35:1–8.

[5] Morris H. Surgical pathology of the lower uterine segment caesarean section scar: is the scar a source of clinical symptoms? Int J Gynecol Pathol 1995;14:16–20.

[6] Monteagudo A, Carreno C, Timor-Tritsch IE. Saline infusion sonohysterography in non-pregnant women with previous cesarean delivery: the "niche" in the scar. J Ultrasound Med 2001;20:1105–15.

[7] Bij de Vaate AJ, Brölmann HA, van der Voet LF, et al. Ultrasound evaluation of the cesarean scar: relation between a niche and postmenstrual spotting. Ultrasound Obstet Gynecol 2011;37:93–9.

[8] Osser OV, Jokubkiene L, Valentin L. High prevalence of defects in Cesarean section scars at transvaginal ultrasound examination. Ultrasound Obstet Gynecol 2009;34:90–7.

[9] Vervoort AJ, Uittenbogaard LB, Hehenkamp WJ, Brolmann HA, Mol BW, Huirne JA. Why do niches develop in Caesarean uterine scars? Hypotheses on the aetiology of niche development. Hum Reprod 2015;30:2695–702.

[10] Diaz SD, Jones JE, Seryakov M, Mann WJ. Uterine rupture and dehiscence: ten-year review and case-control study. South Med J 2002;95:431–5.

[11] Naji O, Wynants L, Smith A, et al. Predicting successful vaginal birth after Cesarean section using a model based on Cesarean scar features examined by transvaginal sonography. Ultrasound Obstet Gynecol 2013;41:672–8.

[12] Tulandi T, Cohen A. Emerging Manifestations of Cesarean Scar Defect in Reproductive-aged Women. J Minim Invasive Gynecol 2016;23:893–902.

[13] Donnez O, Donnez J, Orellana R, Dolmans MM. Gynecological and obstetrical outcomes after laparoscopic repair of a cesarean scar defect in a series of 38 women. Fertil Steril 2017;107:289–296.

[14] Marotta ML, Donnez J, Squifflet J, Jadoul P, Darii N, Donnez O. Laparoscopic repair of post cesarean section uterine scar defects diagnosed in nonpregnant women. J Min Inv Gynecol 2013;20:386–91.

[15] Gurol-Urganci I, Bou-Antoun S, Lim CP, et al. Impact of Caesarean section on subsequent fertility: a systematic review and meta-analysis. Hum Reprod 2013;28:1943–52.

[16] Gurol-Urganci I, Cromwell DA, Mahmood TA, van der Meulen JH, Templeton A. A population-based cohort study of the effect of Caesarean section on subsequent fertility. Hum Reprod 2014;29:1320–6.

[17] CORONIS Collaborative Group, Abalos E, Addo V, Brocklehurst P, et al. Caesarean section surgical techniques (CORONIS): a fractional, factorial, unmasked, randomised controlled trial. Lancet 2013;382:234–48.

[18] Bij de Vaate AJ, van der Voet LF, Naji O, et al. Prevalence, potential risk factors for development and symptoms related to the presence of uterine niches following Cesarean section: systematic review. Ultrasound Obstet Gynecol 2014;43:372–82.

[19] Fabres C, Arriagada P, Fernandez C, Mackenna A, Zegers F, Fernandez E. Surgical treatment and follow-up of women with intermenstrual bleeding due to cesarean section scar defect. J Minim Invasive Gynecol 2005;12:25–8.

[20] Strandell A, Lindhard A. Why does hydrosalpinx reduce fertility? The importance of hydrosalpinx fluid. Hum Reprod 2002;17:1141–5.

[21] Defrere S, Lousse JC, Gonzalez-Ramos R, Colette S, Donnez J, Van Langendonckt A. Potential involvement of iron in the pathogenesis of peritoneal endometriosis. Mol Hum Reprod 2008;14:377–85.

[22] Van Langendonckt A, Casanas-Roux F, Donnez J. Iron overload in the peritoneal cavity of women with pelvic endometriosis. Fertil Steril 2002;78:712–8.

[23] Tanimura S, Funamoto H, Hosono T, et al. New diagnostic criteria and operative strategy for cesarean scar syndrome: endoscopic repair for secondary infertility caused by cesarean scar defect. J Obstet Gynaecol Res 2015;41:1363–9.

[24] Vikhareva Osser O, Valentin L. Clinical importance of appearance of cesarean hysterotomy scar at transvaginal ultrasonography in nonpregnant women. Obstet Gynecol 2011;117:525–32.

[25] Roberge S, Boutin A, Chaillet N, Moore L, Jastrow N, Demers S, et al. Systematic review of cesarean scar assessment in the nonpregnant state: imaging techniques and uterine scar defect. Am J Perinatol 2012;29:465–71.

[26] Naji O, Daemen A, Smith A, et al. Visibility and measurement of cesarean section scars in pregnancy: a reproducibility study. Ultrasound Obstet Gynecol 2012;40:549–56.

[27] van der Voet LF, Vervoort AJ, Veersema S, BijdeVaate AJ, Brölmann HA, Huirne JA. Minimally invasive therapy for gynaecological symptoms related to a niche in the caesarean scar: a systematic review. BJOG. 2014;121:145–56.

[28] Nezhat C, Grace L, Soliemannjad R, Meshkat Razavi G, Nezhat A. Cesarean scar defect: What is it and how should it be treated? OBG Manag 2016;28(4). Available at: http://www.mdedge.com/obgmanagement/article/107745/surgery/cesarean-scar-defect-what-it-and-how-should-it-be-treated/pdf. Accessed October 25, 2016.

[29] Tahara M, Shimizu T, Shimoura H. Preliminary report of treatment with oral contraceptive pills for intermenstrual vaginal bleeding secondary to a cesarean section scar. Fertil Steril. 2006;86:477–9.

[30] Florio P, Gubbini G, Marra E, et al. A retrospective case-control study comparing hysteroscopic resection versus hormonal modulation in treating menstrual disorders due to isthmocele. Gynecol Endocrinol 2011;27:434–8.

[31] Thurmond AS, Harvey WJ, Smith SA. Cesarean section scar as a cause of abnormal vaginal bleeding: diagnosis by sonohysterography. J Ultrasound Med 1999;18:13–6.

[32] Chang Y, Tsai E, Long CY, Lee CL, Kay N. Resectoscopic treatment combined with sonohysterographic evaluation of women with postmenstrual bleeding as a result of previous cesarean delivery scar defects. Am J Obstet Gynecol 2009;200:370.

[33] Fernandez E, Fernandez C, Fabres C, Alam VV. Hysteroscopic correction of cesarean section scars in women with abnormal uterine bleeding. J Am Assoc Gynecol Laparosc. 1996;3(4, Supplement): S13.

[34] Gubbini G, Centini G, Nascetti D, et al. Surgical hysteroscopic treatment of cesarean-induced isthmocele in restoring fertility: prospective study. JMIG 2011;18:234–7.

[35] Florio P, Filippeschi M, Moncini I, Marra E, Franchini M, Gubbini G. Hysteroscopic treatment of the cesarean-induced isthmocele in restoring infertility. Curr Opin Obstet Gynecol 2012;24:180–6.

[36] Feng YL, Li MX, Liang XQ, Li X. Hysteroscopic treatment of postcesarean scar defect. J Minim Invasive Gynecol 2012;19:498–502.

[37] Wang CJ, Huang HJ, Chao A, Lin YP, Pan YJ, Horng SG. Challenges in the transvaginal management of abnormal uterine bleeding secondary to cesarean section scar defect. Eur J Obstet Gynecol Reprod Biol 2011;154:218–22.

[38] Gubbini G, Casadio P, Marra E. Resectoscopic correction of the "isthmocele" in women with postmenstrual abnormal uterine bleeding and secondary infertility. J Minim Invasive Gynecol 2008;15:172–5.

[39] Vervoort A, van der Voet LF, Hehenkamp W, et al. Hysteroscopic resection of a uterine caesarean scar defect (niche) in women with postmenstrual spotting: a randomised controlled trial. BJOG. 2018;125:326–34.

[40] Grace L, Nezhat A. Should cesarean scar defect be treated laparoscopically? A case report and review of the literature. J Minim Invasive Gynecol 2016;23:843.

[41] Jacobson MT, Osias J, Velasco A, Charles R, Nezhat C. Laparoscopic repair of uteroperitoneal fistula. JSLS 2003;7:367–9.

[42] Donnez O, Jadoul P, Squifflet J, Donnez J. Laparoscopic repair of wide and deep uterine scar dehiscence after cesarean section. Fertil Steril. 2008;89:974–80.

[43] Vervoort A, Vissers J, Hehenkamp W, Brölmann H, Huirne J. The effect of laparoscopic resection of large niches in the uterine caesarean scar on symptoms, ultrasound findings and quality of life: a prospective cohort study. BJOG. 2018;125:317–25.

[44] Zhang Y. A comparative study of transvaginal repair and laparoscopic repair in the management of patients with previous cesarean scar defect. J Minim Invasive Gynecol 2016;23:535–41.

[45] Li C, Tang S, Gao X, et al. Efficacy of combined laparoscopic and hysteroscopic repair of post-cesarean section uterine diverticulum: a retrospective analysis. Biomed Res Int; 2016:1765624.

Andrina Kölle, Katharina Rall und Sarah Brucker

15 Laparoscopic surgery for Müllerian anomalies

15.1 Background

The prevalence of Müllerian anomalies in the female population is 0.2% to 0.5%, whereas in patients suffering from infertility, it is 3% to 13%. Women with a history of recurrent miscarriages have a prevalence of up to 38%. A third of the Müllerian anomalies are septate, a third bicornuate uteri, 10% arcuate uterus, 10% didelphis and unicornuate uterus, and <5% uterine and vaginal aplasia [1–3]. They are often associated with non-Müllerian anomalies such as renal and axial skeletal systems' anomalies.

The different forms of malformations can be referred to the embryologic development of the uterus and the vagina. The proximal three quarters of the vagina, the uterus, and the fallopian tubes originate from the Müllerian ducts. In the embryologic development of the female genital tract, the pairs of Müllerian ducts fuse into a tube, followed by the resorption of the inner wall which forms the hollow organs uterus and vagina, whereas the cranial part remains in pairs and forms the fallopian tubes. The reason for Müllerian anomalies is considered to be an arrested development malformation such as aplasia or incomplete fusion of the Müllerian ducts. This leads to a high frequency of combined malformations of the uterus and the proximal vagina.

The distal part of the vagina is formed by the urogenital sinus. Therefore, malformations of the hymen occur in isolation. As the ovaries are not formed by the Müllerian ducts, patients with isolated Müllerian anomalies have normal hormonal activity. They are often diagnosed as late as puberty, when menarche does not appear or sexual activity is not possible, or even later if infertility is the only symptom [4]. The leading symptom of obstructive female genital malformations and uterine aplasia is primary amenorrhea during normal pubertal development, since hormonal development is unimpaired.

15.2 Diagnosis

The correct diagnosis of the malformation is essential for therapy. If there is a suspicion of a genital anomaly, a clinical examination, inspection of the outer genital organs with the examination of the vaginal length, and an ultrasound of the inner genital organs and the kidneys should be performed [5]. For further investigation and in order to exclude associated malformations of the urinary tract, a magnetic resonance imaging (MRI) including urinary tract collection system can be performed. Before the laparoscopic surgery, associated malformations such as duplicated ureters or atypical anatomic locations of the kidneys or the ureters should be assessed to avoid surgical complications.

https://doi.org/10.1515/9783110535204-015

To dissociate Müllerian anomalies from disorders of sexual development (XY, DSD) a chromosome analysis and a hormone status might be necessary.

In addition to the existing ones, a new classification system of female genital malformations was built in 2013 by the European Society of Human Reproduction and Embryology (ESHRE) and the European Society for Gynaecological Endoscopy (ESGE) that provides a clinically useful instrument for the comparability of diagnoses (Fig. 15.1) [6, 7].

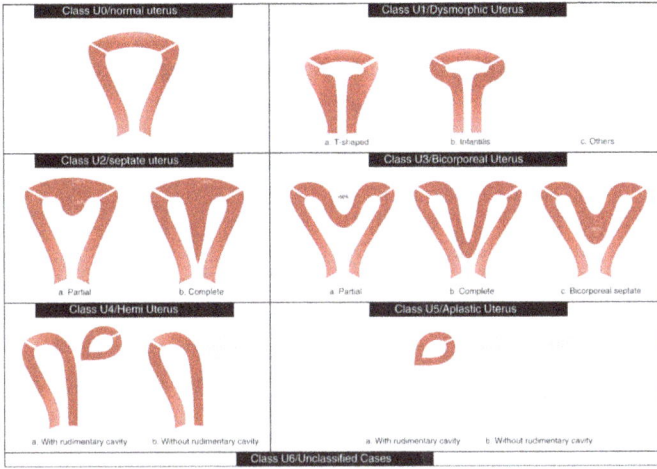

	Uterine anomaly		Cervical/vaginal anomaly	
Main class		**Sub-class**	**Co-existent class**	
U0	Normal uterus		C0	Normal cervix
U1	Dysmorphic uterus	a. T-shaped	C1	Septate cervix
		b. Infantilis		
		c. Others	C2	Double 'normal' cervix
U2	Septate uterus	a. Partial	C3	Unilateral cervical aplasia
		b. Complete		
			C4	Cervical aplasia
U3	Bicorporeal uterus	a. Partial		
		b. Complete		
		c. Bicorporeal septate	V0	Normal vagina
U4	Hemi-uterus	a. With rudimentary cavity (communicating or not horn)	V1	Longitudinal non-obstructing vaginal septum
		b. Without rudimentary cavity (horn without cavity/no horn)	V2	Longitudinal obstructing vaginal septum
U5	Aplastic	a. With rudimentary cavity (bi- or unilateral horn)	V3	Transverse vaginal septum and/or imperforate hymen
		b. Without rudimentary cavity (bi- or unilateral uterine remnants/aplasia)	V4	Vaginal aplasia
U6	Unclassified malformations			
U			C	V

Associated anomalies of non-Müllerian origin:

Fig. 15.1: European Society of Human Reproduction and Embryology/European Society for Gynaecological Endoscopy classification of female genital malformations (2013).

15.3 Congenital vaginal agenesis

Vaginal hypoplasia or vaginal agenesis is seen in complex genital malformations such as the Mayer-Rokitansky-Küster-Hauser (MRKH) syndrome or the complete androgen insensitivity syndrome with chromosome analyses of 46, XY. The incidence of the MRKH syndrome is reported from 1:4000 to 1:5000 in female live births [8].

The main symptom is primary amenorrhea without major abdominal pain. This is due to the combination of an absent vagina with the absence of a functioning uterus. Sexual intercourse is normally not possible or very painful. In some cases, there may be a rudimentary uterus containing functioning endometrium, which can lead to symptomatic hematometra and/or pain without obvious hematometra.

The correction of an absent vagina can be accomplished by different methods, which can be grouped as nonsurgical and surgical.

15.3.1 Nonsurgical method

15.3.1.1 Nonsurgical stretching method

The stretching method developed by Frank involves the prolonged use of a vaginal dilatator by the patient [9]. External pressure is applied regularly to the vaginal dimple with dilators of growing size. The self-dilatation therapy is often considered as the best first-line treatment with a high rate of success and low accompanying risks due its noninvasive nature [10]. Furthermore, the Frank's method is cheap with a success rate from 69 to 95% [11, 12]. The self-dilatation is a therapeutic option in highly motivated patients who refuse a primary surgical therapy.

However, a systematic review concludes that the self-dilatation leads to the shortest vaginal length of 6.65 cm and the lowest Female Sexual Function Index score, which is an objective instrument measuring sexual functioning in women [13]. Moreover, the treatment success depends on the patient's self-discipline and perseverance and could cause considerable physical pain and psychological strain. Apart from being a lengthy procedure, Frank's method is also associated with several medical disadvantages, including vaginal prolapse caused by the absence of vaginal supporting structures and scarring. Other complications include accidental urethral dilatation [14].

15.3.2 Surgical methods

15.3.2.1 Vaginal tunneling—the McIndoe method

The McIndoe method uses skin grafts, e.g., from the buttocks or posterior thigh for the creation of a neovagina. The first step is to make an H-shaped incision in the perineum. A canal is developed with blunt and sharp dissection and by spreading the scissors until the peritoneum of the posterior cul-de-sac is reached. A skin graft is taken and sutured over a vaginal mold, which is then inserted into the created space. The skin graft is secured to the introitus with a few sutures. The mold is removed after 10 to 14 days and a postoperative mold is inserted for 6 more months. A mesh graft may be used to reduce the amount of skin that has to be taken [15].

Complications are partial to total necrosis of the skin graft or development of granulation tissue or even fistula, particularly in those with previous surgical interventions. Postoperative vaginal length is reported between 6 and 9.5 cm, and 78% to 100% of the patients are satisfied with their sexual life [16].

The disadvantages of the mesh graft are shrinkage and long-term need for dilatation. There is also a risk of vaginal prolapse and lack of vaginal lubrication.

The McIndoe method can be recommended to patients with previous major abdominal surgeries and/or other contraindications to the abdominal approach, e.g., after a pouch neobladder. The procedure is more suitable for those women with perineal scarring because the vaginal skin is not required to stretch.

15.3.2.2 Davydov method

The Davydov technique creates a neovagina using the patient's own peritoneum for the lining. To access the peritoneum, a laparoscopy or laparotomy is necessary with their associated trauma and risks. The modified laparoscopic Davydov technique involves a laparoscopic step, followed by a vaginal approach. During the laparoscopic step, the strand that connects the two rudimental uterine horns is lifted, and the peritoneum immediately below is incised transversely for a section of 4–5 cm. Guided by the middle finger, which is inserted in the patient's rectum, this incision is extended in a horseshoe-shaped fashion for approximately 1 cm into the connective tissue beneath, which separates the bladder from the rectum. In order to mobilize the peritoneum, which will constitute the neovaginal walls and vault, the round ligaments are identified by applying traction on the uterine remnants and then are cut bilaterally. The supravesical peritoneum is incised along the apparent line that connects the rudiments. A monofilament is used to create two purse-string sutures for each hemi-pelvis. Each suture is begun from the mobilized peritoneum above the bladder dome by transfixing consecutively the round ligament, the tubal isthmus, the uteroovarian ligament, and the lateral peritoneal leaf. The perineal step creates an anastomosis between the incised pelvic peritoneum and the mucosa of the vaginal dimple. An H-shaped incision is made on the vaginal vestibulum and a dissection between the bladder and rectum is created until the peritoneal margins of the laparoscopically performed transverse incision are identified. After the connection, a vaginal tampon is inserted [17]. Forty-eight hours after surgery, a vaginal obturator is inserted, which has to be used 6 to 8 hours a day until complete vaginal epithelialization is achieved. Intraoperative complications consist of damage to the bladder, the ureters, or the rectum, which can be followed by formation of rectovaginal fistulas, which is rare. Peri- and postoperative complications include peritonitis or insufficient vaginal lubrication [17].

15.3.2.3 Bowel Vaginoplasty

There are many ways of using intestinal segments to create a neovagina. Segments of rectum, ileum, and sigmoid colon have been employed for vaginal replacement. Compared with other segments of the bowel, the sigmoid colon has several advantages: Its location is convenient, it is usually mobile, and its blood supply permits a well-vascularized segment to be isolated.

The laparoscopic procedure releases the sigmoid in the classical manner. A sigmoid transplant is 10 to 15 cm long. It remains vascularized by the inferior sigmoid artery. In a second step, a perineal H-shaped incision is made and a peritoneal opening is made under laparoscopic guidance [18].

Sigmoid grafting offers adequate length, natural lubrication, early coitus, and lack of shrinkage, narrowing, and stenosis at the perineal introitus. Disadvantages are copious vaginal discharge, colitis, or an unpleasant odor. Complications include prolapse of the sigmoid neovagina, insufficiency of the anastomosis, necrosis, or even vaginal malignancy.

The method involves a major operation, including all risks of bowel surgery. This method is not a first-line treatment and should be reserved for highly complex anomalies that have already undergone unsuccessful reconstructive surgery.

15.3.2.4 Surgical Traction methods—laparoscopically-assisted creation of neovagina after Vecchietti and its modifications

Vecchietti developed a method for the creation of a neovagina in patients with congenital vaginal agenesis based on stretching of the vaginal dimple intraabdominally after abdominovaginal dissection of the vesicorectal space. An acrylic dummy (olive) is threaded and inserted in the vaginal dimple. The threads are then passed through the pelvis onto the abdominal wall and connected to a traction device. Using this device, tension is continuously exerted on the vaginal dimple, resulting in the formation of a neovagina by stretching within a matter of days [19]. This method came into widespread use but was associated with the surgical trauma of laparotomy.

To avoid this, an endoscopic approach was established in 1992 at the Department of Obstetrics and Gynaecology at Heidelberg University Hospital, Germany, and was optimized in Tübingen University Hospital, Germany [20].

The advantage of the Vecchietti-based methods is that they create a neovagina with normal anatomy, histomorphology, and functionality [21]. Moreover, there is no need to use exogenous tissues such as skin, peritoneum, or intestine or to perform plastic surgery that causes visible scars. Most importantly, functional results are achieved very quickly. Postoperative vaginal dilatation is essential to prevent vaginal stenosis for up to 6 months or until epithelialization is complete. Initial coitus can take place with the understanding compliance of the partner as soon as 4 weeks after the operation and sexual intercourse is satisfying without the need for additional lubricants.

The advantage over the McIndoe technique is the absence of major scarring from skin grafting in these young patients. The Vecchietti method has good functional results because the neovagina is lined with the typical vaginal epithelium [22].

Surgical steps of creating a laparoscopically assisted neovagina modified from Vecchietti include an initial laparoscopy with simultaneous recto-vaginal palpation. The vaginal dummy (olive) with a central hole for the flow of secretion is inserted in the vaginal dimple, followed by the laparoscopic determination of the perforation point. The vaginal step consists of the perforation of the vaginal membrane through the recto-vesical septum without dissection of the recto-vesical space. The threads that are attached to the vaginal dummy are passed into the peritoneal cavity through perforation of the recto-vesical septum (Fig. 15.2). Following this, the threads are led through the abdominal wall subperitoneally and fixed on a special traction device above the umbilicus. The traction device provides a smooth surface and a stable direction for the tension without unintentional opening or snapping off of the threads and ensures equal tightening of both traction threads [23, 24].

After 5 to 7 days, the traction device is removed and a vaginal dummy (10 × 3 cm) is inserted into the neovaginal space. In the first 4 weeks after surgery, the patients have to wear the vaginal dummy for about 23–24 hours a day. After this period, the time the patients have to wear the dummy is reduced and they can start having sexual intercourse approximately 6 months after the healing of the neovagina is complete. Routine controls are recommended at 1, 3, 6, and 12 months after surgery. After that time, the neovagina stays in adequate size even without regular sexual intercourse.

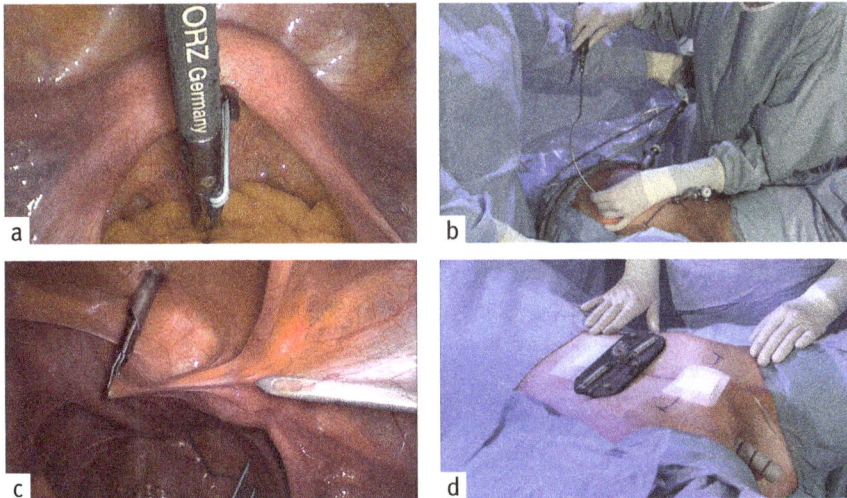

Fig. 15.2: (a) Insertion of the threads through the vaginal dimple under laparoscopic view. (b) Transabdominal insertion of the curved thread guide. (c) Subperitoneal guidance of the threads under laparoscopic view. (d) Abdominal fixation of the traction device.

The procedure is fast, effective, and minimally traumatic, with a low long-term complication rate. Moreover, a good quality of sexual life and sexual satisfaction are reported [24–26].

Surgical vesico-rectal tunneling is not needed and vagino-abdominal blunt perforation of the vaginal dimple is not associated with high complication rates or a poor functional outcome. The improved minimally invasive laparoscopic technique and development of novel instruments have resulted in safer and quicker surgery. In addition, this low-risk procedure creates a vaginal canal in the correct axis that is of adequate size and with secretory capacity. These allow intercourse to take place without the need for continual postoperative dilatation and therefore require minimal care to maintain long-term benefits.

Presently, there is no consensus in the medical literature regarding the best surgical option for the creation of a neovagina. All described procedures should be performed by surgeons with experience in vaginal reconstruction and laparoscopic surgery. It is also important to provide the patient with access to psychological and psychosomatic support. A multidisciplinary approach in all aspects of care cannot be overemphasized [21].

15.4 Uterus bicornis, uterus didelphis (Bicornis, Bicollis)

Müllerian malformations do not necessarily require surgical intervention as long as there is no obstructive malformation causing symptomatic hematometra or hematocolpos, or as long as there is no problem with fertility. It is essential to differentiate between septate uterus and bicornuate uterus (see Fig. 15.1). It is not possible to distinguish between these malformations at hysteroscopy; hence, an MRI, a three-dimensional ultrasound, or a laparoscopy is required for an accurate diagnosis. The possibility of a laparoscopic metroplasty in bicornuate and didelphic uteri under simultaneous hysteroscopy is described. It consists of a gradual incision from the medial aspects of the uterine horns near the region of the fallopian tubes and the subsequent suturing to form a single uterine cavity [27]. Surgical therapy for a bicornuate uterus or uterus didelphis depends on the pregnancy history of the patient and should be performed only if the patient has had recurrent miscarriage or late abortions.

15.5 Uterus unicornis

Fertility is reduced in the presence of a unicornuate uterus. Preterm delivery is reported in between 10% and 44%, and the miscarriage rate is typically between 29% and 58% [28]. A noncommunicating rudimentary horn should be ruled out if a patient with a unicornuate uterus presents with cyclic pain. These patients may also present with dysmenorrhea as a result of endometriosis from retrograde menstrual flow out of the functional endometrium in the horn [29]. Pregnancies can occur in the rudimentary horn. When this happens, this uterus is at risk of rupture. The horn containing the pregnancy should be removed via laparotomy or laparoscopy. Currently, with the good instrumentation and experience, laparoscopic removal of the rudimentary uterus is easily accomplished. If there are no symptoms, the noncommunicating horn can be left untreated [29].

References

[1] Byrne J, Nussbaum-Blask A, Taylor WS, et al. Prevalence of müllerian duct anomalies detected at ultrasound. Am J Med Genet 2000;94(1):9–12.
[2] Brucker SY, Rall K, Campo R, Oppelt P, Isaacson K. Treatment of congenital malformations. Semin Reprod Med 2011;29(2):101–12.
[3] Nahum G. Uterine anomalies. How common are they, and what is their distribution among subtypes? J Peprod Med 1998;43(10):877–87.
[4] Oppelt P, von Have M, Paulsen M, et al. Female genital malformations and their associated abnormalities. Fertil Steril 2007;87(2):335–42.
[5] Oppelt P, Dörr H-G. Kinder- und Jugendgynäkologie (German). 1st ed. Erlangen: Thieme; 2015.
[6] Schöller D, Hölting M, Stefanescu D, et al. Female genital tract congenital malformations and the applicability of the ESHRE/ESGE classification: a systematic retrospective analysis of 920 patients. Arch Gynecol Obstet 2018;297(6):1473–81.
[7] Grimbizis GF, Gordts S, Di Spiezio Sardo A, et al. The ESHRE/ESGE consensus on the classification of female genital tract congenital anomalies. Hum Reprod Oxf Engl 2013;28(8):2032–44.
[8] Aittomäki K, Eroila H, Kajanoja P. A population-based study of the incidence of müllerian aplasia in Finland. Fertil Steril 2001;76(3):624–5.
[9] Frank RT. The formation of an artificial vagina without operation. Am J Obstet Gynecol 1938;35(6):1053–5.
[10] Nakhal RS, Creighton SM. Management of Vaginal Agenesis. J Pediatr Adolesc Gynecol 2012;25(6):352–7.
[11] Callens N, Weyers S, Monstrey S, et al. Vaginal dilation treatment in women with vaginal hypoplasia: a prospective one-year follow-up study. Am J Obstet Gynecol 2014;211(3):228.e1–12.
[12] Edmonds DK, Rose GL, Lipton MG, Quek J. Mayer-Rokitansky-Küster-Hauser syndrome: a review of 245 consecutive cases managed by a multidisciplinary approach with vaginal dilators. Fertil Steril 2012;97(3):686–90.
[13] McQuillan SK, Grover SR. Dilation and surgical management in vaginal agenesis: a systematic review. Int Urogynecology J 2014;25(3):299–311.
[14] Schaffer J, Fabricant C, Carr BR. Vaginal vault prolapse after nonsurgical and surgical treatment of mullerian agenesis. Obstet Gynecol 2002;99(5, Part 2):947–9.
[15] Lang N, Neef I, Blömer A. Surgical management of vaginal aplasia using mesh grafts. 1973;33(7):560–3.
[16] Alessandrescu D, Peltecu GC, Buhimschi CS, Buhimschi IA. Neocolpopoiesis with split-thickness skin graft as a surgical treatment of vaginal agenesis: retrospective review of 201 cases. Am J Obstet Gynecol 1996;175(1):131–8.
[17] Fedele L, Frontino G, Restelli E, Ciappina N, Motta F, Bianchi S. Creation of a neovagina by Davydov's laparoscopic modified technique in patients with Rokitansky syndrome. Am J Obstet Gynecol 2010;202(1):33.e1–6.

[18] Darai E, Toullalan O, Besse O, Potiron L, Delga P. Anatomic and functional results of laparoscopic–perineal neovagina construction by sigmoid colpoplasty in women with Rokitansky's syndrome. Human Reproduction. 2003 Nov 1;18(11):2454–9.

[19] Vecchietti G. Creation of an artificial vagina in Rokitansky-Kuster-Hauser syndrome. Attual Ostet Ginecol. 1965;11(2):131–47.

[20] Gauwerky JFH, Wallwiener D, Bastert G. An endoscopically assisted technique for construction of a neovagina. Arch Gynecol Obstet 1992;252(2):59–63.

[21] Brucker SY, Rall K, Campo R, Oppelt P, Isaacson K. Treatment of congenital malformations. Semin Reprod Med 2011;29(2):101–12.

[22] Fedele L, Bianchi S, Berlanda N, Ciappina N, Motta F, Bianci S. Neovaginal mucosa after Vecchietti's laparoscopic operation for Rokitansky syndrome: structural and ultrastructural study. Am J Obstet Gynecol 2006;195(1):56–61.

[23] Brucker SY, Gegusch M, Zubke W, Rall K, Gauwerky JF, Wallwiener D. Neovagina creation in vaginal agenesis: development of a new laparoscopic Vecchietti-based procedure and optimized instruments in a prospective comparative interventional study in 101 patients. Fertil Steril 2008;90(5):1940–52.

[24] Brucker S, Aydeniz B, Gegusch M, Wallwiener D, Zubke W. Improvement of endoscopically assisted neovagina: new application instruments and traction device. Gynecol Surg 2004;1(2):133–8.

[25] Rall K, Schickner MC, Barresi G, et al. Laparoscopically assisted neovaginoplasty in vaginal agenesis: a long-term outcome study in 240 patients. J Pediatr Adolesc Gynecol 2014;27(6):379–85.

[26] Fliegner Maike, Krupp Kerstin, Brunner Franziska, et al. Sexual life and sexual wellness in individuals with complete androgen insensitivity syndrome (CAIS) and Mayer-Rokitansky-Küster-Hauser syndrome (MRKHS). J Sex Med 2013;11(3):729–42.

[27] Alborzi S, Asadi N, Zolghadri J, Alborzi S, Alborzi M. Laparoscopic metroplasty in bicornuate and didelphic uteri. Fertil Steril 2009;92(1):352–5.

[28] Akar Munire E, Bayar D, Yildiz S, Ozel M, Yilmaz Z. Reproductive outcome of women with unicornuate uterus. Aust N Z J Obstet Gynaecol 2005;45(2):148–50.

[29] Jayasinghe Y, Rane A, Stalewski H, Grover S. The presentation and early diagnosis of the rudimentary uterine horn. Obstet Gynecol [Internet] 2005;105(6). Available at: https://journals. lww.com/greenjournal/Fulltext/2005/06000/The_Presentation_and_Early_Diagnosis_of_ the.29.aspx.

Gokhan Sami Kilic and Ibrahim Alanbay

16 Minimally invasive techniques for urinary incontinence: laparoscopic/robotic-assisted Burch colposuspension (urethropexy)

16.1 Introduction

For many years, open Burch colposuspension (urethropexy), first described in 1961 [1], was accepted as the gold standard in the treatment of incontinence due to urethral mobility [2]. Lapitan *et al.* found a 68.9–88.0% overall cure rate for open retropubic colposuspension, based on their review of 2403 women who underwent the procedure [3]. Its overall continence rates were found to be approximately 85–90% within the first year and 70% after 5 years [3]. Then, in 1991, as the use of minimally invasive surgeries increased in popularity and momentum, the first laparoscopic Burch procedure was described [4]. Laparoscopic colposuspension has its own obvious advantages over open cases, such as improved visualization, shorter hospital stay, and faster recovery [5]. But the introduction of midurethral sling kits to the urogynecology world drew attention away from colposuspension. The kits grew in popularity because they are user-friendly and provide a shorter surgery time. However, mesh-related complications created an abundance of litigation issues that have been highlighted in the media and have led to multiple Food and Drug Administration (FDA) announcements. The FDA announcements do not specifically implement restrictions on midurethral sling use, but the bad publicity surrounding mesh has motivated patients to seek mesh-free alternatives for urinary incontinence [6]. Recently, robotic-assisted surgeries were introduced, and the robotic-assisted colposuspension is now a feasible option to open Burch [7]. This chronology of events has led to the increased use of laparoscopic or robotic-assisted colposuspension in recent years.

Based on the literature [8], the following reasons support choosing laparoscopic/robotic-assisted retropubic colposuspension:

- Concomitant pelvic floor reconstruction together with laparoscopic/robotic-assisted colposuspension and paravaginal repair can correct anterior compartment prolapse [9].
- A laparoscopic/robotic-assisted colposuspension can be performed at the same time as a concomitant hysterectomy, with or without salpingo-oophorectomy.
- Laparoscopic/robotic-assisted colposuspension eliminates the potential, long-term complications of mesh in patients at high risk of mesh erosion due to poor vaginal tissue vascularity, cancer, and history of pelvic radiation.

https://doi.org/10.1515/9783110535204-016

- Laparoscopic/robotic-assisted colposuspension can be offered after a failed vaginal midurethral tape procedure [10]. These patients receive urodynamic testing first to confirm the stress incontinence.
- Laparoscopic/robotic-assisted colposuspension is an alternative for patients seeking options that do not involve mesh.

16.2 Pertinent information

A few related issues need to be addressed before the Burch operation is described:
- Sutures are found to be better than mesh or staples in retropubic colposuspension, and two suspending sutures are better than single sutures in each side [11, 12].
- During the Burch operation, the vaginal anterior wall is pulled forward, and the entire abdominal pressure can be directed to the posterior compartment of the urogenital hiatus. This procedure can cause iatrogenic rectocele or enterocele development in 10–15% of cases [13–15]. Therefore, this risk should be disclosed when informed consent is obtained. To prevent this complication, the use of Halban's culdoplasty or Moschowitz posterior cul-de-sac obliteration is also suggested along with synchronous retropubic suspension operations. This decision should be made with the patient before the surgery.
- If a midurethral sling is planned after a failed retropubic colposuspension, the authors require an operative note from the previous surgeon disclosing whether the peritoneum was closed. If the peritoneum was left open during the previous Burch operation, the bowel loop could potentially get trapped in the retropubic space, and there is a risk that passing needles used for the retropubic midurethral sling may injure the bowel. If a previous operation note cannot be obtained, the authors recommend placing a camera intraperitoneally to pass the sling needle under direct visualization.

16.3 Retropubic space description

The retropubic space (or Retzius) is an extraperitoneal space. It is located behind the pubic symphysis and in front of the urinary bladder, and it extends to the level of the umbilicus. The lateral border of the retropubic space reaches the pelvic sidewall. The structures located at the lateral boundaries are the obturator internus muscle and endopelvic facia (the arcus tendineus fascia of pelvis). The boundaries also include the pubic rami laterally and the symphysis pubis anteriorly. The retropubic space contains anterior aspects of the proximal urethra and extraperitoneal portions of the bladder; these structures lie on the endopelvic fascia. The Cooper's ligament (pectineal ligament) covers the superior pubic ramus and is used as a suture fixation point; a surgeon must know the anatomy of Cooper's ligament relative to other pelvic structures. The major vascular structure in this region, especially in the paraurethral area, is the Santorini complex, which is a venous network that contains vaginal vessels. Thus, the important anatomical landmarks of the retropubic space are the pubic symphysis, Cooper's ligament (pectineal ligament), veins of Santorini, pubocervical fascia, pubourethral ligament, obturator neurovasculer bundle, and external iliac artery and vein. Dissection at the lateral borders of the Retzius space is important, and the surgeon must be careful to avoid the important anatomical structures encountered during this procedure, such as the obturator neurovasculer bundle and aberrant obturatory vessels. Knowledge of the relative locations of these structures is crucial because their close proximity and obscured location could result in inadvertent injury. This knowledge is especially important when performing a minimally invasive procedure (both laparoscopically and robotically) because it can be difficult to maintain perspective and depth of field due to camera magnification and loss of tactile sensation.

In a cadaver study [6], the distances between the major anatomical structures and the suture sites were measured after the classical Burch operation. The paravaginal fascia was dissected using the same technique as in open surgery. The study showed that the mean distance from the most lateral suture in the Cooper's ligament to the obturator bundle was 25.9 ± 7.6 mm, and the distance to the external iliac vessels was 28.9 ± 9.3 mm. Notably, the obturator neurovascular bundle and external iliac vessels lie, on average, less than 3 cm from the most lateral suture through the Cooper's ligament and in some cases are within 1.5 cm.

16.4 Colposuspension procedure

Laparoscopic colposuspension is performed using either a transperitoneal or extraperitoneal approach. The technique described in this chapter is mostly described in terms of robotic surgery:

1. The patient is placed in the modified dorsal lithotomy position to allow vaginal manipulation when the surgeon enters in the retropubic area.
2. After proper entry into the abdominal cavity, the surgeon places a robotic camera 5 to 10 cm above the umbilicus. In addition to the camera, two 8-mm working ports are inserted at the right side of the patient's abdomen, and a third one is inserted in the left lower quadrant, lateral to the rectus muscle, between the symphysis pubis and the umbilicus.
3. Prior to the retropubic dissection, a 22F Foley catheter with a 30-ml balloon is placed in the bladder. The bladder is filled with 300 ml of normal or blue-stained saline (3-ml methylene blue 10 µg/ml in 1000 ml normal saline), facilitating the

identification of the upper limit of the bladder and upper edge of symphysis pubis. The anterior peritoneal incision starts approximately 1 to 3 cm above the upper limit of the bladder.

4. The incision is extended laterally to the medial umbilical ligament on each side. The loose connective tissue in the space is dissected bluntly with the help of intra-peritoneal gas to arrive at the symphysis pubis bone anteriorly with the Cooper's ligaments positioned laterally on each side (Fig. 16.1).

*It should be kept in mind that the aberrant obturator vessels (corona mortis) and obturator neurovascular bundle, and even the external iliac vessels, may be encountered during upper lateral dissection.

5. The bladder is then drained, and the dissection is continued until a lateral position to the pelvic side wall is acquired so that the obturator muscle and the arcus tendineus fascia pelvis (white line) can be seen bilaterally. Experience enables the surgeon to decide if the lateral margin of the dissection has been reached.

6. The adipose tissue behind the symphysis, between the bladder and the pubic bones and between urethrovesical junction (paraurethral tissue) and white line, is gently separated. Attention should be paid to the pubic branches of the aberrant obturator or inferior epigastric vessels near or above the Cooper's ligament.

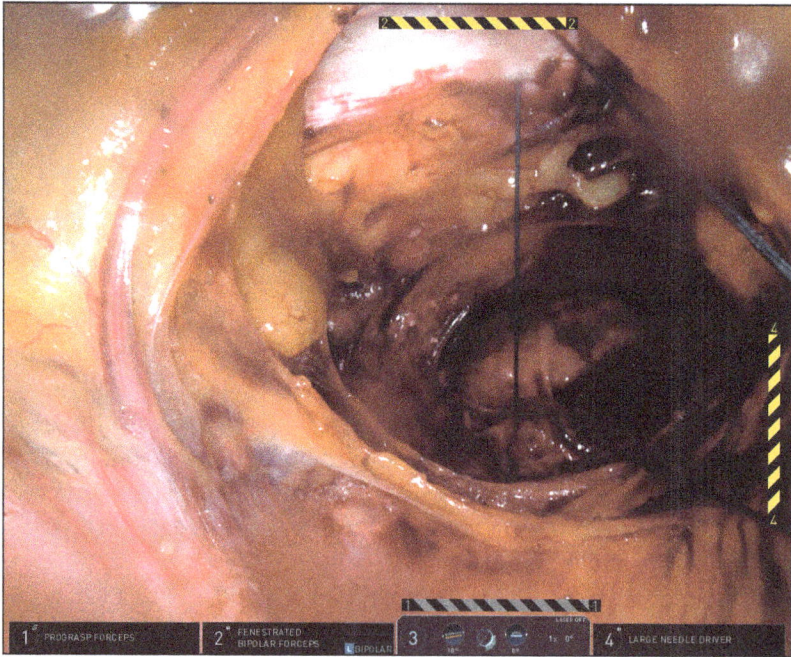

Fig. 16.1: Suturing landmarks of Retzius space.

7. The bladder base is dissected bluntly and pushed medially by the help of the finger in the vagina, elevating the anterior vaginal wall (Fig. 16.2).

*During the dissection, the surgeon should avoid dissecting within 2 cm of the urethrovesical junction to prevent inadvertent bleeding and nerve damage. It is important to remember that there may be internal pudendal and venous plexus from the vaginal vessels.

8. Finally, the pubourethral ligament, urethrovesical junction, and urinary bladder base are revealed clearly within the space of the Retzius.
9. It is absolutely necessary to see the white paravaginal endopelvic fascia and put the sutures here for an effective surgery. Before suturing, all sutures can be placed in the abdomen and on the anterior wall of the abdomen to simplify this part of the operation.
10. The first suture is passed into the paravaginal fascia as a double bite, approximately 2 cm lateral to the midurethra, and a second suture is placed 2 cm distal to the bladder neck without passing through the vaginal epithelium. The sutures should be fixed to the nearest point on the ipsilateral Cooper's ligament. During suturing, two fingers should be placed in the vagina to apply upward pressure to identify the appropriate areas in the lateral vaginal wall to suture.
    a. When using a laparoscopic approach, the authors prefer to place their hands intravaginaly to identify the endopelvic fascia during suturing.

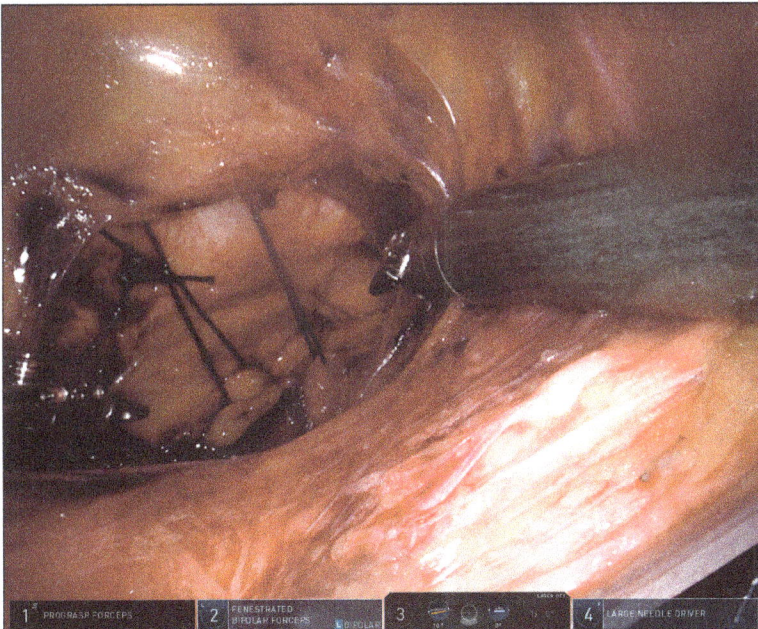

Fig. 16.2: Endopelvic fascia on the left side Retzius space. Air knots in four retropubic sutures.

b. In robotic-assisted cases, the bedside assistant should visualize the fascia, and the console-side surgeon should grasp the fascia with a prograsp before suturing. Traction on the Foley catheter at the same time can fix and help to identify paraurethral fascia and urethrovesical junction.

*It is important to use nonabsorbable monofilament suture material for a successful procedure. Nonabsorbable 2-0 sutures (Ethibond Excel® Polyester, Ethicon Inc. USA) are the authors' preference.

11. When tying the suture, excessive upward tension on the vaginal wall can be avoided using the following two methods:

a. A probe with 1-cm marks for calibration can be used to ensure that the distance between the upper edge of the Foley balloon (filled with 12 ml of water) and the superior border of the symphysis pubis is not less than 2 cm, or

b. There must be a space of at least a two-finger breadth between the suture knot and the Cooper's ligament.

*The intended tension when tying the suture should be enough to bring the stitched vaginal wall to the level of the arcus tendineus fascia pelvis (Fig. 16.2).

*The sliding suture technique is very helpful at this stage to adjust the tension of the suture (Fig. 16.3).

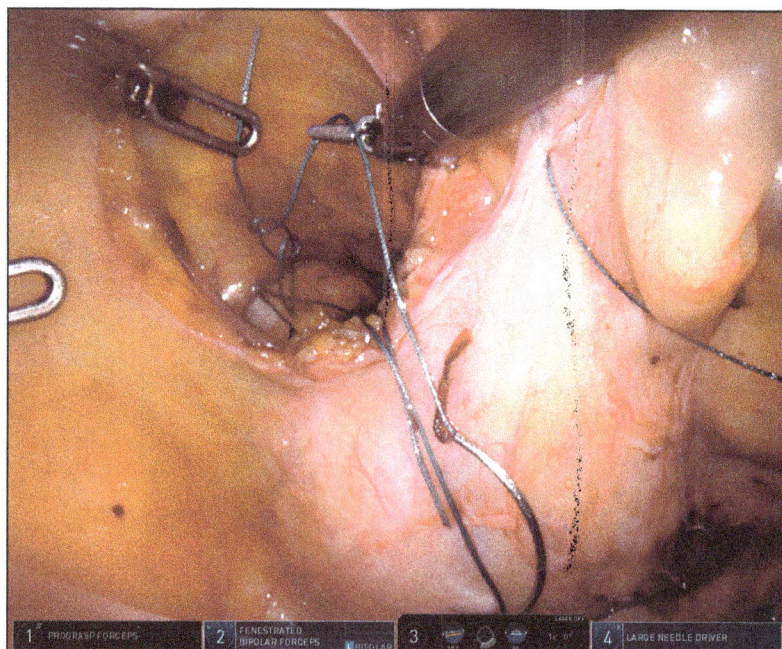

Fig. 16.3: Sliding suture knot.

12. The procedure is repeated on the contralateral side. Bleeding control is performed after the sutures. If needed, hemostasis with chemical agents can be used. Next, the anterior peritoneal incision is closed with polyglactin 910 or barbed sutures so that the bowel does not enter the space.

13. A cystoscopy should then be performed after each case to ensure that the Burch sutures have not gone through the bladder and to confirm normal ureteral efflux.

References

[1] Burch JC. Urethrovaginal fixation to Cooper's ligament for correction of stress incontinence, cystocele, and prolapse. Am J Obstet Gynecol 1961;81:281–90.

[2] Huang WC, Yang JM. Anatomic comparison between laparoscopic and open Burch colposuspension for primary stress urinary incontinence. Urology 2004;63:676–81.

[3] Lapitan MC, Cody DJ, Grant AM. Open retropubic colposuspension for urinary incontinence in women. Cochrane Database Syst Rev 2017;CD002912.

[4] Vancaillie TG. Laparoscopic bladder neck suspension. J Laparoendosc Surg 1991;1:169–73.

[5] Price N, Jackson SR. Advances in laparoscopic techniques in pelvic reconstructive surgery for prolapse and incontinence. Maturitas 2009;62:276–80.

[6] Kinman CL, Agrawal A, Deveneau NE, Meriwether KV, Herring NR, Francis SL. Anatomical Relationships of Burch Colposuspension Sutures. Female Pelvic Med Reconstr Surg 2017;23:72–4.

[7] Patel PR, Borahay MA, Puentes AR, Rodriguez AM, Delaisse J, Kilic GS. Initial experience with robotic retropubic urethropexy compared to open retropubic urethropexy. Obstet Gynecol Int 2013;2013:315680.

[8] Hong J-H, Choo M-S, Lee K-S. Long-term results of laparoscopic Burch colposuspension for stress urinary incontinence in women. J Korean Med Sci 2009;24:1182–6.

[9] Jenkins TR, Liu CY. Laparoscopic Burch colposuspension. Curr Opin Obstet Gynecol 2007;19:314–8.

[10] De Cuyper EM, Ismail R, Maher CF. Laparoscopic Burch colposuspension after failed sub-urethral tape procedures: a retrospective audit. Int Urogynecol J Pelvic Floor Dysfunct 2008;19:681–5.

[11] Moehrer B, Carey M, Wilson D. Laparoscopic colposuspension: a systemic review. Br J Obstet Gynaecol 2003;110:230–5.

[12] Persson J, Wollner-Hanssen P. Laparoscopic Burch colposuspension for stress urinary incontinence: a randomised comparison of one or two sutures on each side of the urethra. Obstet Gynecol 2000;95(1):151–5.

[13] Demirci F, Petri E. Perioperative complications of Burch colposuspension. Int Urogynecol J Pelvic Floor Dysfunct 2000;11:170–5.

[14] Demirci F, Yucel N, Ozden S, Delikara N, Yalti S, Demirci E. A retrospective review of perioperative complications in 360 patients who had Burch colposuspension. Aust N Z J Obstet Gynaecol 1999;39:472–5.

[15] Sun MJ, Ng SC, Tsui KP, Chang NE, Lin KC, Chen GD. Are there any predictors for failed Burch colposuspension? Taiwan J Obstet Gynecol 2006;45:33–8.

Burak Zeybek and Gokhan Sami Kilic

17 Robotic procedures for management of apical compartment prolapse

17.1 Introduction

Pelvic organ prolapse (POP) affects 11% of women in the United States; approximately 200,000 POP surgical procedures are performed annually [1]. It has become a growing public health problem; during a woman's lifetime, the estimated risk of undergoing POP surgery is 11–19%, and it is expected to be higher in the near future due to increased life expectancy [2, 3]. The significant role of level I support (apical support) has been demonstrated in previous studies showing that its loss is a major factor in the development of symptomatic and apical wall prolapse [4, 5]. In addition, neglecting to address the apical compartment in certain patients during prolapse surgery is associated with failure of the POP surgery in the long-term [6]. There are a variety of procedures that can be performed either abdominally (open, minimally invasive) or vaginally for this purpose. The aim of this chapter is to demonstrate the practical aspects of robotic sacrocolpopexy and robotic uterosacral vault suspension in patients with POP.

17.2 Robotic sacrocolpopexy

17.2.1 Anatomy

17.2.1.1 Mechanisms of pelvic organ support

Pelvic organ support depends on the fine balance between the levator ani muscle and connective tissues in the pelvis. The levator ani muscle holds the pelvic floor closed and provides lifting forces to prevent pelvic organ descent, while pelvic support structures attach the uterus and vagina to the pelvic walls. When the muscles are damaged or weakened, or when the endopelvic fascia is not strong enough to hold the organs in place, a downward force vector occurs, causing progressive distress on the pelvic support system, which leads to downward displacement of pelvic structures [7].

17.2.1.2 Levator ani muscle

The levator ani muscle is comprised of three components: the pubovisceral (pubococcygeus), iliococcygeal, and puborectalis muscles [8]. The pubovisceral muscle is further divided into three subcomponents: the pubovaginal, puboperineal, and puboanal, all of which are aspects of one muscle but are not distinct muscles. These

https://doi.org/10.1515/9783110535204-017

subcomponents all run from the pubic bone, but their insertion sites are different: the puboperineal muscle inserts into the perineal body, the pubovaginal muscle inserts in the vaginal wall at mid-urethra level, and the puboanal muscle inserts in the intersphincteric groove between the internal and external anal sphincters. The different insertion sites give these muscles different roles and functions; the puboperineal muscle pulls the perineal body to the pubis, the pubovaginal muscle elevates the vagina to mid-urethra level, and the puboanal muscle elevates the anus and its attached anoderm. The iliococcygeus muscle arises laterally from the arcus tendineous levator ani and provides lifting forces, which course +41 degrees and +33 degrees, respectively, above the horizontal line in the standing posture. The puborectalis muscle also originates from the pubis. It makes a sling around the rectum to form the anorectal angle. However, its course of action is below the horizontal line, with an angle of –19 degrees (Fig. 17.1) [7].

17.2.1.3 Endopelvic fascia

Support structures are formed by the endopelvic fascia, a connective tissue network that surrounds all pelvic organs and connects them loosely to the pelvic musculature and bones. These tissues are divided into three levels, first described by DeLancey, reflecting the type of support, from cranial to caudal [4].

Level I support: Uterosacral / cardinal ligament complex

The upper third of the vagina and cervix are attached to lateral pelvic sidewalls and the sacrum via the uterosacral and cardinal ligaments, which are composed of connective tissues that contain blood vessels, lymphatics, and nerves. The uterosacral ligaments (USLs) originate from the posterolateral aspect of the cervix at the level of the internal cervical os. However, despite their name, they do not end at the sacrum; instead, they insert in the sacrospinous ligament and the coccygeus muscle complex on the pelvic sidewalls in the majority of women. The general consensus is that there is no direct insertion to the bone, and in only 7% of healthy individuals, they insert in the region of S2–S4 presacral fascia [9].

Level 1 support is similar for both the anterior and posterior compartments, except for one important difference in the posterior section. The uterosacral complex consists of two parts: the ventral superficial, which is visible during surgery, and the deep dorsal, which is below the peritoneum and cannot be seen without dissection. The deep dorsal portion of this complex is important for the posterior compartment because the cardinal ligaments are in a relatively vertical orientation in a standing posture, physiologically, and the dorsally oriented sacrouterine complex prevents the uterus/upper vagina from sliding down the inclined plane of the levator plate.

Loss of level 1 support is correlated with the prolapse of all compartments (apical, anterior, and posterior). However, the answer to the question of which component

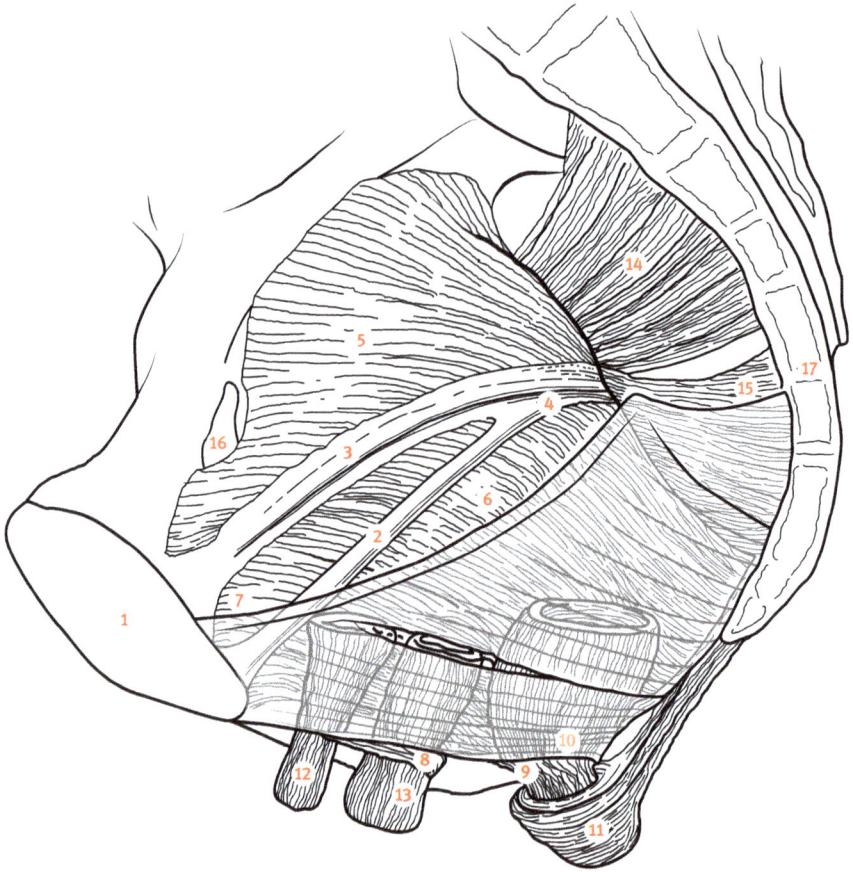

Fig. 17.1: Schematic view of the pelvis from left lateral side: 1. symphysis pubis, 2. arcus tendineus fascia pelvis, 3. arcus tendineus levator ani, 4. ischial spine, 5. obturator internus muscle, 6. iliococcygeus muscle, 7. pubovaginalis muscle, 8. puboperinealis muscle, 9. puboanalis muscle, 10. puborectalis muscle, 11. external anal sphincter, 12. urethra, 13. vagina, 14. priformis muscle, 15. cocygeus muscle, 16. obturator canal, 17. sacrum.

Note that the levator ani consists of three parts: pubovisceralis muscle (also termed as pubococcygeus), puborectalis muscle, and iliococcygeus muscle. The pubovisceralis muscle has also three components: puboperinealis, pubovaginalis, and puboanalis. All of these parts of the levator ani have different lines of action.

The anterior attachment of the arcus tendineus fascia pelvis is to the caudal inner surface of the pubic bone, which is at approximately 4 mm lateral to the pubic symphysis.

(levator ani muscle injury or connective tissue support loss) is more significant in the pathogenesis of POP lies within the fact that the cervix may easily be pulled down to the level of the hymen or pushed up to the level of the sacrum in healthy women with no descensus or prolapse. The pubovisceral portion of levator ani muscle injury has been proven to be the main causative factor in POP (Fig. 17.2) [10–12].

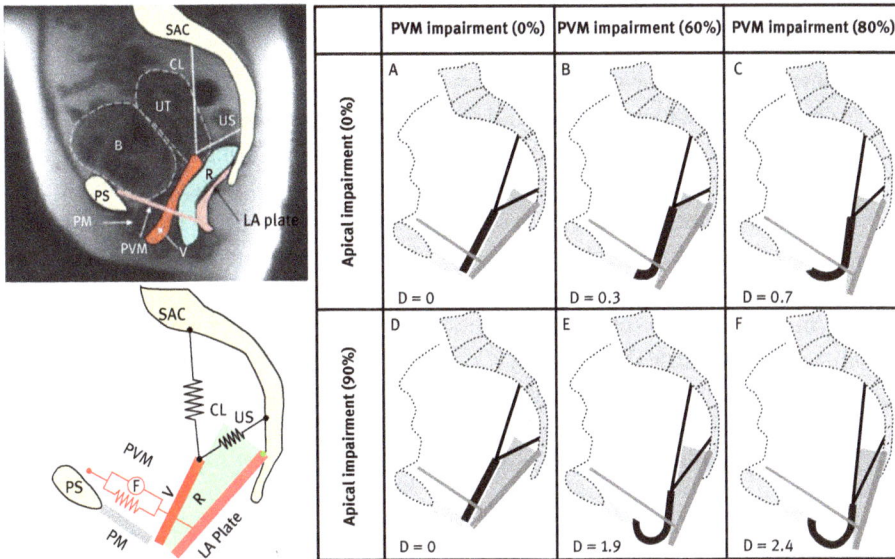

Fig. 17.2: Two-dimensional magnetic resonance (MR) imaging-based biomechanical model showing the effects of pubovisceral muscle impairment and apical (uterosacral/cardinal ligament complex) impairment in the pathogenesis of POP. Left panels show model development: midsagittal MR image and biomechanical model. Right panels show a simulated magnitude of anterior vaginal wall prolapse under maximum Valsalva with various degrees of pubovisceral muscle (PVM) and cardinal / uterosacral complex impairment (indicated in percentage). D represents the size of prolapse measured as the descent of the most dependent point of vaginal wall from the end of the perineal membrane. PVM: Pubovisceral muscle; PS: Pubic symphysis; SAC: Sacrum; PM: Perineal membrane; LA plate: Levator plate; R: Rectum; V: Vagina; CL: Cardinal ligament; US: Uterosacral ligament; B: Bladder; UT: Uterus (Complimentary sharing from Dr. John DeLancey work).

Level II support

This level of support is the continuation of the cardinal ligament complex at the level of the ischial spine, where the middle third of the vagina is attached to the arcus tendineous fasciae pelvis (ATFP) or the "white line." ATFP originates from the ischial spine and ends on the inferior edge of the symphysis pubis, creating a bar-like structure on each side of the pelvic wall for the anterior part of the vagina to attach. At this level, the posterior part of the vagina is attached to the aponeurosis of the levator ani between the ischial spine and perineal body. The loss of level II support results in paravaginal defects and anterior compartment prolapse.

Level III support

This is the most distal part of the support, where the distal third of the vagina and urethra are attached to the perineal membrane and the perineal body and its surrounding structures. The loss of level III support can result in urethral hypermobility, urinary incontinence, and rectocele.

17.2.2 Procedure

The following is a step-by-step description of the procedure:

1. Prepping and positioning: Prep and drape the patient in the dorsal lithotomy posi-
    tion with her legs padded in stirrups. Tuck and pad her arms to minimize nerve
    injury. Despite the fact that the port placements vary from patient to patient, and
    surgeon to surgeon, we prefer to use a three-arm system (three robotic arms and
    one robotic camera = total of four robotic ports) and a 12-mm assistant port. Align
    all ports within about 5–15 degrees and at least 8–10 cm apart when using the
    DaVinci Si® surgical system; an advantage of using the Xi® system is it allows port
    alignment in a straight line with a narrower space between the ports (approxi-
    mately 8 cm). Place the camera port 5–10 cm above the umbilicus for a proper
    view of the sacral promontory. Fig. 17.3 demonstrates the port placements for both
    the DaVinci (Intuitive Surgical, Sunnyvale, CA) Si® and Xi® systems.

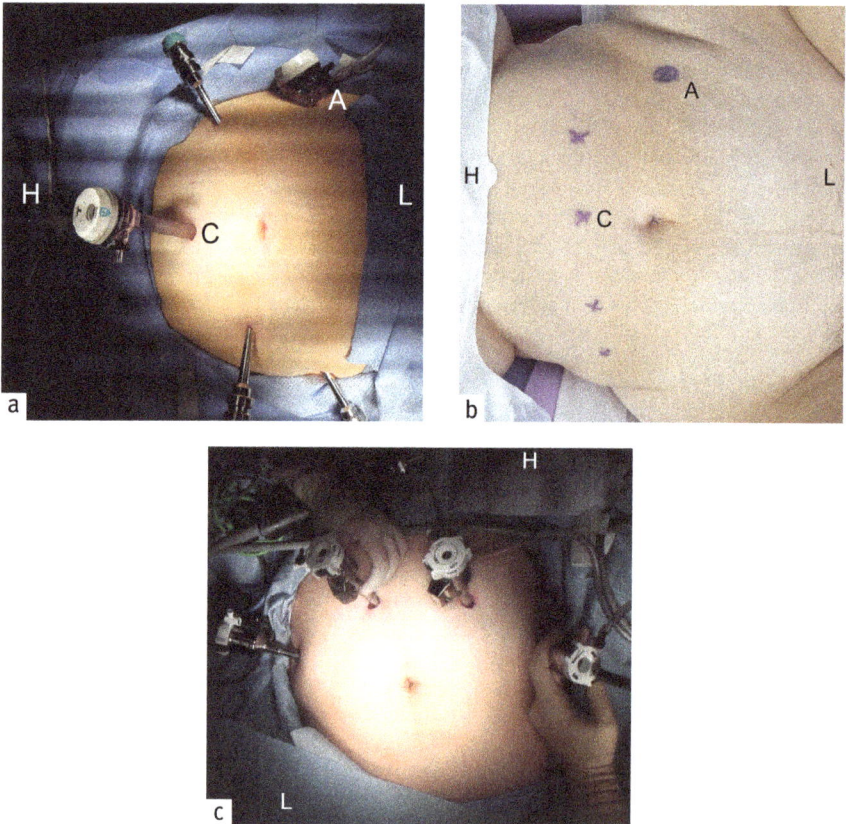

Fig. 17.3: Port placements for the DaVinci (Intuitive Surgical, Sunnyvale, CA) Si® and Xi® systems.
(a) Port placements for the Si® system. (b & c) Port placements for the Xi® system.

2. Creating vesicovaginal and rectovaginal spaces for mesh placement: In a patient with a prior hysterectomy, an EEA™ sizer (Medtronic Inc., MN, USA) may be used by the assistant to manipulate the vaginal cuff. After inspecting the cuff within the pelvis, dissect the peritoneum overlying the cuff with the da Vinci PK™ Dissecting Forceps (advanced bipolar) and monopolar scissors. If a hysterectomy is planned at the time of the procedure, these spaces can be created after uterine vessels are ligated prior to colpotomy, when the uterine manipulator is already in place.

3. Placing the mesh: Place the Y-shaped prolene type 1 mesh in the abdomen and suture it into the anterior and posterior vaginal walls through the previously dissected vesicovaginal and rectovaginal spaces with two barbed sutures on each side in a running fashion. In our practice, we start suturing at the very distal end of the vaginal wall and move proximally. Keep in mind that the sheared forces are strongest at the proximal parts of the "Y," so make sure to appropriately suture the proximal portion of the vaginal walls close to the vaginal apex. We prefer to adjust the arms of "Y" to 6 cm in patients with stage 2 prolapse per the POP-Q system. In patients with stage ≥3 prolapse, we adjust this length to 8 cm. Particular caution must be taken for dissections >8 cm because this area contains periurethral nerves and the vascular plexus.

4. Preparing the sacral promontory: This step requires particular attention since this area includes significant anatomical landmarks. To improve visualization when using a traditional laparoscopy or Xi® robotic system, airplane the patient to the left (10 degrees). The Si® system has to be undocked before repositioning the patient. Through the assistant port, the bedside assistant can sweep the sigmoid colon out of the field using a laparoscopic bowel retractor. Then, identify the track of the right ureter. Next, identify and ligate the middle sacral artery on the sacral promontory. The right common iliac vein is more laterally located from the center of the promontorium than the left common iliac vein (24.00 ± 4.65 vs. 19.00 ± 6.44 mm) [13], and this close proximity of the left common iliac vein to the sacral promontory deserves special attention to avoid major vessel injury at the time of suture placement (Fig. 17.4).

5. Dissecting between the vaginal cuff and sacrum: Once the promontorium is identified, dissect away the peritoneum overlying the sacrum. At this point, you may use one of two techniques (tunneling vs. nontunneling). (1) Using the nontunneling technique, incise the peritoneum between the sacral promontory and the vaginal cuff with sharp scissors to place the mesh under the peritoneum. Then, close the peritoneum in a running fashion at the end of the procedure. (2) Using the tunneling technique, create a peritoneal tunnel between the vaginal cuff and the sacrum without incising the peritoneum. Then, feed the mesh through the tunnel and lay it flat, free of tension. There are two potential advantages of using the tunneling vs. the nontunneling technique. First, less injury to the inferior hypogastric plexus can be anticipated since there is no peritoneal incision. Second, the risk of ureteral kinking can be avoided since there is no need for peritoneal closure. Although there are no published data comparing these two

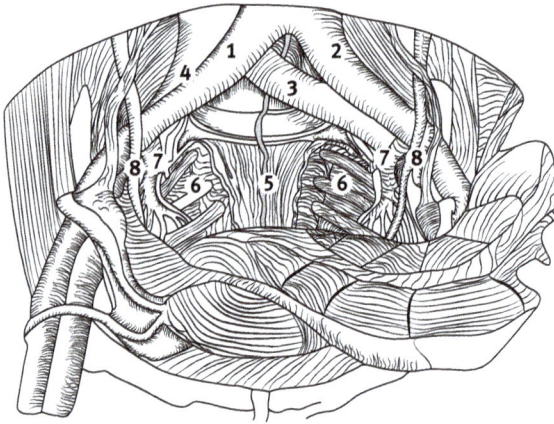

Fig. 17.4: Demonstration of anatomical structures around the sacral promontorium. The close proximity of the left common iliac vein deserves special attention at the time of suture placement. 1. Right common iliac artery; 2. Left common iliac artery; 3. Left common iliac vein; 4. Right common iliac vein; 5. Middle sacral artery; 6. Sacral nerve roots; 7. Internal iliac arteries; 8. Ureters.

methods, our preliminary results show significant improvement in urinary function in patients who underwent surgery via the tunneling technique (Fig. 17.5; unpublished data).

6. Pulling the vaginal cuff: The decision of how much to pull the vaginal cuff depends on the patient's maximum vaginal length and her age. In our practice, we pull the mesh up to two-thirds of the maximum vaginal length in patients younger than 60 years old, but only up to one-half of the maximum vaginal length in patients older than 60 years old. With the assistant's aid, perform this procedure by pushing the EEA™ sizer (Medtronic Inc., MN, USA) into the vagina to measure the maximum length and pulling out one-third to one-half based on the patient's age.

7. Placing sutures in the sacral promontory: Suture the mesh to the anterior longitudinal ligament at the promontorium with a nonabsorbable suture. We prefer to use Gore-Tex® CVO2 (Gore Medical, Newark, USA) or Ethibond® (Ethicon, Somerville, NJ, USA) 2-0 sutures at this stage. Place a minimum of two sutures. On rare occasions, it might be difficult to identify the sacral promontory due to morbid obesity or history of multiple abdominal surgeries. These patients should be counseled about alternative options of apical prolapse surgery, such as high uterosacral vault suspension, as a back-up plan.

17.2.3 Women who would benefit from sacrocolpopexy

Abdominal sacrocolpopexy provides better objective anatomical long-term outcomes when compared to vaginal repairs [14, 15]. Therefore, women with increased

**Improvement in Urinary Function in
Tunneled vs Non-Tunneled SCP**

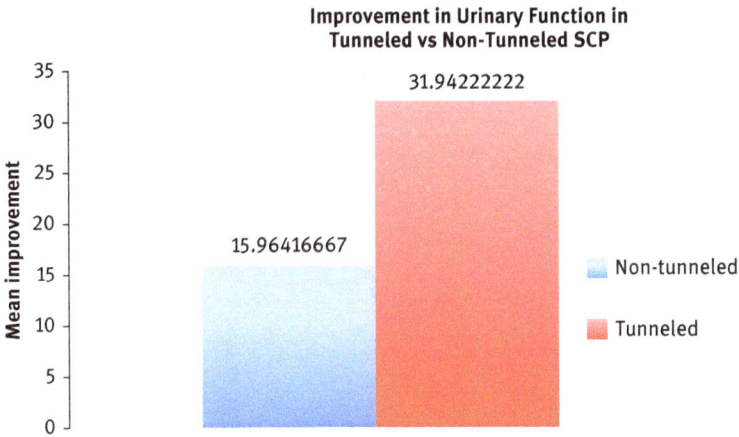

Fig. 17.5: Surgical outcomes of urinary function after tunneled vs. nontunneled robotic sacrocolpopexy.

risk of recurrent prolapse would benefit from sacrocolpopexy. This group includes those with:

– Young age
– Obesity
– Stage IV POP
– Previous failed POP surgery

17.2.4 Surgical outcomes

The long-term outcomes for abdominal sacrocolpopexy have been reported in the extended Colpopexy and Urinary Reduction Efforts (eCARE) trial [16]. This study was initially designed as a randomized controlled trial in women without stress urinary incontinence who underwent abdominal sacrocolpopexy to investigate whether adding a prophylactic Burch urethropexy affects the incidence of *de novo* stress urinary incontinence after POP surgery. The original study's follow-up period was extended to assess the long-term anatomic and symptomatic recurrence of POP. At the 7-year follow-up, the anatomic failure rate was reported as 22% and 27% in patients with and without urethropexy, respectively. Symptomatic failure rates were 24% and 29% and composite failure rates were 34% and 48%, respectively, within the groups. In a systematic review and meta-analysis that included 577 patients who underwent robotic sacrocolpopexy, the anatomic cure rate was reported to be 88.4–100% in a mean follow-up period of 26.9 (range 7–59) months [17]. Patients should be counseled that the long-term reoperation rates for POP after sacrocolpopexy ranges between 2% and 26%, based on long-term study results [18].

17.2.5 Complications

The complication rates from robotic sacrocolpopexy data are reported as follows [17]:

- Mesh exposure/erosion: 4.1% (posterior vagina is the most common site of erosion/exposure, followed by apex and anterior vagina, with a mean follow-up of 26.9 months)
- Reoperation for mesh revision: 1.7%
- Reoperation rate for apical prolapse: 0.8%
- Reoperation rate for nonapical prolapse: 2.5%
- Bladder injury: 2.8%
- Wound infection: 2.4%

The mesh exposure rate after robotic sacrocolpopexy is reported to be slightly higher than open (3.4%) [19] and laparoscopic (2.7%) [20] sacrocolpopexies. The most common site of mesh exposure is the posterior vaginal wall, followed by the apex and anterior vaginal wall. The type of mesh is also important for exposure; the lowest rate was reported for polypropylene (0.5%), followed by polyethylene and polytetrafluoroethylene (3.1% to 5%). The most common reason for reoperation is recurrent prolapse, followed by mesh revision. The majority of the prolapse recurrences occur at the posterior vaginal wall, which suggests that in patients with significant posterior vaginal wall defects, a concomitant posterior repair might be offered in addition to sacrocolpopexy to decrease the risk of possible future reoperation.

In the eCARE trial, the reoperation rate for recurrent prolapse was reported to be 5% and the mesh erosion rate was 10.5% at 7 years [16]. The cases were performed by 25 surgeons from seven different sites, which makes the outcomes more generalizable; however, the types, sizes, configurations of mesh type, numbers of sutures, and procedure techniques were not standardized.

17.3 High uterosacral vault suspension

Understanding the anatomy and dynamics of level 1 support for the uterus and upper vagina is essential, not only because these ligaments are responsible for providing apical support but also because they are strongly related to anterior wall prolapse [21]. Knowing that anterior wall descent is the most common form of POP in almost 85% of cases [22] and the anterior wall is the most common site of failure in the long-term after POP surgery (72% of recurrences) [23] has led us realize that anterior and apical defects are one phenomenon instead of two separate ones. In this section, anatomical relationships and the histology of the USLs will be presented, and practical considerations of high uterosacral vault suspension will be described.

17.3.1 Anatomical considerations

USLs consist of fibroelastic and smooth muscle tissue containing autonomic nerves. They represent the lateral boundaries of the posterior cul-de-sac and are positioned lateral to the rectum. The ligament has a fan-shaped structure with mean widths of 5.2 ± 0.9 cm at its cranial (sacral) portion, 2.7 ± 1.0 cm at its intermediate portion, and 2.0 ± 0.5 cm at its caudal (cervical) portion [24, 25]. Its length has been measured between 12 and 14 cm in cadaver studies [26]; however, magnetic resonance (MR) images of living women reported much shorter measurements, with a mean craniocaudal distance of 2.1 ± 0.8 cm (range 1–5 cm) [9]. This discrepancy could be attributed to the fact that the measurements during MR imaging (MRI) represent the lengths at rest, while cadaver studies require dissections. MRI also aided in understanding the insertion locations of the ligaments. The most common proximal insertion point is the sacrospinous ligament-coccygeus muscle complex (82%), followed by the sacrum (7%). Rarely, the insertion point is at the piriformis muscle, sciatic foramen, or ischial spine. These variations are partly due to the two architectural compartments of the USLs:

- The superficial compartment is the visible portion that is covered by peritoneum and is visible during surgery within the pelvic cavity.
- The deep compartment requires retroperitoneal dissection to be exposed during surgery. It includes parasympathetic fibers from the S2–S4 sacral nerve roots, which join to the superior hypogastric plexus to form the inferior hypogastric plexus or pelvic plexus.

Distal attachments of the ligament are noted to be cervix alone in 33% of individuals, both cervix and vagina in 63%, and only vagina in 4%.

17.3.2 Histology and mechanical characteristics of the USLs

The content and texture of USLs are not uniform along their length; three different histologic regions have been identified [27]. At the one-third distal portion (cervical), the ligament consists of closely packed bundles of smooth muscle, along with medium- and small-sized blood vessels and small nerve bundles. The intermediate third of the ligament is predominantly composed of connective tissue with few nerve elements and blood vessels. This portion includes less smooth muscle when compared to the distal third. The proximal third (sacral) is almost entirely composed of loose connective tissue with intermingled fat, a few vessels, nerves, and lymphatics. This histological architecture gives different tensile strengths to these portions, making the distal part the strongest, followed by the intermediate part. The proximal portion is the weakest. In a cadaver study, the distal portion was shown to support a weight of >37.4 lbs (17 kg) before it failed at the level of the cervix and ischial spines, whereas the sacral portion failed at 11 lbs (5 kg) [24]. Studies in living women show that a much smaller amount of force is needed to move the uterus and stretch the ligament: 1 lb (0.45 kg) of force is enough to move the uterus 12 mm *in vivo* [28]. This difference might be explained by the fact that the tissues are pre-conditioned in *in vitro* trials, wherein they are tensioned a few times prior to actual measurement, which might affect the tensile strength. More studies are needed to clarify this discrepancy.

Opposed to general belief, USLs are not elastic structures, and ligament stiffness is not correlated with POP [29]. However, ligament length is noted to be a strong predictor of POP-Q, supporting the logic behind the uterosacral vault suspension—the shorter the ligament, the stronger the apical support, and the lesser the risk of pelvic descent.

17.3.3 Lines of action of pelvic support structures

As previously mentioned, the levator ani muscle, the main support system, has sub-divisons with different functions. The pubovisceral fibers course +41 degrees and the iliococygeus fibers course +33 degrees above the horizontal line in a standing posture, whereas this line is −19 degrees for the puborectal muscle [7]. The anal sphincter's line of action is also below the horizontal line. Also, the pubovisceral, iliococcygeus, and puborectal muscles have horizontal fibers that work together as a horizontal force that closes the levator hiatus. Regarding connective tissues, the cardinal liga-ment has almost a vertical direction in a standing position, whereas the USLs has an angle of +18 degrees above the horizontal line [7]. The vectoral summary for the lines of action of these structures is as follows:

– Vertical vectors: The pubovisceral and iliococcygeus muscles and the cardinal ligament together act as lifting forces to prevent pelvic descent.
– Horizontal vectors: The horizontal fibers of the pubovisceral, iliococcygeus, and puborectal muscles work as a closing force, as noted above, while the USLs act as a rope that ties the ship (the uterus and upper vagina) to the deck (the presacral fascia), preventing these structures from sliding down the inclined plane of the levator plate.

17.3.4 Procedure

Identify the ureters: Identify the ureters, and make a 2–3-cm peritoneal incision between the USL and the ureter on each side with scissors (Fig. 17.6a,b).
1. *Lateralize the ureters*: Once the peritoneal incision is made, laterally dissect the ureters to avoid ureteral kinking (Fig. 17.6b).

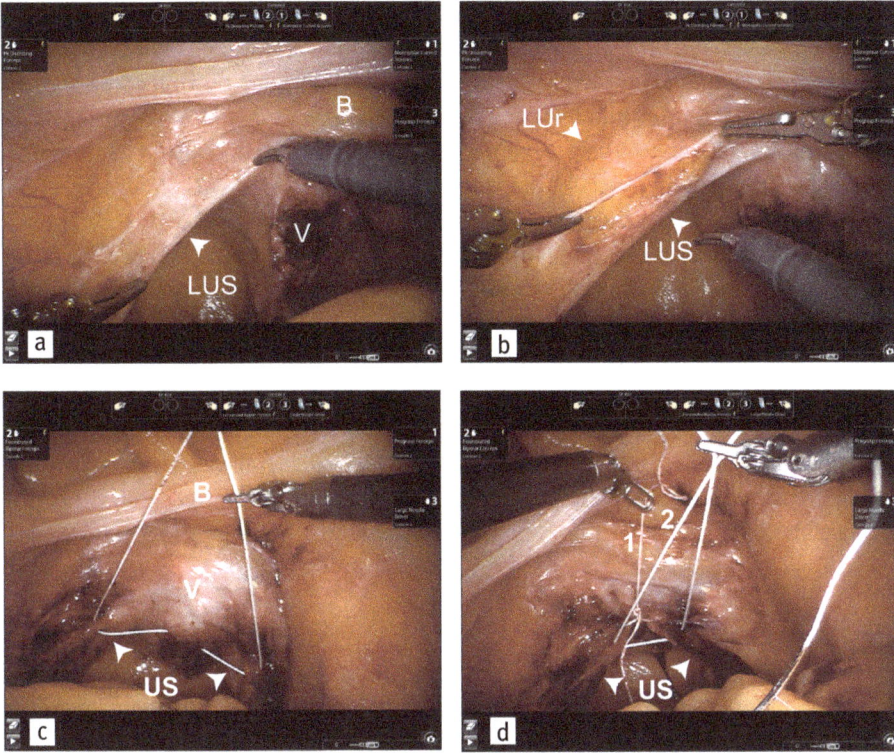

Fig. 17.6: Demonstration of robotic high uterosacral vault suspension. (a) Identification of the ureters. (b) A 2–3-cm peritoneal incision is made between the uterosacral ligament and the ureter on each side with scissors. Once the peritoneal incision is made, the ureters are dissected laterally to avoid ureteral kinking. (c) Placement of the first suture. (d) Placement of the second suture. LUS: Left uterosacral ligament; V: Vaginal cuff; B: Bladder; LUr: Left ureter; US: Bilateral uterosacrals.

2. Place a 2/0 nonabsorbable suture in the midportion of the right USL, and attach it to the midline vaginal apex, including both posterior and anterior vaginal walls. Incorporate the left side mid-USL with the same suture, and tie it (Fig. 17.6c).
3. Place another 2/0 nonabsorbable suture approximately 1 cm proximal to the first suture, which includes both USLs. The aim of this suture is to relieve the tension and support the first suture (Fig. 17.6d).
4. Perform a cystoscopy at the end of the procedure to confirm bilateral ureteral efflux.

17.3.5 Outcomes

Data regarding surgical outcomes for USL suspension are mostly from vaginal route procedures, but studies comparing vaginal and laparoscopic routes showed similar success and complication rates [30, 31]. A systematic review and meta-analysis of

11 studies that included 930 patients with a median follow-up of 25 months reported pooled success rates of 81.1%, 98.3%, and 87.4% for the anterior, apical, and posterior compartments, respectively [32]. A successful anatomic outcome was defined as POP-Q stage 0 or 1 in this review. The higher degree of POP-Q stage in the anterior compartment prior to the procedure was related to less successful postoperative outcomes (92% success rate with preoperative stage 2 anterior wall prolapse vs. 67% success rate with preoperative stage 3). The results regarding subjective symptoms were reassuring, with a rate of 82–100% for symptom relief; however, the data could not be pooled due to methodological differences between the studies. The reoperation rate for symptomatic prolapse or stress incontinence was reported to be 9% (only four studies reported data). Improvement in bowel symptoms was modest but did not reach statistical significance. Dyspareunia was relieved in 68–100% of patients (only in two studies), but 25% of patients still reported mild or severe dyspareunia postoperatively. Data regarding the effect of the uterosacral vault suspension on ≥stage 3 posterior vaginal wall prolapse are lacking, and further research is needed for clarification.

17.3.6 Complications

The most common, but also the most worrisome, complication of the procedure is ureteral kinking, which is approximately 11%, based on previous reports [33, 34]. This occurrence is not surprising when the close proximity of the ureters, USLs, and suspension sutures is taken into account. In a study of 15 embalmed female cadavers, in which the distance between the ureter and the USL was investigated, mean distances of 0.9 ± 0.4, 2.3 ± 0.9, and 4.1 ± 0.6 cm were measured in the cervical, intermediate, and sacral portions of the USLs, respectively [24]. The ischial spine was consistently beneath the intermediate portion, and the distance from the ischial spine to the ureter was 4.9 ± 2.0 cm. In another study, in which 15 unembalmed female cadavers were included, the distance between uterosacral vault suspension sutures to the ureter was measured and the mean distance was noted to be 14 mm for both proximal and distal sutures [35]. The discrepancy between these two studies could be explained by the different tissue characteristics in embalmed vs. unembalmed cadavers and the pliability of the fresh tissue potentially affecting ureteral position. To prevent this complication, ureteral patency should be checked via cystoscopy after both sutures are tied. If both ureters do not efflux briskly, the sutures should be removed, starting with the proximal one.

Another complication is sacral nerve entrapment. In the study by Wieslander *et al.* [35], suspension sutures were noted to be at the level of the S1 in 43.8%, the S2 in 33.3%, and the S3 in 22.9% of specimens. One of the 48 sutures entrapped the third sacral nerve. The proximal sutures were located at a level medial to the sacral foramina in 38.5% of the specimens, anterior in 42.3%, and lateral in 19.2%.

The distal sutures were located at a level medial to the sacral foramina in 31.8% of the specimens, anterior in 10.9%, and lateral in only 27.3%. These findings were in line with the study by Siddique *et al.*, in which the anatomical relationship of USLs to the sacral plexus was investigated in six embalmed female cadavers [36]. The authors demonstrated that the mean distances between USLs and the S4, S3, S2, and S1 trunks superior to the ischial spine (the level of intermediate portion of USLs where sutures are commonly placed) were 0.9 cm, 1.5 cm, 2.6 cm, and 3.9 cm, respectively, placing S2–S4 at more risk to nerve injury during uterosacral vault suspension. These observations from cadaver studies are supported by case series and retrospective reviews of patients who underwent uterosacral vault suspension. Flynn *et al.*, in a review of 182 patients, identified seven women with sensory neuropathy and pain in the S2–S3 dermatomes immediately during the postoperative period (substantial sharp buttock pain and numbness that radiated down the center of the posterior thigh to the popliteal fossa in one or both lower extremities) [37]. Pelvic examinations were nonspecific in four women; however, in the other three women, the pain was exacerbated by pulling on the ipsilateral uterosacral suture, suggesting nerve entrapment in these patients. Therefore, the authors decided to remove the ipsilateral USL sutures (within 4 days of the procedure) in three women; these women experienced immediate subjective pain reduction and complete resolution of pain by 6 weeks. The remaining four women were treated conservatively (physical therapy, nonsteroidal anti-inflammatory drugs, gabapentin) and had symptom resolution up to 6 months postoperatively.

Acknowledgment: Authors thank Dr. John DeLancey for graciously sharing his work used on Figure 17.2

References

[1] Jones KA, Shepherd JP, Oliphant SS, Wang L, Bunker CH, Lowder JL. Trends in inpatient prolapse procedures in the United States, 1979–2006. Am J Obstet Gynecol 2010; 202:501.e1–7.

[2] Olsen AL, Smith VJ, Bergstrom JO, Colling JC, Clark AL. Epidemiology of surgically managed pelvic organ prolapse and urinary incontinence. Obstet Gynecol 1997;89:501–6.

[3] Kurkijärvi K, Aaltonen R, Gissler M, Mäkinen J. Pelvic organ prolapse surgery in Finland from 1987 to 2009: A national register based study. Eur J Obstet Gynecol Reprod Biol 2017;214:71–7.

[4] DeLancey JO. Anatomic aspects of vaginal eversion after hysterectomy. Am J Obstet Gynecol 1992;166:1717–24.

[5] Summers A, Winkel LA, Kussain H, DeLancey JOL. The relationship between anterior and apical compartment support. Am J Obstet Gynecol 2006;194:1438–43.

[6] Eilber KS, Alperin M, Khan A, et al. Outcomes of vaginal prolapse surgery among female Medicare beneficiaries: the role of apical support. Obstet Gynecol. 2013;122:981–7.

[7] DeLancey JO. What's new in the functional anatomy of pelvic organ prolapse? Curr Opin Obstet Gynecol. 2016;28:420–9.

[8] Kearney R, Sawhney R, DeLancey JO. Levator ani muscle anatomy evaluated by origin-insertion pairs. Obstet Gynecol 2004;104:168–73.

[9] Umek WH, Morgan DM, Ashton-Miller JA, DeLancey JO. Quantitative analysis of uterosacral ligament origin and insertion points by magnetic resonance imaging. Obstet Gynecol 2004;103:447–51.

[10] DeLancey JO, Morgan DM, Fenner DE, et al. Comparison of levator ani muscle defects and function in women with and without pelvic organ prolapse. Obstet Gynecol 2007;109:295–302.

[11] Dietz HP, Simpson JM. Levator trauma is associated with pelvic organ prolapse. BJOG 2008;115:979–84.

[12] DeLancey JO, Sørensen HC, Lewicky-Gaupp C, Smith TM. Comparison of the puborectal muscle on MRI in women with POP and levator ani defects with those with normal support and no defect. Int Urogynecol J 2012;23:73–7.

[13] Akhgar J, Terai H, Suhrab Rahmani M, et al. Anatomical location of the common iliac veins at the level of the sacrum: relationship between perforation risk and the trajectory angle of the screw. Biomed Res Int 2016;2016:1457219.

[14] Maher C, Feiner B, Baessler K, Schmid C. Surgical management of pelvic organ prolapse in women. Cochrane Database Syst Rev 2013;4:CD004014.

[15] Siddiqui NY, Grimes CL, Casiano ER, et al. Mesh sacrocolpopexy compared with native tissue vaginal repair: a systematic review and meta-analysis. Obstet Gynecol 2015;125:44–55.

[16] Nygaard I, Brubaker L, Zyczynski HM, et al. Long-term outcomes following abdominal sacrocolpopexy for pelvic organ prolapse. JAMA 2013;309:2016–24.

[17] Hudson CO, Northington GM, Lyles RH, Karp DR. Outcomes of robotic sacrocolpopexy: a systematic review and meta-analysis. Female Pelvic Med Reconstr Surg 2014;20:252–60.

[18] Hilger WS, Poulson M, Norton PA. Long-term results of abdominal sacrocolpopexy. Am J Obstet Gynecol 2003;189:1610–1.

[19] Nygaard IE, McCreery R, Brubaker L, et al. Abdominal sacrocolpopexy: a comprehensive review. Obstet Gynecol 2004;104:805–23.

[20] Ganatra AM, Rozet F, Sanchez-Salas R, et al. The current status of laparoscopic sacrocolpopexy: a review. Eur Urol 2009;55:1089–103.

[21] Rooney K, Kenton K, Mueller ER, FitzGerald MP, Brubaker L. Advanced anterior vaginal wall prolapse is highly correlated with apical prolapse. Am J Obstet Gynecol 2006;195:1837–40.

[22] Hendrix SL, Clark A, Nygaard I, Aragaki A, Barnabei V, McTiernan A. Pelvic organ prolapse in Women's Health Initiative: gravity and gravidity. Am J Obstet Gynecol 2002;186:1160–6.

[23] Fialkow MF, Newton KM, Weiss NS. Incidence of recurrent pelvic organ prolapse 10 years following primary surgical management: a retrospective cohort study. Int Urogynecol J Pelvic Floor Dysfunct 2008;19:1483–7.

[24] Buller JL, Thomson JR, Cundiff GR, Krueger Sullivan L, Schön Ybarra MA, Bent AE. Uterosacral ligament: description of anatomic relationships to optimize surgical safety. Obstet Gynecol 2001;97:873–9.

[25] Ramanah R, Berger MB, Parratte BM, DeLancey JO. Anatomy and histology of apical support: a literature review concerning cardinal and uterosacral ligaments. Int Urogynecol J 2012;23:1483–94.

[26] Vu D, Haylen BT, Tse K, Farnsworth A. Surgical anatomy of the uterosacral ligament. Int Urogynecol J 2010;21:1123–8.

[27] Campbell RM. The anatomy and histology of the sacrouterine ligaments. Am J Obstet Gynecol 1950;59:1–12.

[28] Bartscht KD, DeLancey JO. A technique to study the passive supports of the uterus. Obstet Gynecol 1988;72:940–3.

[29] Smith TM, Luo J, Hsu Y, Ashton-Miller J, Delancey JO. A novel technique to measure in vivo uterine suspensory ligament stiffness. Am J Obstet Gynecol 2013;209:484.e1–7.

[30] Lin LL, Phelps JY, Liu CY. Laparoscopic vaginal vault suspension using uterosacral ligaments: a review of 133 cases. J Minim Invasive Gynecol. 2005;12:216–20.

[31] Rardin CR, Erekson EA, Sung VW, Ward RM, Myers DL. Uterosacral colpopexy at the time of vaginal hysterectomy: comparison of laparoscopic and vaginal approaches. J Reprod Med 2009;54:273–80.

[32] Margulies RU, Rogers MA, Morgan DM. Outcomes of transvaginal uterosacral ligament suspension: systematic review and metaanalysis. Am J Obstet Gynecol 2010;202:124–34.

[33] Barber MD, Visco AG, Weidner AC, Amundsen CL, Bump RC. Bilateral uterosacral ligament vaginal vault suspension with site-specific endopelvic fascia defect repair for treatment of pelvic organ prolapse. Am J Obstet Gynecol 2000;183:1402–11.

[34] Karram M, Goldwasser S, Kleeman S, Steele A, Vassallo B, Walsh P. High uterosacral vaginal vault suspension with fascial reconstruction for vaginal repair of enterocele and vaginal vault prolapse. Am J Obstet Gynecol 2001;185:1339–43.

[35] Wieslander CK, Roshanravan SM, Wai CY, Schaffer JI, Corton MM. Uterosacral ligament suspension sutures: Anatomic relationships in unembalmed female cadavers. Am J Obstet Gynecol. 2007;197:672.e1–6.

[36] Siddique SA, Gutman RE, Schön Ybarra MA, Rojas F, Handa VL. Relationship of the uterosacral ligament to the sacral plexus and to the pudendal nerve. Int Urogynecol J Pelvic Floor Dysfunct 2006;17:642–5.

[37] Flynn MK, Weidner AC, Amundsen CL. Sensory nerve injury after uterosacral ligament suspension. Am J Obstet Gynecol 2006; 195: 1869–72.

Rufus Cartwright and Natalia Price

18 Laparoscopic management of mesh complications

18.1 Introduction

Despite serious safety concerns, rates of incontinence and prolapse surgeries incorporating polypropylene meshes have increased over the last two decades [1, 2]. A large majority of current incontinence procedures utilize either retropubic or transobturator synthetic polypropylene slings [3–5], with increasing adoption of abdominal polypropylene mesh procedures including hysteropexy for uterine prolapse and sacrocolpopexy for vault prolapse [6, 7]. Use of vaginal prolapse mesh was rapidly adopted, reaching more than 40% of vaginal prolapse procedures in the United States by 2009 [8], but this proportion has fallen sharply in the United States [9, 10] and many other countries [11, 12] after the Food and Drug Administration warnings of 2008 and 2011. Despite European consensus guidance [13], also urging caution, vaginal prolapse mesh use remains common across many parts of Europe [5], with worrying variation in practice both between [5] and within different countries [14].

The earliest studies using polypropylene slings and meshes [15, 16] identified few complications. Subsequent studies have identified serious complications including mesh exposure or extrusion through the vaginal mucosa; erosion into the bladder, urethra, or bowel; negative impacts on bladder or bowel function; and pelvic pain or dyspareunia caused by mesh shrinkage or direct nerve impingement. In medium-to long-term follow-up, polypropylene incontinence slings have been found to have 10% risk of hospitalization for complications [17, 18] and 3–10% reoperation rates [17, 19–21]. Vaginal prolapse meshes have been associated with an 11% risk of mesh erosion and 7% risk of reoperation for mesh erosion in randomized trials [22]. Outside of trial settings, complications have been even more common, as demonstrated in a large Scottish population-based study [18], where vaginal prolapse mesh was associated with a 20% risk of hospitalization for complications and a 20% risk of reoperation. This difference can perhaps be accounted for by the observation that mesh complications are more common for low volume surgeons and where prolapse and incontinence meshes are used together [23]. Abdominal open or laparoscopic sacrocolpopexy is associated with around a 3% risk of mesh erosion [24], around an 11% risk of hospitalization for complications [18], and a 5% risk of reoperation for complications [25]. Rates of chronic pain and dyspareunia in real-world practice are not well characterized for any of these types of mesh procedure, but in trial settings have ranged from as low as 2% for incontinence slings [26], up to a 40% risk with vaginal prolapse meshes in some studies [22]. While reoperations for pain remain relatively uncommon, persistent pain remains one of the leading causes of litigation.

https://doi.org/10.1515/9783110535204-018

Most mesh erosions into the vagina, urethra, or bladder, and most cases of dyspareunia associated with mesh, can be dealt with using an entirely vaginal approach, and techniques for this are described elsewhere [27]. However, as media attention has highlighted safety concerns about mesh, more women are requesting complete excision of mesh, which cannot typically be achieved vaginally. This chapter describes primarily the laparoscopic techniques for dealing with these mesh-related complications, including excision of the abdominal portion of retropubic mesh slings, as well as abdominally placed meshes for hysteropexy and sacrocolpopexy. In the following sections, we address the indications for such complete mesh excision, the preoperative work-up, specific surgical approaches and considerations, and, where available, the patient outcomes.

18.2 Indications

Media coverage of mesh complications has led some patients to attribute very diverse symptoms to insertion of mesh, including chronic fatigue, fibromyalgia, and chronic pain distant from the pelvis. Patients may also have psychological morbidity, rooted in anxieties about long-term harms of mesh. While polypropylene mesh may cause significant chronic inflammation [28] with associated local pain, there is little evidence for systemic effects of mesh [29], and certainly no evidence for human carcinogenesis [30, 31]. As discussed later in the chapter, there is moderate evidence for resolution of pelvic pain following mesh excision for some, but not all, patients. Mesh erosions into vagina, bladder, or urethra can also be effectively addressed, but there is little evidence for other benefits of mesh removal. Preoperative counseling must address patients' expectations for the surgery and set realistic goals for improvement. Patients must understand the alternatives to operative management including vaginal estrogens, specialist physiotherapy, and medications to optimize bladder and bowel function. Patients must be made aware that mesh excision can be associated with major immediate complications, and potential for recurrent prolapse or incontinence, depending on which portion of mesh is excised. While some surgeons are performing simultaneous mesh excision and reimplantation of either mesh [17] or autologous fascia [32], recurrence of either prolapse or incontinence is difficult to predict. In our own center, we would typically favor a second stage nonmesh procedure only if patients do develop *de novo* symptoms, a strategy supported by other expert opinion [27].

18.3 Preoperative investigations

There remains very little evidence to rationalize preoperative investigation before mesh excision. Vaginal erosions should be excluded with careful examination, if necessary under anesthesia. Where erosion into the lower urinary tract is suspected, consider cystoscopy before definitive surgery to enable surgical planning. Similarly, when bowel involvement is suspected, consider rectosigmoidoscopy. Pelvic imaging including translabial or transvaginal ultrasound or pelvic MRI scan may be particularly informative where previous attempts have been made to partially excise the mesh, or when chronic infection or abscess is suspected, and can help exclude other causes of pelvic pain. Urodynamics or defecating proctography may also be indicated depending on the nature of the patient's symptoms.

18.4 Laparoscopic techniques for excision of retropubic midurethral slings

A three-port laparoscopy is performed using a 0-degree laparoscope. The bladder is instilled with 300 ml of normal saline with methylene blue, to help delineate the dome of the bladder. With the patient in the Trendelenburg position, the retropubic space is opened using a monopolar hook at 2 cm above the bladder reflection. A plane of loose areolar tissue can be easily developed from this correct incision point. With careful blunt dissection the space of Retzius is developed, and the bladder is reflected down bilaterally to expose the urethra and sphincter complex in the midline, and the obturator vessels and nerves bilaterally, similar to the dissection for a laparoscopic colposuspension. The arms of the mesh can then be identified, and the relation of the mesh to the important structures in the retropubic space can be assessed at this stage. The mesh arms may sometimes be found deviated from what would be an optimal insertion. For a retropubic sling, the most proximal portion visible can be dissected from the abdominal wall using monopolar hook or scissors. The free edge is then grasped with a toothed grasper, and under traction, the mesh can be sharply dissected out from the surrounding structures. This can be continued down to the level of the vagina where the tape is divided. If a patient opts for total excision, the vaginal portion of the tape is best excised first before undertaking the laparoscopy as this helps define the limit of the laparoscopic dissection. Once hemostasis is assured in retropubic space, the peritoneal edges can be sutured using a single continuous polyglactin suture. Excised portions of mesh should be retained for microbiological culture [33] and histological examination [34]. Many meshes excised for vaginal erosion will show bacterial colonization [33], but there is occasional evidence of infection of meshes that have not eroded [35].

18.5 Laparoscopic techniques for excision of apical meshes

Again, a minimum three-port laparoscopy is performed using a 0-degree laparoscope. With the patient in Trendelenburg position any adhesions are divided, and a careful assessment is made of adhesions or bowel herniation related to the mesh. The bowel

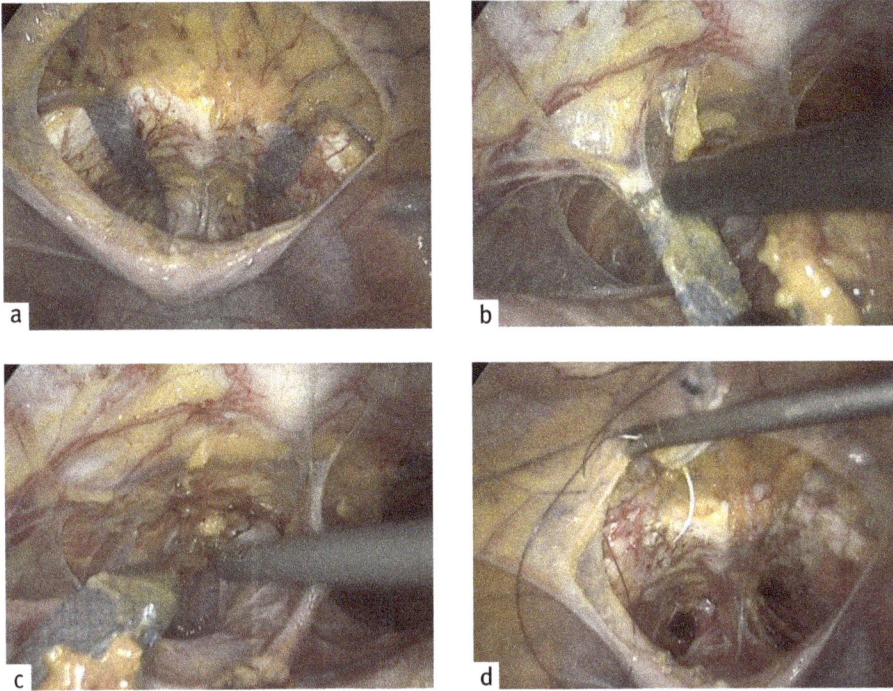

Fig. 18.1: Laparoscopic excision of retropubic sling arm. (a) The cave of Retzius is opened showing the course of both arms. (b) With traction on the end of one arm, dissection commences using monopolar hook. (c) The dissection is extended to the suburethral portion. (d) The peritoneal incision is closed using monofilament suture.

is mobilized to expose the promontory and right pelvic sidewall. The peritoneum over the promontory is lifted with a grasper and opened using diathermy. With traction on the mesh, sharp and blunt dissection can be used to free the mesh and any capsule from the surrounding tissue. Devices used to fix the mesh to the promontory, such as Pro-Tack staples, may be difficult to remove, but this should be attempted if there is suspicion of sacral osteomyelitis. The mesh itself can be followed toward the vault or cervix, with dissection proceeding with constant awareness of the path of the right ureter, rectosigmoid colon, and vessels, which may be dragged toward the mesh by chronic inflammatory processes. Again, excised portions of the mesh should be reserved for microbiological and histological analysis.

18.6 Laparoscopic techniques for excision of meshes eroding into the bladder or urethra

Various vaginal and cystoscopic techniques have been described for excision of mesh eroding the urethra or bladder, including use of cystoscopic trimming [36], or ablation with a holmium laser [37], all of which carry a high risk of recurrence of erosions. Several small case series have described vesicoscopic approaches to vesical mesh erosions. The earliest technique described by Maher and colleagues [38] does not require bladder insufflation but uses a large 5-cm cystotomy for adequate access. In the technique described by Grange and colleagues [39], the bladder is filled with CO_2 using a urethral catheter and then suspended from the anterior abdominal wall, before an incision is made at the dome. Sarlos and colleagues [40] recommend filling the bladder to 200 ml, and routinely place bilateral ureteric stents before entering at the dome. This approach may provide optimal exposure for mesh erosions close to or within the trigone, as may be typical with vaginal prolapse meshes, or the anterior arm of a sacrocolpopexy mesh. These techniques allow removal of intraluminal and submucosal mesh but leave the intramural portion of the mesh, with a risk of recurrence of mesh erosion.

Midurethral slings typically erode more laterally in the bladder. A modification of these techniques for retropubic slings can be used for total laparoscopic excision of an eroding sling without cystotomy at the dome (Fig. 18.2). One case series has recommended combined cystoscopy and laparoscopy, to help avert ureteric

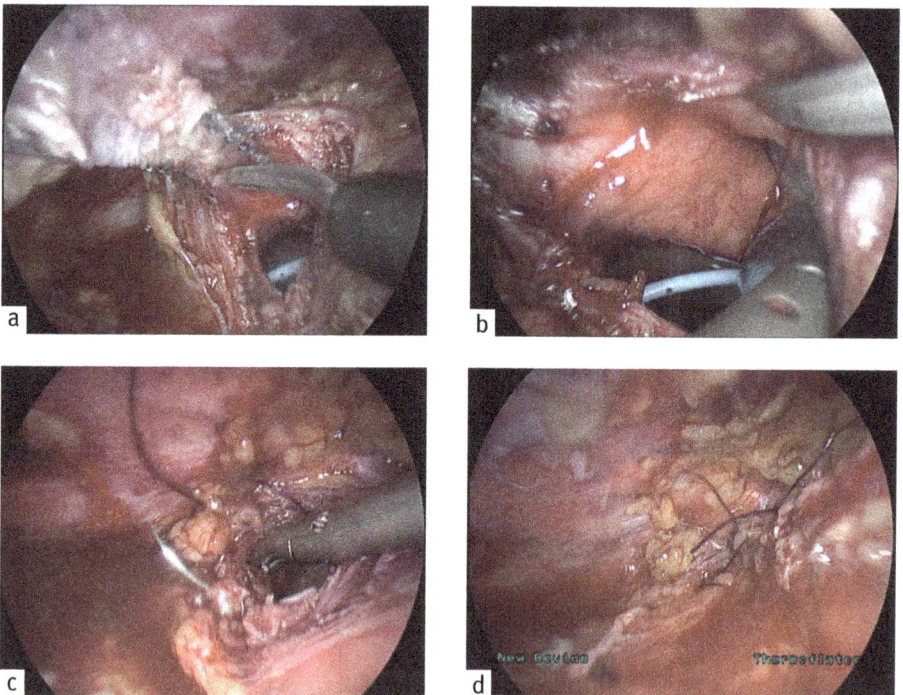

Fig. 18.2: Laparoscopic excision of mesh eroding into the bladder. (a) A cystotomy is made where the tape breaches the bladder wall. (b) The tape is completely freed from the bladder using scissors. (c) The cystotomy is sutured in two layers with polyglactin suture. (d) A check for watertight closure is made.

injury [41] with a lateral cystotomy. Our own group uses ureteric stenting to help avoid such injuries. We use the same extra peritoneal approach as for excision of noneroding midurethral slings. The sling arms are dissected down to the bladder wall. The cystotomy is then made where the sling erodes into the bladder, minimizing the trauma to the bladder still further. In contrast to the earlier techniques, this method allows complete excision of the intramural portion of the mesh, preventing any recurrence of erosion. The same technique can be used to dissect slings that have eroded the urethra. Some authors have combined laparoscopic excision with a midline vaginal division of the tape [41] to help free the mesh from the urethra. If possible, a total laparoscopic approach is always preferable, as it eliminates the risk of urethrovaginal fistulas. As in the other techniques, the cystotomy is closed in two layers using a polyglactin suture. An indwelling catheter is left for 2 weeks to allow bladder healing, with a cystogram performed at 2 weeks postoperation, prior to the catheter removal.

18.7 Patient outcomes after laparoscopic mesh excision

The few available case series suggest that total laparoscopic excision of mesh is typically safe and feasible, but the evidence regarding patient outcomes is less clear [42] and may vary by indication. A handful of case reports describe the excision of mesh for sacral osteomyelitis, with apparently good outcomes [24, 43, 44]. Similarly, where the major concern is erosion into the lower urinary tract, the few small case series of laparoscopic management [38, 39, 45] suggest approximately a 10% risk of recurrent erosion, which compares favorably to cystoscopic approaches. Improvement in pain is variable [46]. The largest available laparoscopic series, while still providing only low-quality evidence, suggest that 68–100% of patients will experience improvement in pain [35, 47], which provides some basis on which to counsel patients. Some evidence suggests that obturator neuralgia is much more likely to improve than pudendal neuralgia [48], but otherwise, factors predicting improvement in pain are unclear. It is also difficult to counsel patients about the risk of recurrent stress incontinence after removal of slings, with estimates of new-onset stress incontinence ranging from 22% to 53% [35, 47], with an additional risk of new onset urgency incontinence.

18.8 Conclusion

The laparoscopic approach for excision of retropubic tapes and apical prolapse meshes has numerous advantages over vaginal or open approaches. These include precise dissection under direct vision, which gives better exposure and identification of anatomical structures, and the opportunity for a complete excision to prevent recurrence. Despite these advantages, patient outcomes remain very difficult to predict. Resolution of pain cannot be guaranteed, and the impact of surgery on lower urinary tract symptoms is also variable. The key to successful surgery is therefore careful pre-operative counseling, so that patients have realistic expectations for improvement.

References

[1] Wu JM, Gandhi MP, Shah AD, Shah JY, Fulton RG, Weidner AC. Trends in inpatient urinary incontinence surgery in the USA, 1998–2007. Int Urogynecol J 2011;22:1437–43.

[2] Jonsson Funk M, Edenfield AL, Pate V, Visco AG, Weidner AC, Wu JM. Trends in use of surgical mesh for pelvic organ prolapse. Am J Obstet Gynecol 2013;208:79.e1–7.

[3] Gibson W, Wagg A. Are older women more likely to receive surgical treatment for stress urinary incontinence since the introduction of the mid-urethral sling? An examination of Hospital Episode Statistics data. BJOG 2016;123:1386–92.

[4] Kurkijärvi K, Aaltonen R, Gissler M, Mäkinen J. Surgery for stress urinary incontinence in Finland 1987–2009. Int Urogynecol J 2016;27:1021–7.

[5] Haya N, Baessler K, Christmann-Schmid C, et al. Prolapse and continence surgery in countries of the Organization for Economic Cooperation and Development in 2012. Am J Obstet Gynecol 2015;212:755.e1–7.

[6] Elterman DS, Chughtai BI, Vertosick E, Maschino A, Eastham JA, Sandhu JS. Changes in pelvic organ prolapse surgery in the last decade among United States urologists. J Urol 2014;191:1022–7.

[7] Madsen AM, Raker C, Sung VW. Trends in hysteropexy and apical support for uterovaginal prolapse in the United States from 2002 to 2012. Female Pelvic Med Reconstr Surg 2017;23:365–71.

[8] Khan AA, Eilber KS, Clemens JQ, Wu N, Pashos CL, Anger JT. Trends in management of pelvic organ prolapse among female Medicare beneficiaries. Am J Obstet Gynecol 2015;212:463.e1–8.

[9] Sedrakyan A, Chughtai B, Mao J. Regulatory warnings and use of surgical mesh in pelvic organ prolapse. JAMA Intern Med 2016;176:275–7.

[10] Younger A, Rac G, Clemens JQ, et al. Pelvic organ prolapse surgery in academic female pelvic medicine and reconstructive surgery urology practice in the setting of the food and drug administration public health notifications. Urology 2016;91:46–51.

[11] Jha S, Cutner A, Moran P. The UK National Prolapse Survey: 10 years on. Int Urogynecol J 2017;26:325–7.

[12] Plata M, Bravo-Balado A, Robledo D. Trends in pelvic organ prolapse management in Latin America. Neurourol Urodyn 2017;194:1455.

[13] Chapple CR, Cruz F, Deffieux X, et al. Consensus statement of the European Urology Association and the European Urogynaecological Association on the use of implanted materials for treating pelvic organ prolapse and stress urinary incontinence. Eur Urol 2017;72:424–31.

[14] van IJsselmuiden MN, Detollenaere RJ, Kampen MY, Engberts MK, van Eijndhoven HWF. Practice pattern variation in surgical management of pelvic organ prolapse and urinary incontinence in the Netherlands. Int Urogynecol J 2015;26:1649–56.

[15] Ulmsten U, Falconer C, Johnson P, et al. A multicenter study of tension-free vaginal tape (TVT) for surgical treatment of stress urinary incontinence. Int Urogynecol J Pelvic Floor Dysfunct 2998;9:210–3.

[16] Bader G, Fauconnier A, Roger N, Heitz D, Ville Y. [Cystocele repair by vaginal approach with a tension-free transversal polypropylene mesh. Technique and results]. Gynecol Obstet Fertil 20014;32:280–4.

[17] Keltie K, Elneil S, Monga A, et al. Complications following vaginal mesh procedures for stress urinary incontinence: an 8 year study of 92,246 women. Sci Rep 2017;7:12015.

[18] Morling JR, McAllister DA, Agur W, et al. Adverse events after first, single, mesh and non-mesh surgical procedures for stress urinary incontinence and pelvic organ prolapse in Scotland, 1997–2016: a population-based cohort study. Lancet 2017;389:629–40.

[19] Welk B, Al-Hothi H, Winick-Ng J. Removal or revision of vaginal mesh used for the treatment of stress urinary incontinence. JAMA Surg 2015;150:1167–75.

[20] Jonsson Funk M, Siddiqui NY, Pate V, Amundsen CL, Wu JM. Sling revision/removal for mesh erosion and urinary retention: long-term risk and predictors. Am J Obstet Gynecol 2013;208: 73.e1–7.

[21] Fusco F, Abdel-Fattah M, Chapple CR, et al. Updated systematic review and meta-analysis of the comparative data on colposuspensions, pubovaginal slings, and midurethral tapes in the surgical treatment of female stress urinary incontinence. Eur. Urol. 2017;72:567–91.

[22] Maher C, Feiner B, Baessler K, Feiner B, Baessler K. Surgery for women with anterior compartment prolapse. Cochrane Database Syst Rev 2016;11:CD004014.

[23] Chughtai B, Barber MD, Mao J, Forde JC, Normand S-LT, Sedrakyan A. Association between the amount of vaginal mesh used with mesh erosions and repeated surgery after repairing pelvic organ prolapse and stress urinary incontinence. Jama Surg 2017;152:257–63.

[24] Unger CA, Paraiso MFR, Jelovsek JE, Barber MD, Ridgeway B. Perioperative adverse events after minimally invasive abdominal sacrocolpopexy. Am. J. Obstet. Gynecol. 2014;211:547.e1–8.

[25] Diwadkar GB, Barber MD, Feiner B, Maher C, Jelovsek JE. Complication and reoperation rates after apical vaginal prolapse surgical repair: a systematic review. Obstet Gynecol 2009;113:367–73.

[26] Brubaker L, Norton PA, Albo ME. Adverse events over two years after retropubic or transobturator midurethral sling surgery: findings from the Trial of Midurethral Slings (TOMUS) study. Am. J. Obstet. Gynecol. 2011;205:498.e1–6.

[27] Barber MD. Surgical techniques for removing problematic mesh. Clin Obstet Gynecol 2013;56:289–302.

[28] Nolfi AL, Brown BN, Liang R, et al. Host response to synthetic mesh in women with mesh complications. Am. J. Obstet. Gynecol. 2016;215:206.e1–8.

[29] Chughtai B, Sedrakyan A, Mao J, Eilber KS, Anger JT, Clemens JQ. Is vaginal mesh a stimulus of autoimmune disease? Am. J. Obstet. Gynecol. 2017;216:495.e1–495.e7.

[30] Chughtai B, Sedrakyan A, Mao J, et al. Challenging the myth: transvaginal mesh is not associated with carcinogenesis. J. Urol. 2017;198:884–89.

[31] Moalli P, Brown B, Reitman MTF, Nager CW. Polypropylene mesh: evidence for lack of carcinogenicity. Int Urogynecol J 2014;25:573–76.

[32] Oliver JL, Chaudhry ZQ, Medendorp AR, et al. Complete excision of sacrocolpopexy mesh with autologous fascia sacrocolpopexy. Urology 2017;106:65–69.

[33] Boulanger L, Boukerrou M, Rubod C, et al. Bacteriological analysis of meshes removed for complications after surgical management of urinary incontinence or pelvic organ prolapse. Int Urogynecol J Pelvic Floor Dysfunct 2008;19:827–31.

[34] Li L, Wang X, Park JY, Chen H, Wang Y, Zheng W. Pathological findings in explanted vaginal mesh. Hum. Pathol. 2017. doi:10.1016/j.humpath.2017.07.020

[35] Rouprêt M, Misraï V, Vaessen C, Cour F, Haertig A, Chartier-Kastler E. Laparoscopic surgical complete sling resection for tension-free vaginal tape-related complications refractory to first-line conservative management: a single-centre experience. Eur. Urol. 2010;58:270–74.

[36] Frenkl TL, Rackley RR, Vasavada SP, Goldman HB. Management of iatrogenic foreign bodies of the bladder and urethra following pelvic floor surgery. Neurourol. Urodyn. 2008;27:491–95.

[37] Doumouchtsis SK, Lee FYK, Bramwell D, Fynes MM. Evaluation of holmium laser for managing mesh/suture complications of continence surgery. BJU Int. 2011;108:1472–78.

[38] Maher C, Feiner B. Laparoscopic removal of intravesical mesh following pelvic organ prolapse mesh surgery. Int Urogynecol J 2011;22:1593–95.

[39] Grange P, Kouriefs C, Georgiades F, Charalambous S, Robinson D, Cardozo L. Eroded tape: a case of an early vesicoscopy rather than laser melting. Urology 2017;102:247–51.

[40] Sarlos D, Aigmueller T, Schaer G. A technique of laparoscopic mesh excision from the bladder after sacrocolpopexy. Am. J. Obstet. Gynecol. 2015;212:403.e1–3.

[41] Pikaart DP, Miklos JR, Moore RD. Laparoscopic removal of pubovaginal polypropylene tension-free tape slings. JSLS 2006;10:220–25.

[42] Wolff GF, Winters JC, Krlin RM. Mesh excision: is total mesh excision necessary? Curr Urol Rep 2016;17:34.

[43] Apostolis CA, Heiselman C. Sacral osteomyelitis after laparoscopic sacral colpopexy performed after a recent dental extraction: a case report. Female Pelvic Med Reconstr Surg 2014;20:e5–7.

[44] Feng TS, Thum DJ, Anger JT, Eilber KS. Sacral osteomyelitis after robotic sacrocolpopexy. Female Pelvic Med Reconstr Surg 2016;22:e6–7.

[45] Roslan M, Markuszewski MM. Transvesical laparoendoscopic single site surgery to remove surgical materials penetrating the bladder: initial clinical experience in 9 female patients. J. Urol. 2013;190:909–15.

[46] Giannitsas K, Costantini E. How to deal with pain following a vaginal mesh insertion. Eur Urol Focus 2016;2:268–71.

[47] Rigaud J, Pothin P, Labat JJ, et al. Functional results after tape removal for chronic pelvic pain following tension-free vaginal tape or transobturator tape. J. Urol. 2010;184:610–15.

[48] Marcus-Braun N, Bourret A, Theobald von P. Persistent pelvic pain following transvaginal mesh surgery: a cause for mesh removal. Eur. J. Obstet. Gynecol. Reprod. Biol. 2012;162:224–28.

Rainer Kimmig

19 Laparoscopic surgery for cervical cancer

19.1 Introduction

Cervical cancer is still the fourth most common malignancy in women worldwide, despite all attempts in screening, early detection, and even HPV vaccination, cervical cancer was responsible of 250,000 deaths in 2012 [1]. Generally, treatment consists of surgery and/or radiochemotherapy [2]. Surgery is mainly recommended in early cervical cancer, primarily stage Ia and Ib1 according to The International Federation of Gynecology and Obstetrics (FIGO) [3], although surgical treatment of Stage Ib2–II is also still routinely performed in specialized centers [4]. Currently, there is no evidence that favors surgery or radiochemotherapy in Ib2 tumors [5]. Although recommended in most guidelines to abandon radical hysterectomy in case of positive pelvic nodes to reduce morbidity due to adjuvant radiochemotherapy, it is not clear whether this may potentially improve recurrence free survival [6]. In addition, evidence was found that pelvic lymphadenectomy in addition to paraaortic node dissection was beneficial in cases of positive bulky nodes prior to primary radiochemotherapy of advanced cervical cancer [7].

In this chapter, radical hysterectomy, pelvic systematic lymphadenectomy, paraaortic systematic lymphadenectomy, sentinel node dissection, radical trachelectomy, and less invasive procedures will be discussed with respect to the laparoscopic approach. In principal, the term laparoscopy means in this context all laparoscopic procedures including robotic surgery.

19.2 Radical hysterectomy and systematic pelvic lymphadenectomy

Following the introduction of laparoscopy into surgical treatment of cervical cancer by Dargent and Querleu in the early 1990s [8, 9], minimally invasive surgery (MIS) has been implemented more or less entirely in the subsequent decades. As summarized in [10], "laparoscopic or robotic radical hysterectomy and pelvic lymphadenectomy are likely non-inferior to laparotomy with respect to surgical outcomes and survival" [11–17]. There was also no evidence of compromising the oncological outcome and the minimal invasive approach became widely accepted [18–20]. However, in 2018, the prospective randomized the Laparoscopic Approach to Cervical Cancer (LACC) Trial has been published that reported a significantly less recurrence-free survival (97.1% vs. 91.0%) and lower rate of overall survival (99.0% vs. 93.8%) in stage Ia and Ib1 treated by laparoscopy compared to laparotomy [21]. On parallel, the data of an epidemiologic cohort study seemed to support these findings [22].

https://doi.org/10.1515/9783110535204-019

Currently, there is a an ongoing debate about the validity and the impact of these data on our practice with respect to minimal invasive therapy [19, 23–25]. However, at present, it is difficult to draw final conclusions. But we may say that the results refer to The International Federation of Gynecology and Obstetrics (FIGO) Ib1 tumors ≥2 cm in size. Thus, for tumors less than 2 cm, stage Ia, at least no statistical difference between the groups has been reported in either report. Hence, these results predominantly apply to tumors between 2 and 4 cm in size.

Second, although not proven, as long as cell or tissue dissemination (spilling) cannot be ruled out as a cause for recurrence, we should cautiously prevent any contact of the tumor to the surgical field. This can be achieved by closing the vagina preoperatively as described by Dargent for vaginal radical hysterectomy or potentially by using a stapler before dissection.

If a decision for minimal invasive radical hysterectomy is made, there are different strategies.

19.3 Tailoring radicality according to tumor size/stage versus resection of the entire ontogenetic compartment

Up to now, the most common approach to minimize morbidity in smaller tumors was to limit the resection borders according to the tumor size just to achieve free margins. There was a lot of effort to define different classes of radical hysterectomy for standardization, which in newer classifications also included "nerve-sparing" techniques [26, 27]. The problem of this tailored approach is that it refers on macroscopic tumor extension rather than the tissue at risk. Ideally, all the tissue at risk should be removed by respecting the borders of neighboring tissue to reduce morbidity to a minimum. This is the approach of the entire resection of ontogenetic tissue compartments. In case of cervical cancer, this means the Müllerian compartment, consisting of the uterus, the vascular (Fig. 19.1), and the ligamentous mesometrium (Fig. 19.2), including the first regional lymph compartments. This total mesometrial resection (TMMR) is sufficient for all organ confined cancers. In case of tumors extending beyond the compartment borders, the procedure has to be extended to the neighboring compartments (EMMR). The principles and clinical results of this concept of TMMR/EMMR were previously published by Höckel [28–31]. Surgery and surgical anatomy were consecutively described and illustrated for laparoscopy step by step in [32].

Pelvic lymphadenectomy has been less well defined. Usually, lymph nodes along the external and internal iliac artery and the common iliac artery will be removed more or less completely. From the studies of Höckel, it is evident that the first nodes involved are usually those along the uterine artery (mesometrial) and the paravisceral nodes reached by the connecting lymph vessels to the nodes along the vascular and ligamentous mesometrium below the common iliac bifurcation of

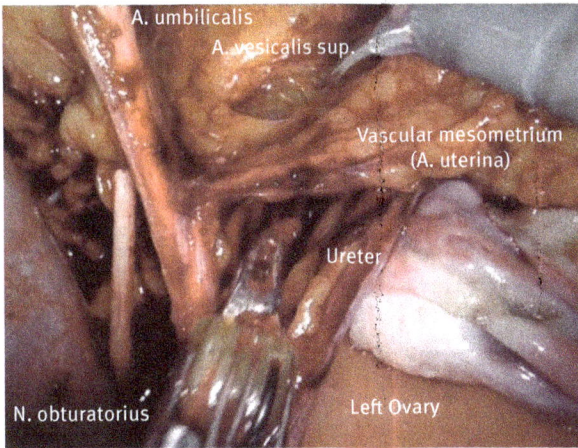

Fig. 19.1: Uterine vascular mesometrium on the left.

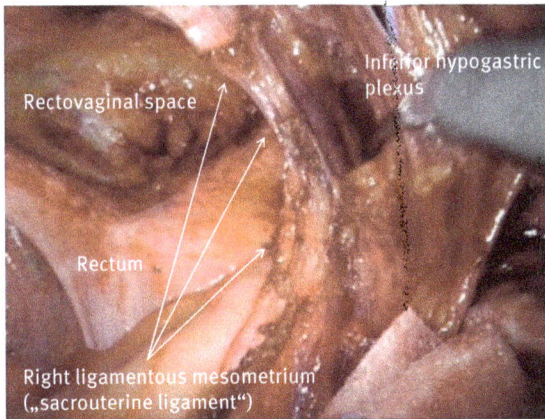

Fig. 19.2: Uterine ligamentous mesometrium on the right.

the artery (ventrally) and vein (dorsally) (Figs. 19.3 and 19.4). Thus, the prespinal, preischial, and presacral lymph nodes have to be resected in addition to the obturator, internal, and external iliac nodes as the primary lymph node compartment in cervical cancer (Fig. 19.5). The common iliac nodes represent the secondary lymph node compartment and should be resected for safety, but are usually not involved, if the first compartment is free of disease. The tertiary lymphatic compartment is the lumbar inframesenteric paraaortic region. If these nodes are negative, there is no substantial risk of higher lymph node involvement [33, 34]. However, there is one exception; if there is tumor infiltration of the isthmus or corpus uteri, there may be involvement of the paraaortic nodes drained via the ovarian lymphatic vessels

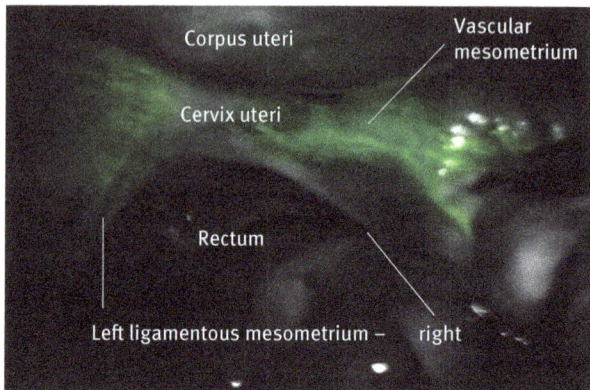

Fig. 19.3: Lymphatic drainage along the uterine vascular and ligamentous mesometrium.

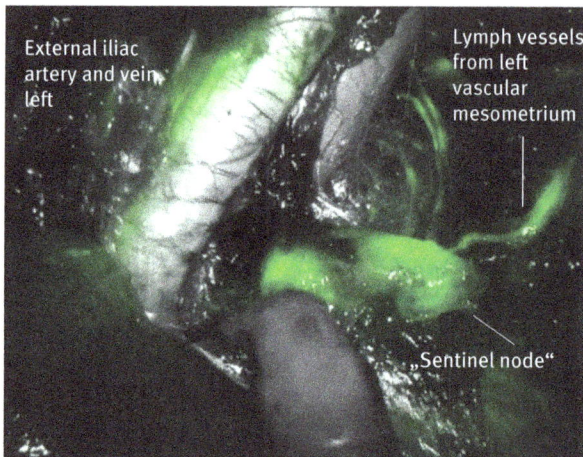

Fig. 19.4: Uterine sentinel node in the left iliac region following indocyanine green (ICG) application.

(Fig. 19.6), as it is known from endometrial cancer (M. Höckel, 2018, personal communication). These have to be removed as primary lymph compartment in this situation. The principles of lymphatic drainage of the uterine cervix and corpus have been investigated using indocyanine green (ICG) injection [35].

For laparoscopy, the different lymph node compartments and technique of resection have been described systematically [36]. In addition, the technique of laparoscopic surgery for TMMR and pelvic and paraaortic lymphadenectomy has been demonstrated in numerous video presentations with and without ICG. These are available either as open access (PubMed, YouTube) or in ESGO eAcademy [37–47]. Hence, the reader is advised to refer to these resources for further details.

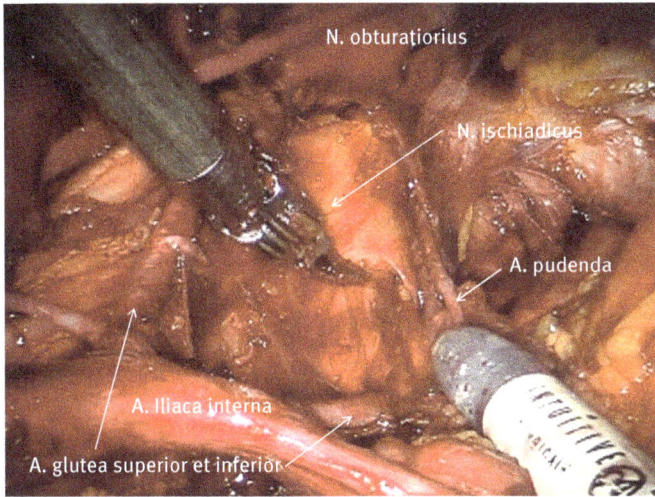

Fig. 19.5: Prespinal and gluteal region ventro-medially to the ischiadic nerve, left.

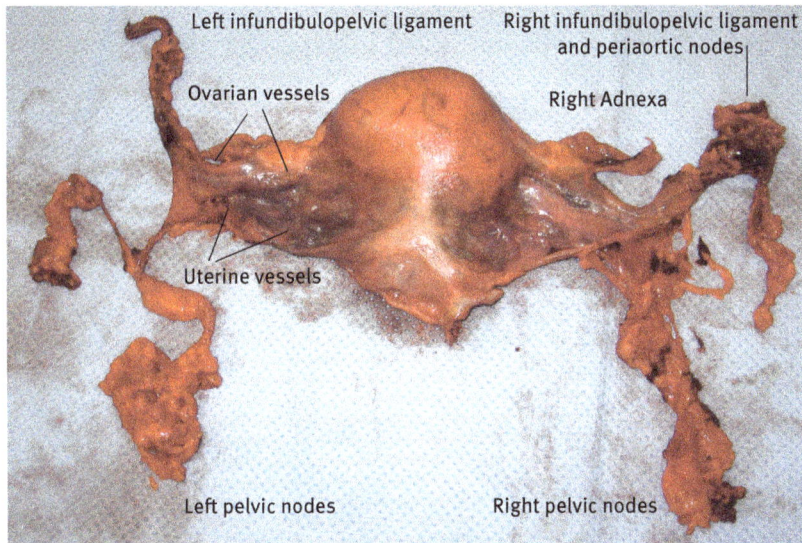

Fig. 19.6: Surgical specimen of a peritoneal mesometrial resection (PMMR) with pelvic nodes.

19.4 Sentinel node dissection in cervical cancer

There is consensus that tumor infiltration of more than 3 mm in depth and/or additional risk factors carry an increased risk for pelvic lymph node metastases and nodes should be evaluated [48]. However, 80–85% of the patients are expected to be node negative and would be overtreated by systematic lymphadenectomy [49]. To reduce morbidity—mainly lymphedema, lymphocele, and vessel injury—whether patients with positive nodes may be accurately identified by sentinel node biopsy has been evaluated. Although initial studies with blue dye and technetium showed accuracy for tumors <2 cm only [50], others [10] reported a high bilateral detection rate and a false-negative rate close to 0 for early cervical cancer. It has also been shown that ICG seems to be superior to blue dye and radioactive tracers. Isolated sentinel node excision reduced morbidity and did not increase the risk of recurrence compared to complete pelvic lymphadenectomy in node negative disease [51–55]. Thus, sentinel node excision is a less invasive alternative to diagnostic pelvic lymph node resection, usually performed laparoscopically.

An interesting variant with respect to diagnostic and therapeutic aspects could be the "targeted compartmental lymphadenectomy," first described for treatment of endometrial and ovarian cancer [56, 57]. With this method, the vascular and ligamentous mesometria will be resected in continuity with the lymph vessels marked by ICG, including the sentinel nodes of each channel "en bloc" (Fig. 19.6).

19.5 Paraaortic lymph node staging in advanced cervical cancer

In cases of planned primary radiochemotherapy, paraaortic lymph node staging is usually recommended prior to final treatment decision [58]. As outlined earlier, in tumors with no infiltration of the isthmus or corpus uteri, the removal of inframesenteric paraaortic nodes, including the lumbar chain (Fig. 19.7), is sufficient to preclude higher node involvement if histologically negative [59]. Only in the case of

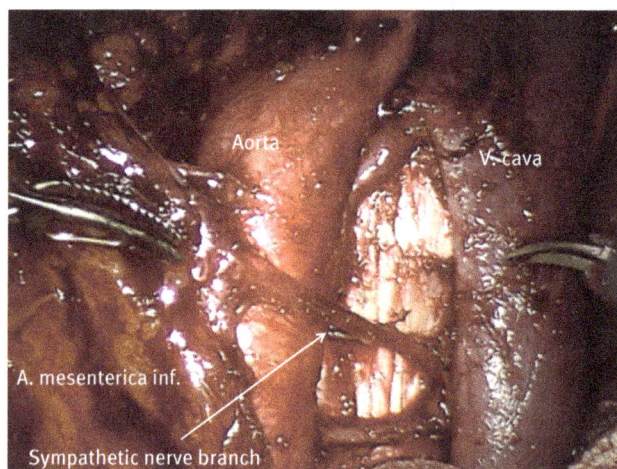

Fig. 19.7: Inframesenteric paraaortic region (right) with removal of the lumbar chain.

uterine infiltration beyond the cervix should infrarenal paraaortic node dissection be performed for staging as it is for positive inframesenteric nodes (see 19.2 Radical hysterectomy and systematic pelvic lymphadenectomy section).

19.6 Cone biopsy or simple hysterectomy

At present, there is agreement that in cervical cancers with stage Ia1 with no lympho-vascular space involvement (LVSI), cone biopsy is sufficient. There is a very low risk in parametrial involvement in tumors >2 cm with surgically staged negative nodes [10, 60, 61]. Thus, it may be justified to perform extrafascial hysterectomy instead of radical hysterectomy in these situations. To evaluate the safety of less radical surgery in early cervical cancer, there is one randomized trial (SHAPE trial: NCT01658930) and two prospective cohort studies (ConCerv: NCT01048853 and GOG278:NCT01649089) that are ongoing at present [62–64].

19.7 Fertility sparing surgery

Since cervical cancer occurs during reproductive age, the question of fertility preservation is important. As already outlined, in Ia1 with no LVSI, cone biopsy is sufficient. In Ia2 to Ib1 (<2 cm) tumors with negative nodes, no LVSI, no neuroen-docrine subtype, and invasion less than 10 mm, a recurrence rate of <1% following cone biopsy or simple trachelectomy has been reported [65]. In an excellent review Covens *et al.* report a crude recurrence and survival rate of 4.5% vs. 1.7% for tumors less than 2 cm and 11% vs. 4.2% in tumors >2 cm in diameter for radical trachelec-tomy with pelvic node dissection. In patients who had neoadjuvant chemotherapy for tumor reduction, the numbers were 6.3% vs. 1.3% [10, 66]. Thus, it seems justifiable to offer patients fertility-sparing treatment, depending on their individual situation. Whether radical trachelectomy as introduced by Dargent an Schneider [67, 68], less radical methods of cone biopsy and simple trachelectomy, or more radical approaches such as fertility preserving mesometrial resection [69] will be combined with lymph node assessment in the future has to be evaluated in further trials.

In summary, laparoscopic surgery in cervical cancer is widely used for different indications. It has been shown that with respect to morbidity, recovery, and life quality, MIS is beneficial compared to open surgery. With respect to the LACC data, oncological safety has to be assessed further and results have to be thoroughly observed. Patients have to be informed about these data to give informed consent prior to MIS. However, we have to remember that for tumors less than 2 cm and no additional risk factors, MIS has not been shown disadvantageous in this study and tumors higher than stage Ib1 have not been investigated.

References

[1] Bray F, Ferlay J, Soerjomataram I, Siegel RL, Torre LA, Jemal A. Global cancer statistics 2018: GLOBOCAN estimates of incidence and mortality worldwide for 36 cancers in 185 countries.CA Cancer J Clin 2018 September 12 [Epub ahead of print].

[2] Koh WJ, Greer BE, Abu-Rustum NR, et al. Cervical Cancer, Version 2.2015. J Natl Compr Canc Netw 2015 Apr;13(4):395–404; quiz 404.

[3] Pecorelli S, Zigliani L, Odicino F. Revised FIGO staging for carcinoma of the cervix. Int J Gynaecol Obstet 2009;105(2):107–8. doi:10.1016/j.ijgo.2009.02.009.

[4] Derks M, van der Velden J, de Kroon CD, et al. Surgical treatment of early-stage cervical cancer: a multi-institution experience in 2124 cases in the Netherlands over a 30-year period. Int J Gynecol Cancer 2018 May;28(4):757–63. doi: 10.1097/IGC.0000000000001228.

[5] Nama V, Angelopoulos G, Twigg J, Murdoch JB, Bailey J, Lawrie TA. Type II or type III radical hysterectomy compared to chemoradiotherapy as a primary intervention for stage IB2 cervical cancer [review]. Cochrane Database Syst Rev 2018 Oct 12;10:CD011478. doi:10.1002/14651858. CD011478.pub2.

[6] Derks M, Groenman FA, van Lonkhuijzen LRCW, et al. completing or abandoning radical hysterectomy in early-stage lymph node-positive cervical cancer: impact on disease-free survival and treatment-related toxicity. Int J Gynecol Cancer 2017 Jun;27(5):1015–20. doi: 10.1097/IGC.0000000000000974.

[7] Bendifallah S, de Foucher T, Ouldamer L, et al.; Groupe de Recherche FRANCOGYN. Comparison of pelvic and para-aortic lymphadenectomy versus para-aortic lymphadenectomy alone for locally advanced FIGO stage IB2 to IIB cervical cancer using a propensity score matching analysis: Results from the FRANCOGYN study group. Eur J Surg Oncol 2018 Aug 30. pii: S0748-7983(18)31287-3. doi: 10.1016/j.ejso.2018.08.013 [Epub ahead of print].

[8] Dargent D, Mathevet P. [Radical laparoscopic vaginal hysterectomy]. J Gynecol Obstet Biol Reprod (Paris) 1992;21(6):709–10.

[9] Querleu D. Laparoscopically assisted radical vaginal hysterectomy. Gynecol Oncol 1993 Nov;51(2):248–54.

[10] Zigras T, Lennox G, Willows K, Covens A. Early cervical cancer: current dilemmas of staging and surgery [review]. Curr Oncol Rep 2017 Aug;19(8):51. doi: 10.1007/s11912-017-0614-5.

[11] Steed H, Rosen B, Murphy J, Laframboise S, De Petrillo D, Covens A. A comparison of laparoscopic-assisted radical vaginal hysterectomy and radical abdominal hysterectomy in the treatment of cervical cancer. Gynecol Oncol 2004;93(3):588–93. doi:10.1016/j. ygyno.2004.04.003.

[12] Li G, Yan X, Shang H, Wang G, Chen L, Han Y. A comparison of laparoscopic radical hysterectomy and pelvic lymphadenectomy and laparotomy in the treatment of Ib–IIa cervical cancer. Gynecol Oncol 2007;105(1):176–80. doi:10.1016/j.ygyno.2006.11.011.

[13] Taylor SE, McBee WC Jr, Richard SD, Edwards RP. Radical hysterectomy for early stage cervical cancer: laparoscopy versus laparotomy. JSLS 2011;15(2):213–7. doi:10.4293/108 680811X13022985132218.

[14] Wright JD, Herzog TJ, Neugut AI, et al. Comparative effectiveness of minimally invasive and abdominal radical hysterectomy for cervical cancer. Gynecol Oncol 2012;127(1):11–7. doi:10.1016/j.ygyno.2012.06.031.

[15] Hong JH, Choi JS, Lee JH, et al. Comparison of survival and adverse events between women with stage IB1 and stage IB2 cervical cancer treated by laparoscopic radical vaginal hysterectomy. Ann Surg Oncol 2012;19(2):605–11. doi:10.1245/s10434-011-1904-z.

[16] Park JY, Kim DY, Kim JH, Kim YM, Kim YT, Nam JH. Laparoscopic compared with open radical hysterectomy in obese women with early-stage cervical cancer. Obstet Gynecol 2012;119(6):1201–9. doi:10.1097/AOG.0b013e318256ccc5.

[17] van de Lande J, von Mensdorff-Pouilly S, Lettinga RG, Piek JM, Verheijen RH. Open versus laparoscopic pelvic lymph node dissection in early stage cervical cancer: no difference in surgical or disease outcome. Int J Gynecol Cancer 2012;22(1):107–14. doi:10.1097/IGC.0b013e31822c273d.

[18] Conrad LB, Ramirez PT, Burke W, et al. Role of minimally invasive surgery in gynecologic oncology: an updated survey of members of the Society of Gynecologic Oncology. Int J Gynecol Cancer 2015;25:1121–7.

[19] Wang YZ, Deng L, Xu HC, Zhang Y, Liang ZQ. Laparoscopy versus laparotomy for the management of early stage cervical cancer. BMC Cancer 2015;15:928.

[20] Fader AN. Surgery in cervical cancer. N Engl J Med 2018 Oct 31. doi: 10.1056/NEJMe1814034.

[21] Ramirez PT, Frumovitz M, Pareja R, et al. Minimally invasive versus abdominal radical hysterectomy for cervical cancer. N Engl J Med 2018 Oct 31. doi: 10.1056/NEJMoa1806395.

[22] Melamed A, Margul DJ, Chen L, et al. Survival after minimally invasive radical hysterectomy for early-stage cervical cancer. N Engl J Med 2018 Oct 31. doi: 10.1056/NEJMoa1804923.

[23] Kimmig R, Ind T. Minimally invasive surgery for cervical cancer: consequences for treatment after LACC Study. J Gynecol Oncol 2018 Jul;29(4):e75. doi: 10.3802/jgo.2018.29.e75 [Epub ahead of print May 14, 2018].

[24] Park JY, Nam JH. How should gynecologic oncologists react to the unexpected results of LACC trial? J Gynecol Oncol 2018 Jul;29(4):e74. doi: 10.3802/jgo.2018.29.e74. No abstract available.

[25] Leitao MM Jr. The LACC Trial: has minimally invasive surgery for early-stage cervical cancer been dealt a knockout punch? Int J Gynecol Cancer 2018 Sep;28(7):1248–50. doi: 10.1097/IGC.0000000000001342. No abstract available.

[26] Piver MS, Rutledge F, Smith JP. Five classes of extended hysterectomy for women with cervical cancer. Obstet Gynecol 1974 Aug;44(2):265–72. No abstract available.

[27] Querleu D, Morrow CP. Classification of radical hysterectomy [review]. Lancet Oncol 2008 Mar;9(3):297–303. doi: 10.1016/S1470-2045(08)70074-3.

[28] Höckel M, Horn LC, Manthey N, et al. Resection of the embryologically defined uterovaginal (Müllerian) compartment and pelvic control in patients with cervical cancer: a prospective analysis. Lancet Oncol 2009 Jul;10(7):683–92. doi: 10.1016/S1470-2045(09)70100-7 [Epub ahead of print May 29, 2009].

[29] Höckel M, Horn LC, Einenkel J. (Laterally) extended endopelvic resection: surgical treatment of locally advanced and recurrent cancer of the uterine cervix and vagina based on ontogenetic anatomy. Gynecol Oncol 2012 Nov;127(2):297–302. doi: 10.1016/j.ygyno.2012.07.120 [Epub ahead of print August 1, 2012].

[30] Höckel M Morphogenetic fields of embryonic development in locoregional cancer spread. Lancet Oncol 2015 Mar;16(3):e148–51. doi: 10.1016/S1470-2045(14)71028-9.

[31] Wolf B, Ganzer R, Stolzenburg JU, Hentschel B, Horn LC, Höckel M. Extended mesometrial resection (EMMR): surgical approach to the treatment of locally advanced cervical cancer based on the theory of ontogenetic cancer fields. Gynecol Oncol 2017 Aug;146(2):292–8. doi: 10.1016/j.ygyno.2017.05.007 [Epub ahead of print May 16, 2017].

[32] Kimmig R, Wimberger P, Buderath P, Aktas B, Iannaccone A, Heubner M. Definition of compartment-based radical surgery in uterine cancer: radical hysterectomy in cervical cancer as 'total mesometrial resection (TMMR)' by M Höckel translated to robotic surgery (rTMMR). World J Surg Oncol 2013 Aug 26;11:211. doi: 10.1186/1477-7819-11-211.

[33] Höckel M, Horn LC, Tetsch E, Einenkel J. Pattern analysis of regional spread and therapeutic lymph node dissection in cervical cancer based on ontogenetic anatomy. Gynecol Oncol 2012 Apr;125(1):168–74. doi: 10.1016/j.ygyno.2011.12.419 [Epub ahead of print December 2011].

[34] Höckel M, Einenkel J, Horn LC. Paraaortic lymphatic spread in cervical cancer. Gynecol Oncol 2012 Dec;127(3):677; author reply 677–8. doi: 10.1016/j.ygyno.2012.07.122 [Epub ahead of print August 3, 2012].

[35] Kimmig R, Aktas B, Buderath P, Rusch P, Heubner M. Intraoperative navigation in robotically assisted compartmental surgery of uterine cancer by visualisation of embryologically derived lymphatic networks with indocyanine-green (ICG). J Surg Oncol 2016 Apr;113(5):554–59. doi: 10.1002/jso.24174 [Epub ahead of print January 21, 2016].

[36] Kimmig R, Iannaccone A, Buderath P, Aktas B, Wimberger P, Heubner M. Definition of compartment based radical surgery in uterine cancer-part I: therapeutic pelvic and periaortic lymphadenectomy by Michael Höckel translated to robotic surgery. ISRN Obstet Gynecol 2013 Mar 25;2013:297921. doi: 10.1155/2013/297921. Print 2013.

[37] Video 1: Kimmig K. Laparoscopic Robotically Assisted Total Mesometrial Resection and Therapeutic Lymphadenectomy (TMMR) according to Michal Hoeckel's Technique—Part Two. ESGO eAcademy. August 2, 2012; 33615. Available at: http://eacademy.esgo.org/esgo/2000/dvds/33615/k.rainer.kimmig.laparoscopic.robotically.assisted.total.medometrial.resection.html?f=p14s49121m10.

[38] Video 2: Kimmig K. Robotic Surgery in Gynaecology—Therapeutic Lymphadenectomy of the Pelvic Nodes (TPL1)—Module I: Common Iliac, Subaortic and Presacral Nodes. ESGO eAcademy. October 10, 2013; 38736. Available at: http://eacademy.esgo.org/esgo/2000/dvds/38736/k.rainer.kimmig.robotic.surgery.in.gynaecology.-.therapeutic.lymphadenectomy.html?f=l5987m10.

[39] Video 3. Kimmig K. Robotic Surgery in Gynaecology—Therapeutic Lymphadenectomy of the Pelvic Nodes (TPL1)—Module II: Lower Paravisceral and External Iliac Nodes. ESGO eAcademy. October 3, 2013; 38737. Available at: http://eacademy.esgo.org/esgo/2000/dvds/38737/k.rainer.kimmig.robotic.surgery.in.gynaecology.-.therapeutic.lymphadenectomy.html?f=s49121m10. 39.

[40] Video 4: Kimmig K. Robotic Surgery in Gynecology—Therapeutic Lymphadenectomy of the Pelvic Nodes (TPL1)—Module III: Upper Paravisceral—Prespinal and Preischaidic Nodes. ESGO eAcademy. October 10, 2013; 38738. Available at: http://eacademy.esgo.org/esgo/2000/dvds/38738/k.rainer.kimmig.robotic.surgery.in.gynecology.-.therapeutic.lymphadenectomy.of.html?f=l5987m10.

[41] Video 5: Kimmig K. Robotic Surgery in Gynaecology—Therapeutic Paraaortic Lymphadenectomy (TPL2)—Module IV: Inframesenteric Periaortic Nodes. ESGO eAcademy. October 8, 2013; 95407. Available at: http://eacademy.esgo.org/esgo/2000/dvds/95407/k.rainer.kimmig.robotic.surgery.in.gynaecology.-.therapeutic.paraaortic.html?f=l5987m10.

[42] Video 6: Kimmig K. Robotic Surgery in Gynaecology—Therapeutic Paraaortic Lymphadenectomy (TPL2)—Module V1: Infrarenal/Supramesenteric Periaortic Nodes. ESGO eAcademy. June 6, 2013; 95405. Available at: http://eacademy.esgo.org/esgo/2000/dvds/95405/k.rainer.kimmig.robotic.surgery.in.gynaecology.-.therapeutic.paraaortic.html?f=s49121m10.

[43] Video 7: Kimmig K. Robotic Surgery in Gynecology—Therapeutic Paraaortic Lymphadenectomy (TPL2)—Module V2: Infrarenal Periaortic Nodes with Resection of 'Mesonephric' Compartment of Ovarian Vessels. ESGO eAcademy. June 3, 2014; 95406. Available at: http://eacademy.esgo.org/esgo/2000/dvds/95406/k.rainer.kimmig.robotic.surgery.in.gynecology.-.therapeutic.paraaortic.html?f=s49121m10.

[44] Video 8: Kimmig R, Buderath P, Rusch P and Aktas B Surgical anatomy of the ligamentous mesometrium and robotically assisted ICG-guided resection in cervical cancer. Educational video. Gynecol Oncol Rep 2016. Submitted.

[45] Video 9: Kimmig R, Rusch P, Buderath P, Aktas B. Left paraaortic, inframesenteric lymphadenectomy preserving the superior hypogastric plexus supported by indocyanine green (ICG) labeling of the lymphatic compartment in cervical cancer. Gynecol Oncol Rep 2016 Sep 14;18:14. doi: 10.1016/j.gore.2016.09.002.

[46] Video 10: Kimmig R, Rusch P, Buderath P, Aktas B. Aortic utero-ovarian sentinel nodes and left infrarenal aortic lymph node dissection by ICG supported navigation. Gynecol Oncol Rep 2017 Feb 9;20:22–23. doi: 10.1016/j.gore.2017.02.003. eCollection May 2017.

[47] Video 11: Kimmig R, Buderath P, Mach P, Rusch P, Aktas B. Surgical treatment of early ovarian cancer with compartmental resection of regional lymphatic network and indocyanine-green-guided targeted compartmental lymphadenectomy (TCL, paraaortic part). J Gynecol Oncol 2017 May;28(3):e41. doi: 10.3802/jgo.2017.28.e41 [Epub ahead of print March 21, 2017].

[48] National Comprehensive Cancer Network. NCCN clinical practice guidelines in oncology (NCCN Guidelines): cervical cancer. Version I. 2016. Available at: https://www.nccn.org/professionals/physician_gls/PDF/cervical.pdf.

[49] Kadkhodayan S, Hasanzadeh M, Treglia G, et al. Sentinel node biopsy for lymph nodal staging of uterine cervix cancer: a systematic review and meta-analysis of the pertinent literature [review]. Eur J Surg Oncol 2015 Jan;41(1):1–20. doi: 10.1016/j.ejso.2014.09.010 [Epub ahead of print October 23, 2014].

[50] Altgassen C, Hertel H, Brandstädt A, Köhler C, Dürst M, Schneider A; AGO Study Group. Multicenter validation study of the sentinel lymph node concept in cervical cancer: AGO Study Group. J Clin Oncol 2008 Jun 20;26(18):2943–51. doi: 10.1200/JCO.2007.13.8933.

[51] Gortzak-Uzan L, Jimenez W, Nofech-Mozes S, et al. Sentinel lymph node biopsy vs. pelvic lymphadenectomy in early stage cervical cancer: is it time to change the gold standard? Gynecol Oncol 2010;116(1):28–32. doi:10.1016/j.ygyno.2009.10.049.

[52] Lécuru F, Mathevet P, Querleu D, et al. Bilateral negative sentinel nodes accurately predict absence of lymph node metastasis in early cervical cancer: results of the SENTICOL study. J Clin Oncol 2011;29(13):1686–91. doi:10.1200/JCO.2010.32.0432.

[53] Mathevet P, Lécuru F, eds. Effect of Sentinel Lymph-Node Biopsy Alone on the Morbidity of the Surgical Treatment of Early Cervical Cancer: Results From the Prospective Randomized Study Senticol 2. ASCO Annual Meeting Proceedings. 2015. DOI: 10.1200/jco.2015.33.15_suppl.5521 Journal of Clinical Oncology 33, no. 15_suppl (May 20, 2015):5521–5521.

[54] Ruscito I, Gasparri ML, Braicu EI, et al. Sentinel node mapping in cervical and endometrial cancer: indocyanine green versus other conventional dyes—a meta-analysis. Ann Surg Oncol 2016;23(11):3749–56. doi:10.1245/s10434-016-5236-x.

[55] Lennox GK, Covens A. Can sentinel lymph node biopsy replace pelvic lymphadenectomy for early cervical cancer? Gynecol Oncol 2017;144(1):16–20. doi:10.1016/j.ygyno.2016.08.337.

[56] Kimmig R, Buderath P, Rusch P, Aktas B. Technique of ICG-guided targeted compartmental pelvic lymphadenectomy (TCL) combined with pelvic peritoneal mesometrial resection (PMMR) for locoregional control of endometrial cancer—a proposal. Gynecol Oncol Rep 2017 Apr 6;20:125–126. doi: 10.1016/j.gore.2017.04.002. eCollection May 2017.

[57] Kimmig R, Buderath P, Mach P, Rusch P, Aktas B. Surgical treatment of early ovarian cancer with compartmental resection of regional lymphatic network and indocyanine-green-guided targeted compartmental lymphadenectomy (TCL, paraaortic part). J Gynecol Oncol 2017 May;28(3):e41. doi: 10.3802/jgo.2017.28.e41 [Epub ahead of print March 21, 2017].

[58] Angeles MA, Martínez-Gómez C, Migliorelli F, et al. Novel surgical strategies in the treatment of gynecological malignancies [review]. Curr Treat Options Oncol 2018 Nov 9;19(12):73. doi: 10.1007/s11864-018-0582-5.

[59] Azaïs H, Ghesquière L, Petitnicolas C, et al. Pretherapeutic staging of locally advanced cervical cancer: Inframesenteric paraaortic lymphadenectomy accuracy to detect paraaortic metastases in comparison with infrarenal paraaortic lymphadenectomy. Gynecol Oncol 2017 Nov;147(2):340–4. doi: 10.1016/j.ygyno.2017.09.012 [Epub ahead of print September 14, 2017].

[60] Covens A, Rosen B, Murphy J, et al. How important is removal of the parametrium at surgery for carcinoma of the cervix? Gynecol Oncol 2002;84(1):145–9. doi:10.1006/gyno.2001.6493.

[61] Gemer O, Eitan R, Gdalevich M, et al. Can parametrectomy be avoided in early cervical cancer? An algorithm for the identification of patients at low risk for parametrial involvement. Eur J Surg Oncol 2013;39(1):76–80.doi:10.1016/j.ejso.2012.10.013.

[62] Plante M. Radical versus simple hysterectomy and pelvic node dissection in patients with low-risk early stage cervical cancer (SHAPE). ClinicalTrials.gov Identifier: NCT01658930. Available at: https://clinicaltrials.gov/ct2/show/NCT01658930. Accessed November 11, 2018.

[63] MD Anderson Cancer Center. Conservative surgery for women with cervical cancer. ClinicalTrials.gov Identifier: NCT01048853. Available at: https://clinicaltrials.gov/ct2/show/NCT01048853. Accessed November 11, 2018.

[64] Covens A. Studying the physical function and quality of life before and after surgery in patients with stage 1 cervical cancer. ClinicalTrials.gov Identifier: NCT01649089. Available at: https://clinicaltrials. gov/ct2/show/NCT01649089. Accessed November 11, 2018.

[65] Bentivegna E, Gouy S, Maulard A, Chargari C, Leary A, Morice P. Oncological outcomes after fertility-sparing surgery for cervical cancer: a systematic review. Lancet Oncol 2016;17(6):e240–53. doi:10.1016/S1470-2045(16)30032-8.

[66] Willows K, Lennox G, Covens A. Fertility-sparing management in cervical cancer: balancing oncologic outcomes with reproductive success. Gynecol Oncol Res Pract 2016;3:9. doi:10.1186/s40661-016-0030-9.

[67] Dargent D, Mathevet P. Schauta's vaginal hysterectomy combined with laparoscopic lymphadenectomy. Baillieres Clin Obstet Gynaecol 1995 Dec;9(4):691–705.

[68] Schneider A, Krause N, Kühne-Heid R, Nöschel H. [Preserving fertility in early cervix carcinoma: trachelectomy with laparoscopic lymphadenectomy]. Zentralbl Gynakol 1996;118(1):6–8. German.

[69] Kimmig R, Aktas B, Heubner M. Chapter 23. Compartment-based radical surgery: The TMMR, FMMR and PMMR family in uterine cancer. In: Hrsg v Kilic SG, Ertan K, Kose MF, eds. Robotic Surgery. Practical Examples in Gynecology. De Gruyter Berlin/Boston; 2013:287–318. ISBN 978-3-11-030657-6.

Kirsten Huebner, Alexander di Liberto, Catharina Luck
and Kubilay Ertan

20 Minimal invasive surgery for endometrial cancer

20.1 Introduction

Endometrial cancer (EC) is the fifth most prevalent cancer worldwide in women up
to the age of 65 years. The risk of getting diagnosed with EC by this age varies from
0.46% (in developing countries) to 0.92% (in developed countries) [1]. The incidences
of EC worldwide are constantly rising. It is primarily the cancer of the postmenopausal woman, with a mean age of diagnosis at 62 years (age-standardized incidence is
9.5 to 15 per 100,000 women [2]), and a mean age at death of 70 years [3]. Seventy-
one percent of the patients are diagnosed at stage 1 of the disease. The overall 5-year
disease-free interval of stage 1 EC is high (>90%) after adequate surgical and adjuvant
treatment, if needed [4].

EC is classified into two histological subtypes presenting with different risk factors,
molecular genetic profiles [5], pathways of carcinogenesis, and clinico-oncological
outcome [6, 7]. According to this concept, endometrioid type 1 carcinoma evolves from
an atypical hyperplastic precursor, undergoes a malignant transformation by estrogenic stimulation, and develops into endometrioid adenocarcinoma [8]. Therefore,
exposure to unopposed estrogen is the strongest risk factor, as seen in chronic ano-
vulation as in the polycystic ovary syndrome, estrogen replacement therapy (even if
decreased by the use of progestins) [9, 10], high endogenous estrogen production in
adipose tissue or by estrogen-secreting tumors, as well as seen in the estrogen-agonist
effect of tamoxifen on endometrial tissue [11]. Furthermore, a history of nulliparity,
infertility, early menarche, and late menopause, as well as diabetes mellitus, as an
independent factor or associated with obesity is also related to a higher EC risk. This
subtype 1 accounts for 80–90% of cases, is predominantly seen in younger and/or
obese patients, is generally diagnosed at an early stage, appears in a better differentiation (grade 2–3), and seems to have a better prognosis compared to the subtype 2 EC.

The latter, also known as nonendometrioid subtype 2 carcinoma (10–20%
of ECs), develops on the grounds of an atrophic endometrium, without estrogenic
stimulation [8], into a uterine papillary serous carcinoma or clear cell carcinoma.
Frequently, carcinosarcoma (malignant mixed-Mullerian tumor) is assigned to this
group due to its similar clinical characteristics [12]. Generally, type 2 ECs are related
to a more aggressive tumor behavior, often diagnosed at an advanced stage and
higher grade, leading to a disproportionally higher mortality (40%). Therefore, they
are considered a uterine high-risk factor for recurrence (GOG 99, subchapter 2), and
with regard to a worse oncological outcome, grade 3 endometrioid cancer is often
allocated to this group. Upon other studies, the LAP2 study showed that subtype 2 EC

https://doi.org/10.1515/9783110535204-020

carcinomas appear predominantly in the elderly population with a lower body mass index (BMI) [13], demonstrating that age is an important general risk factor. The dilemma of a more aggressive tumor nature in elderly patients on the one hand but with an increased surgical risk due frailty and a higher comorbidity index on the other hand may lead clinicians to an understaging of this patient group with worse oncological outcomes (see chapter 20.3).

Hence, the above-mentioned populations of elderly and obese patients represent the majority of patients with EC. From a surgeon's point of view, both are considered surgical high-risk groups requiring adequate and oncologically feasible operative techniques, which will be discussed below.

Lately, another risk factor has been looked at more closely, which is diabetes mellitus. The mechanisms are multiple; insulin and insulin-like growth factors are known to enhance directly the proliferation of EC cells, and insulin reduces the levels of sex hormone binding globulin, which augments the biological availability of estradiol [14]. It is assumed that in EC genesis, diabetes counts as an independent predictor for an aggressive tumor nature and poor oncological outcome, as similarly seen in colorectal [15] and pancreatic [16] cancer. Not only is this silent disease strongly associated with obesity, but also, interestingly, two recent studies could show that diabetes specifically in nonobese patients (BMI $<30/<25$ kg/m^2) led to a significantly higher all-cause, cancer-specific and non-cancer-related mortality compared to the obese diabetic EC patient group [17, 18]. It therefore seems to be a strong risk factor. In this context, low BMI is even discussed to be a marker for the severity and type of diabetes and existence of comorbidity [17].

Apart from diabetes, medical comorbidities in general are considered another risk factor as they have been shown to not only negatively affect the overall EC survival [19] but also aggravate the EC-specific outcome, predominantly in nonobese patients with subtype 2 EC [18]. This may be explained by the fact that women with a high comorbidity index seem to present at a more advanced EC stage and subsequently receive surgical and adjuvant undertreatment [20].

Lastly, whereas most ECs are thought to emerge sporadically, a small group of patients with EC shows a genetic predisposition. The Lynch syndrome (hereditary nonpolyposis colorectal cancer syndrome [HNPCC]) accounts for 2–5% of all ECs, and endometrioid EC is the most frequent extracolonic manifestation. In fact, in half of predisposed families, the detection EC was sentinel, revealing the genetic predisposition for HNPCC [21]. Early onset of EC (the risk rises significantly at the age of >40) and low BMI should therefore alert in patients with or without a family history fulfilling the Amsterdam criteria II (according to the International Collaborative group on HNPCC, 1999).

To date, the association between germline mutations in BRCA genes and the risk of EC could not be proven. However, a prospective study could demonstrate that women with genetic mutations for BRCA 1/2 showed a high relative risk for EC (11.6) when under tamoxifen therapy compared to untreated carriers ($p = 0.17$)

within the observational period of 3.3 years [22]. Conversely to the risk factors named above, protective factors such as the use of combined oral contraceptive pills, depot medroxyprogesterone acetate, or progestin-releasing intrauterine-uterine devices could be identified. Unexpectedly, smoking could reduce EC risk, particularly in postmenopausal women [23].

For the prognosis and oncological outcome of EC, not only the histological subtype has relevance but also other risk factors such as intermediate or high tumor grade, deep myometrial invasion, lymphovascular space involvement (LVSI), cervical stroma invasion, adnexal involvement, malignant peritoneal cytology, pelvic and para-aortic lymph node involvement, respectively, vaginal, inguinal, or distant metastasis, in general. Among the above-mentioned, the most important prognostic factors for stage 1 EC remains the depth of myometrial invasion >50% (stage), positive LVSI, as well as an intermediate or high tumor grade. These were the identified postoperative criteria, also called "uterine risk factors," classifying patients of stage 1 carcinoma into the high-intermediate risk group (HI-R EC) for recurrence by the GOG 99 study in 2004. Patients of this group were found to benefit from a comprehensive surgical staging including complete pelvic and para-aortic lymphonodectomy (LNE) in order to select them for adjuvant therapy or avoid overtreatment in the case of a negative lymph node status.

The typical symptoms of EC are abnormal uterine bleeding, postmenopausal bleeding, suspicious vaginal discharge, and rarely none of them. Symptoms of the later stage might be similar to those of ovarian cancer such as abdominal/pelvic pain, abdominal distension, feeling of early abdominal fullness, change of bowel, and bladder function.

The standard evaluation of EC consists of transvaginal sonography, endometrial biopsy, or dilatation and curettage (D&C) with or without hysteroscopy, whereas the gold standard continues to be the D&C combined with diagnostic hysteroscopy as this yields higher accuracy than blind D&C [24].

With regard to preoperative metastatic evaluation, EC primarily remains a surgical staged disease (GOG 33, 1987, see chapter 20.3). A computed tomography (CT) scan, magnetic resonance imaging (MRI), or positron emission tomography/CT can be useful for deciding upon the mode of surgical approach, triaging poor surgical candidates, or in case of symptoms indicating possible metastasis to atypical sites [25]. Among the above-mentioned, imaging by MRI seems to have the highest interobserver concordance [26]. In the assumption of an advanced cancer stage, cystoscopy, rectoscopy, and rectal endosonography, as well as a chest X-ray and an abdominal ultrasound, can be considered individually as part of the preoperative workup.

The CA 125 tumor marker is selectively used in patients whose comorbidities do not allow comprehensive staging surgery or have a high-risk cancer histology, such as papillary serous EC [27]. Interestingly, a prospective Danish study could show that not only CA 125 but also the marker human epididymis protein 4 (HE 4) was significantly increased in patients with the prognostic high-risk factors of high histological grade, affected LN, deep myometrial invasion, cervical involvement, and increased FIGO stage [28].

After the FIGO staging system was revised in 2009, the recommendation of how to perform a comprehensive staging surgery in EC patients continues to be total hysterectomy with bilateral salpingo-oophorectomy, with or without bilateral pelvic and para-aortic lymph node dissection, as well as omentectomy and peritoneal biopsies when indicated (Tab. 20.1, modified according to [29]). Even though a positive peritoneal cytology is no longer an upstaging factor, it is still an essential component of the 2009 FIGO staging system.

Alterations of the procedure can be considered with regard to conserving the ovaries in premenopausal women with early-stage and low-risk EC or in a same group with fertility-preserving wishes by a uterus-conserving, progestin-based approach. However, this is not the standard of care and needs thorough pretherapeutical assessment, follow-ups, and ultimately the hysterectomy as the curative treatment [30].

Traditionally, the surgical treatment of EC has been performed by laparotomy. However, not only the GOG LAP 2 study but also multiple clinical studies of the previous two decades have demonstrated that EC should be initially approached with a minimally invasive surgical technique conferring reduced surgical risk to patients at identical oncological outcome (see chapter 20.3). Robotic-assisted laparoscopy is a safe and feasible minimally invasive alternative for patients with EC, ideal in obese and elderly patients or complex cases, as discussed below.

Limitations of the minimally invasive surgery (MIS) approach would be grossly metastatic manifestations of EC outside the uterus, disseminated involvement of lymph nodes in preoperative imaging, extremely large-sized uterus that cannot

Tab. 20.1: Overview of the stage-adjusted surgical intervention in EC patients.

Tumor stage	Surgical intervention
pT1a, G1, G2	Laparoscopic hysterectomy (extent of hysterectomy is not defined: range between simple HE vs. radical hysterectomy) with BSO; optional pelvic and para-aortic lymphonodectomy (LNE)
pT1a, G3, and pT1b, G1-3	TLH with BSO and pelvic and para-aortic LNE, if applicable: omentectomy
pT2	(Radical) hysterectomy, BSO + pelvic and para-aortic LNE
pT3a	Radical hysterectomy, BSO + pelvic and para-aortic LNE, omentectomy, tumor debulking
pT3b, pT3c	If applicable: radical hysterectomy, BSO + colpectomy, pelvic and para-aortic LNE
pT4a	If applicable: pelvic exenteration + pelvic and para-aortic LNE
N1	Total hysterectomy with BSO + pelvic and para-aortic LNE
M1	If applicable: palliative hysterectomy and tumor debulking

be vaginally evacuated without bisecting, and evidence of deep infiltration of the uterine wall with the risk of perioperative perforation [31].

Vaginal hysterectomy can be appropriate in patients with a high comorbidity index and at high surgical risk for early-stage EC, with similar oncological outcomes [32].

Standard pelvic LNE is characterized by the dissection of the nodal tissue of the common iliac arteries, the anterior and medial aspect of the cranial half of the external iliac vessels, and the nodal tissue plane anteriorly to the obturator nerve. Para-aortic lymph node dissection comprises the removal of lymphatic tissue anterior of the caudal inferior vena cava between the renal vessels and the mid-right common iliac artery. Likewise, on the left, the plane of lymph node resection extends between the aorta and left ureter from the renal vessels to the mid-left common iliac artery [30]. Despite the fact that the GOG 33 study demonstrated the benefit of harvesting the para-aortic lymph nodes up to the renal vessels [33], some authors suggest LNE only up to the inferior mesenteric artery. According to a recent study by Mariani et al., as much as 38–46% of patients with para-aortic lymph node involvement would be missed due to isolated positive lymph nodes in this area [34].

A comprehensive staging with a complete pelvic and para-aortic lymph node dissection has the advantage of knowing the exact diagnosis, evaluating the prognosis, and triaging patients for the adequate adjuvant therapy. There is overall consensus that the complete procedure, including pelvic and para-aortic LNE, is indicated in the high-intermediate risk group (HI-R EC, GOG 99) of stage 1 EC and higher FIGO stages. Apart from the above-mentioned benefits, it is even believed by many authors to have a therapeutic effect [35–37]. In this context, the ASTEC trial should be mentioned, although controversy exists due to some of its weaknesses. In contrast to the above consensus, this large randomized, multicenter trial showed the same oncological outcome of early-stage EC of high-intermediate risk patients who were randomized to a complete surgical staging with LNE or to the group without LNE, after both groups had received pelvic external beam radiotherapy (pelvic EBRT). On the grounds of these findings, the authors questioned the efficacy of LNE in early-stage intermediate-high risk EC [38], given that pelvic EBRT is performed. Interestingly, the cotrial ASTEC/EN.5 demonstrated that the overall survival in intermediate-high risk early-stage EC patients postoperatively was likewise not improved after adjuvant pelvic EBRT compared to the group who did not receive radiotherapy. Unfortunately, in the ASTEC/EN.5, the number of women in the group who had LNE for their primary surgery was low; hence, it was difficult to draw a firm conclusion on a possible interaction between lymphadenectomy and postoperative adjuvant pelvic EBRT. Taking also the high toxicity of radiotherapy into consideration, the authors concluded that pelvic EBRT "cannot be recommended as part of routine treatment for women with intermediate-risk or high-risk early-stage EC with the aim of improving survival" [39].

Definitive guidelines for a complete lymph node dissection in patients of early-stage EC of low-risk for recurrence (L-R EC, GOG 99) remain unclear, and the procedure might not be warranted, as concluded by Mariani *et al.* [34] and Todo *et al.* [35] and others.

Ultimately, the sentinel lymph node (SLN) dissection technique may offer the solution to this dilemma determining which early-stage low-risk patient might benefit from a complete lymphadenectomy. In fact, 10% of early-stage low-risk patients and 15% of patients in the intermediate-risk group were shown to be upstaged after SLN dissection [40]. A very recent Japanese study confirmed the applicability of early-stage EC in low-risk patients and demonstrated high detection rates, sensitivity, and negative predictive value in intermediate-/high-risk patients, in both pelvic and para-aortic SLN biopsy [41].

Particularly patient groups of high surgical risk such as elderly, obese, and multimorbid women, would take advantage of the SLN biopsy, the associated reduced operation time, and decreased perioperative morbidity and mortality [42].

The adjuvant treatment of vaginal brachytherapy in patients with stage I/II EC with high-intermediate risk showed an equivalent reduction of the locoregional recurrence rate compared to the pelvic EBRT, although neither of them affected the overall survival [39]. Yet, compared to pelvic EBRT, vaginal brachytherapie has fewer gastrointestinal side effects and shows better quality of life and is therefore deemed the adjuvant treatment of choice [43]. Whereas only 10–15% of all new diagnosed EC are found to be in FIGO stage III/IV, they constitute for 50% of all uterine cancer-related deaths. In these cases and in recurrent EC, the most crucial aspect, and an independent prognostic factor, for progression-free and overall survival is radical surgical treatment with maximal cytoreduction [44], going as far as pelvic exenteration particularly in previously irradiated patients. Adjuvant treatment with combined radiochemotherapy (pelvic EBRT and paclitaxel/carboplatin) completes the multi-modal approach to advanced EC.

Selected women diagnosed with EC who are unsuitable for surgery can be treated with primary radiation followed by chemotherapy [30].

20.2 History of minimal invasive surgery in EC

Historically, EC has been treated by abdominal hysterectomy and bilateral salpingo-oophorectomy, until in 1987, the GOG 33 trial described the benefits of surgical staging, including the pelvic and para-aortic LNE [33]. It was the first trial to demonstrate that clinically diagnosed stage 1 EC postoperatively had pathologi-cally proven risk factors for recurrence; 22% had myometrial invasion of the outer third, 71% had grade 2 or 3 disease, and 15% were positive for lymphovascular space invasion. Furthermore, among the clinically stage 1 patients, 9% showed pelvic LN metastases, 6% had para-aortic nodal dissemination, 5% had adnexal involvement, and 6% had other extrauterine metastases, meaning an upstage after surgery for this patient group. Growing evidence had suggested that extrauterine disease was related to a poorer prognosis and that adjuvant treatment was required for a complete therapy in order to improve the oncological outcome. Thus, the surgical staging procedure was deemed the key to properly diagnosing EC in order to triage patients for adjuvant therapy if applicable. As a consequence, in 1988, the FIGO officially converted EC to a surgically staged disease with pelvic and para-aortic LNE included.

Within the same year (1987), the first laparoscopic hysterectomy was performed by Reich *et al.* [45], and the first extraperitoneal endoscopic pelvic LNE, by Dargent *et al.* [46]. In 1992, the first laparoscopic hysterectomy for EC and the first laparoscopic para-aortic LNE for a gynecological malignancy were completed by Childers *et al.* [47]. A year later, the same group released a case series of 59 patients who underwent laparoscopically assisted surgical staging for their stage 1 EC, rating this procedure as an "attractive alternative to the traditional surgical approach in patients with stage I endometrial carcinoma" [48].

In 1993, Reich conducted the first total laparoscopic hysterectomy [49], and in the same decade, multiple studies proved the feasibility of the laparoscopic approach in EC.

In 2004, another landmark study was completed by the GOG. The GOG 99 study demonstrated that adjuvant external beam radiation therapy (pelvic EBRT) could only lower the rate of recurrence in women with IB, IC, and II stage EC in the presence of high-intermediate risk factors (HI-R EC) such as grade 2 or 3, positive for LVSI, and depth of invasion to the outer one-third of the myometrium combined with age. In low-risk cases, recurrence was anyhow low and EBRT showed no further benefit; hence, unnecessary overtreatment with corresponding side effects can be avoided in this patient population. Overall survival was not affected in either group [50].

In the meantime, the robotic-assisted system was implemented, matured, and in 2005 approved by the Food and Drug Administration for gynecological surgery in the US.

In 2009, a cooperation of multiple European medical institutions released the results of the ASTEC trial assessing the therapeutic effect of LNE on overall survival in early-stage EC [38]. A total of 1408 women with stage 1 EC had been randomly allocated to surgical staging with LNE vs. without LNE (but palpation of the para-aortic lymph nodes). All women with high-intermediate uterine risk factors such as FIGO IA or IB with high-grade pathology of G3, papillary serous or clear cell, as well as FIGO IC and FIGO IIA, and independent of lymph node status, received radiotherapy. The results showed equal progression-free interval and overall survival in both groups, so the therapeutic benefit of systematic lymphadenectomy for

Tab. 20.2: FIGO classification for staging of endometrial cancer before and after 2009.

Stage	Classification up to 2009	Classification after 2009
I	IA: Endometrium	IA: No or <50% of myometrium
	IB: Inner half of myometrium	IB: ≥50% of myometrium
	IC: Outer half of myometrium	*
II	IIA: Endocervical mucosa	II: Cervical stroma
	IIB: Endocervical stroma	
III	IIIA: Serosa, adnexa, cytology	IIIA: Serosa, adnexa*
	IIIB: Vaginal metastasis	IIIB: Vaginal/Parametrium
	IIIC: Nodal metastasis	IIIC: Nodal metastases IIIC1: pelvic nodes +*
		IIIC2: para-aortic nodes +*
IV	IVA: Bladder or rectal mucosa	IVA: Bladder or rectal mucosa
	IVB: Distant metastases	IVB: Distant metastases

Changes are indicated with *. FIGO classification 1988–2009, revised in 2009.

oncological outcome in early EC was doubted. Although the ASTEC trial is one of the largest reported surgical trials in gynecological oncology, providing some of the best data regarding comprehensive surgical staging, it has ever since been debated due to high rates of crossover to radiotherapy and selection bias.

In the same year, the GOG completed the GOG LAP2 trial comparing the laparoscopic approach to the standard abdominal surgery in EC patients and showed superiority of laparoscopy in terms of fewer moderate to severe postoperative complications, length of hospital stay, and quality of life within 6 postoperative weeks [51].

In 2009, the FIGO staging classification was revised, with four main adjustments (Tab. 20.2).

In 2011, the American Association of Gynecologic Laparoscopists released a position statement claiming that hysterectomies for benign disease shall be performed by vaginal or MIS approach [52].

20.3 Indication for minimal invasive surgery in EC

The MIS approach to the surgical management of early EC has been established as the treatment of choice for many years. Multiple studies could prove the benefit over open surgery with regard to peri- and postoperative complications as well as perioperative data such as rates of blood loss and blood transfusion, hospital stay, return to full activity or work, and quality of life [51, 53–55].

Oncological outcome after laparoscopic staging surgery has also shown comparable results to laparotomy [51, 53, 55, 56], as well as the number of lymph nodes resected in pelvic and para-aortic LNE [56]. While the rates of recurrence within

3 years in the GOG LAP 2 were significantly higher in the laparoscopic group, the overall survival after 5 years was then similar. A large single-arm retrospective study (n = 288 patients) by Lee *et al.* in Taiwan in 2016 revealed overall survival rates for laparoscopically operated early-stage EC as high as 94% in 5 years and 92.7% in a 20-year follow-up [37]. They significantly surpassed the expected overall survival not only for the above-mentioned laparoscopic study results but also for the open surgery procedure, justifying again this method from an oncological aspect.

Even in cases with high-risk histologic subtypes such as uterine serous, clear cell, and carcinosarcoma [57], as well as high-grade endometrioid EC [57, 58], the choice of surgical technique had no impact on the recurrence and survival pattern.

The implementation of the robotic system has been a further milestone in the development of the MIS techniques by alleviating not only the actual surgery. Recent studies have shown that robotic surgery was even surpassing conventional laparoscopy in terms of intra-/postoperative complications, conversion rates, hospital stay, reinterventions, blood loss, or transfusion rate [54, 59–62], with equivalent oncological outcomes [54, 59, 62]. Yet, there are only observational studies to prove this.

The formerly assumed disadvantages of MIS of prolonged operation time and the risk of conversion in early literature were shown to be highly impacted by the learning curve of the MIS team [37]. In fact, the study of Guy *et al.* showed that laparoscopy in general can have shorter operation times compared to robotics and OS [63]. Moreover, robotics, having a much shorter learning curve, was clearly demonstrated to have shorter operation times than conventional laparoscopy after the same surgeon had performed more than 40 cases [64].

The robotic system with high upfront costs at purchase and continued expenses for maintenance and disposable equipment still poses a challenge to the health system. However, a correct cost analysis should take into account the decrease in intra- and postoperative complications with fewer conversion rates, readmissions, and reinterventions and the lowering of laparotomy rates in general as robotic surgery facilitates complex cases as well as surgery in the obese patient [65].

In addition, the costs of robotic surgery decrease in the long-term with increasing hospital volume and procedures [66].

Lastly, having found a surgical method that can avoid abdominal midline incisions from infrasternal to suprapubical, tackling even highly complex cases with fewer perioperative complications and lower rates of blood loss in a decent operation timespan is priceless. Furthermore, women describe their experience with surgery as "easy to overcome" and "feeling recovered shortly after surgery and reporting their health-related quality of life was restored to the preoperative level within 5 weeks after RH" [67].

Ultimately, the choice between the two MIS systems depends on the surgeon's preference and experience as well as to the accessibility of the robotic system.

The two growing population groups of (morbidly) obese and elderly patients show a high incidence of EC and pose group-specific challenges to the MIS surgeon. Reasons for higher risks in the obese patient group with EC are mainly related to higher rates of comorbidities (cardiovascular disease, diabetes mellitus, renal disorders), leading in the long-term to a higher overall mortality, as well as significantly increased peri- and postoperative complications (higher rates of blood loss, wound infection especially aggravated in coexisting diabetes, wound dehiscence, ileus, arrhythmias, acute cardiac events, and venous thrombotic events).

In order to reduce these surgical risks, the laparoscopic approach has become the surgical technique of choice, as long as the compromised cardiopulmonary function due to increased intraabdominal pressure in steep Trendelenburg is manageable. Thus, peri-and postoperative complications, such as transfusion rate, injury of neighboring organs, wound closure or infection, and deep vein thrombosis events, have been significantly lowered by MIS, and return to baseline function is significantly earlier compared to open surgery [68]. In fact, open surgery is considered an independent indicator for surgical complications in morbidly obese women, showing a three times higher rate of such compared to the MIS approach [68]. In addition, OP equipment has been perfected by vacuum mattresses, shoulder holders and surgical stirrups to overcome the concern of inadvertently sliding on the operation table. The solution to the remaining problem of reduced vision in laparoscopic surgery for the (morbidly) obese patient commonly resulting in conversion to laparotomy in order to achieve adequate treatment [51, 69–71] is the implementation of the robotic surgery [72]. This advanced MIS technique is considered a milestone for this surgical high-risk patient group to make their minimal invasive procedure safe, easier, and feasible while allowing a more ergonomic positioning for the surgeon and providing higher instrumental mobility [73]. Compared to conventional laparoscopy, the robotic-assisted surgery was shown to have comparable peri- and postoperative complications rates in the obese patient group, if not lower [72]. With increasing BMI (30–57 [73] and 17.5–69 [74]) and number of comorbidities [74], peri- and postoperative complications rates remained stable when performed by robotic surgery. Yet, it was demonstrated that obese patients with a greater number of comorbidities (three or more) had a higher rate of postoperative complications, specifically cardiac and renal related, even if statistically nonsignificant [74].

As mentioned above, the high costs of the robotic system have always been a topic since its implementation. However, particularly in the patient group of morbidly obese, a recent study showed that the total hospital charges for robotic surgery were only 10% higher than conventional laparoscopy or open surgery in EC [68]. The cost difference is lower in morbidly obese patients as all surgeries in the morbidly obese patient group require more operation time and in addition have higher peri- and postoperative complications; therefore, readmission and reintervention rates after robotic-assisted surgery are fewer. Thus, the advantage of the robotic-assisted system becomes more effective in these higher complex surgeries. However, this study refers to the US medical system, and the costs can be very diverse in different national health systems.

As much as the peri- and postoperative complications in the obese patient group could be lowered, too many of these women still die from the complications of their comorbidities, also in the long run. Obesity is the second most common cause of preventable death, after smoking [75]. It continues to be on us physicians and surgeons to counsel our patients for a healthier lifestyle and weight reduction along with making sure they are handed over to regular follow-ups of their chronic diseases.

EC is also considered the cancer of the elderly, postmenopausal woman being diagnosed at a mean age of 68. With the aging of our population, the prevalences of EC in the elderly patient population are steadily rising. As a matter of fact, EC in elderly patients has a much higher rate of recurrence and lower rate of 5-year cancer-specific survival compared to younger patients [76–78].

Reasons are multifactorial. Data showed that EC in elderly women appears to be more aggressive in terms of histological characteristics, with significantly higher rates of serous and clear cell histology as well as increased rates of grade 2–3 [77, 79, 80] and lymphovascular space invasion [13]. All features are typically found in the histological subtype 2 of EC, underlining the alternative pathway as the predominant carcinogenesis in this patient group. This assumption is supported by the observation that elderly with EC have a significant lower BMI than do younger patients, which correlates inversely with increasing age [13, 79, 81].

Furthermore, elderly patients typically presented with a higher FIGO stage [82], which is known to correlate with the 5-year survival. On the one hand, this might be related to the aggressiveness of the carcinoma in this patient group. On the other hand, it was observed that elderly generally present late with their symptoms (20% wait at least 1 year [83]) and a delayed management of the medical institutions might contribute likewise.

By any means, all mentioned factors seem to be related to a poorer prognosis; in fact, age over 70 years is considered a significant and independent predictor of poorer survival [13, 76]. Looking at a growing high-risk group with regards to recurrence rate and cancer-specific mortality, this calls for the most optimal surgical technique and appropriate radicality. However, studies show that this patient group in particular receives less surgical and adjuvant treatment compared to younger patients [78, 84]. And although MIS is considered the technique of first choice for surgical staging in EC patients in general, it has not yet been converted to the group of elderly patients.

Yet, there is no obvious reason for this. A systematic review of 16 trials comparing perioperative data in the elderly treated with MIS versus open surgery could show lower rates of blood loss, shorter hospital stay, similar rates of operation time, and perioperative complications in the MIS arm [84]. Postoperative complications were either fewer (grade I/II) or similar (grade III/IV) in the MIS arm compared to open surgery. Furthermore, comparing the elderly with the younger patient group treated with MIS, there were no significant differences in operation time, blood loss, hospital stay, perioperative complications, and conversion rates [84].

Looking at complication rates according to surgical approach and age, a subanalysis of the LAP2 study underlines the finding of the above: the rates of postoperative complications of the open surgery group significantly increased with age starting at 60 years old compared to a much more gently inclining rate for the laparoscopic arm [13]. It has to be pointed out that in the LAP2 trial, one of the inclusion criteria was a "good performance status" (GOG performance status <4) with relatively healthy elderly patients, so a low overall rate of complications was expected. Another recent Surveillance, Epidemiology, and End Results Analysis comparing open surgery vs. robotic approach in elderly patient populations showed that with increasing age, perioperative complications also increased in both groups. However, in a subanalysis of the older patient group ($n = 7142$), there were lower rates of perioperative complications and death, shorter hospital stays, and a higher rate of discharge to home in the robotic compared to the open surgery group [63]. This was confirmed by several other retrospective studies [85–87]. To conclude, elderly women with EC seem to benefit from the MIS approach, from as early as the age of 60. Also in this patient group, the implementation of the robotic system contributes to achieve a minimally invasive procedure even in complex cases and prevents unnecessary laparotomies with increased perioperative morbidity.

In terms of oncological outcome, there is limited information in the current literature and no randomized controlled trials with regard to the elderly patient group comparing MIS to open surgery.

Knowing that EC of elderly women has more aggressive tumor characteristics lymph node dissection is a crucial part of a complete staging surgery. In the above-mentioned systematic review [84], the lymph node count was the same for MIS versus open surgery and it was similar in the elderly and younger age group with the exception of two studies showing a significant lower rate of LNE in the elderly group [88, 89]. Similarly, although nonsignificant, a substudy of the GOG LAP2 [13] found out that the largest group of patients having no lymph node dissection was the >80 years old group.

These findings raise the question if surgeons adequately perform LNE in elderly patients when it is indicated, even though laparoscopic LNE appears to be a feasible and safe technique. It is known that in general oncological surgery, the elderly are often undertreated [90] as LNE extends operation time, which is an independent predictor for morbidity in patients above the age of 80 [91]. In addition, it increases perioperative (vascular and neural injury) and postoperative (lymphedema and neurological defects) morbidity. Thus, the hesitation to perform a complete surgical staging in a woman of 80 years is understandable, even though elderly patients "desire radical surgery and disease cure as strongly as the young" [92].

Apart from applying the MIS approach and especially robotics to the group of elderly as a standard of care, another solution to this dilemma could be the standardized application of an oncogeriatric score to predict perioperative morbidity. This has strongly been advocated by the group of Bourgin *et al.* [93] and evaluates frailty rather than the commonly used predictive factor age. The geriatric concept of frailty identifies a patient's physical reserve of coping with a stress situation of a long surgery predicting not only the peri- and postoperative complications but also the domino effect on postoperative morbidity that might follow. It shall ultimately provide help in the decision making of who would benefit from a radical surgical intervention and who is at high risk for complications so preoperative counseling of the elderly woman can quantitatively be objectified. Clinically, the frailty index looks at weight loss, reduction in grip strength, exhaustion, low physical activity, and slowing of walking speed [94] and is considered better performing than other scores (ASA, ECOG, and Charlson Comorbidity index [95, 96]). Besides, postoperative complications specific to this age group can present atypically with falls and confusion for instance and need to be identified as such by the clinicians [97].

Another breakthrough for the surgical high-risk group of elderly women with EC seems to be the implementation of the SLN biopsy when it becomes the standard of care. Once matured and implemented, a complete lymph node staging is performed only when truly indicated so unnecessary perioperative morbidity can be avoided in this frail patient group. At last, it is important to acknowledge that not only the obese but also elderly woman with EC typically have a certain spectrum of comorbidities. If we want to improve their life expectancy, an interdisciplinary approach to control these is a crucial step to make our contribution effective.

20.4 Robotics for EC

In the current literature, the anatomical structures and the steps of the surgical staging procedure in EC patients have been presented many times. In the following section, we go through the procedure of a radical hysterectomy with bilateral salpingo-oophorectomy, para-aortic, then pelvic LNE and infracolic omentectomy, emphasizing on the use of the three robotic arms (Tab. 20.3) and comparing it to the surgical steps of conventional laparoscopy. The description is based on the standard surgical procedure performed in the department of the authors of this chapter.

The preoperative assessment of the size and mobility of the uterus as well as the condition of the vagina and introitus is crucial to achieve the removal of the uterus and adnexa in toto. A large uterus can be cored in a bag and delivered per vaginam, and very large specimens can be placed in an endobag and retrieved via a minilaparotomy at the end of the procedure. The application of an Alexis® wound retractor can facilitate this maneuver. Preoperative bowel prep is useful to optimize intraoperative visualization.

In advanced-stage EC, an initial maximal cytoreduction was demonstrated to have a direct and significant impact on the progression-free and overall survival and

Tab. 20.3: Tabular listing of the steps for the surgical staging procedure in EC by robotics, assigned to the three robotic arms.

Procedure component	Robotic arm 3	Robotic arm 2	Robotic arm 1
Radical hysterectomy	Retracts the lateral third of the round ligament	Coagulates and transects the round ligament	Coagulates and transects the round ligament
Access to parametrium:	Grabs the uterus and retracts it to cephalad	Grasps lateral pedicle of round lig for c-traction	Transects anterior leaf of round lig to ant. midline
– Perivesical and pararectal spaces	Grabs the medial stump of the round ligament	Stays at the lateral stump of the round ligament	Develop the perivesical and pararectal spaces
– Uterine vessels			Uterine vessels are transected
– Medial parametrium			Medial part of the parametrium is dissected and the
Mobilization of ureter			Ureter is mobilized and exposed to the point of its insertion into the bladder
Vesicouterine lig			Vesicouterine ligament is transected laterally
Rectovaginal space	Grabs the uterus and anteverts	Tractions the inferior part of posterior peritoneum	Dissects horizontally to expose rectovag space
Uteracral lig			Uterosacral ligaments are divided
IP lig			IP lig divided 2 cm or more above the iliacs
Colpotomy	Tractions the uterus cephalad	Holds up the bladder flap	Colpotomizes
Para-aortic LND			
Access:	Elevates the peritoneum overlying the distal aorta	Lifting the third portion of the duodenum	Transects the peritoneum vertically
Left area of the aorta and above	Retracts the left leaf of the peritoneum	Lifts the peri- and inter-aorto-caval LN	Dissects LN tissue
Right area of the vena cava	Pulls right ureter + right leaf of peritoneum to right	Lifts the lymphatic tissue	Dissects LN tissue
Pelvic LND			
Access:	Elevates round lig		Incises the post broad lig
External to common iliac LNE	Elevates round lig	Lifts lymphatic tissue under the IP ligament	Dissects external iliac lymphatic nodes
Tracking of the ureter	Applies traction toward medially or laterally		

Tab. 20.3 (continued)

Procedure component	Robotic arm 3	Robotic arm 2	Robotic arm 1
Obturator LNE	Elevates round lig	Traction of LN plane toward medially	Dissects LN
Adhesiolysis of physiol. adhesion of the sigmoid	Gives traction on the round lig	Drags the colon gently toward medially	Performs the adhesiolysis
Omentectomy	Retracts the omentum at the distal end	Lifts the transverse colon for countertraction	Dissects the omentum
Vaginal vault suture	Lifts up the bladder flap	Grasps the anterior then posterior lip of the vagina	Secures the sutures

should be an important surgical goal [98, 99]. In certain situations, additional omentectomy and peritoneal biopsies are recommended, such as in patients with the high risk EC types of clear cell, papillary serous, and carcinosarcoma histology.

In metastatic disease, conversion to laparotomy is often necessary but is dependent on the surgeon's skills and experience.

The patient is placed in a dorsal lithotomy position on a vacuum mattress to reduce sliding during steep Trendelenburg position. Patient positioning is similar in traditional and robotic laparoscopy. Padded shoulder braces with additional gel pads shall prevent neural damage as well as upholstered boot stirrups. First, the abdominal cavity is accessed with the Veres needle at the inferior crease of the umbilicus and a capnoperitoneum is created, then the camera port is placed at the Lee-Huang point or at the Palmers point in case of previous surgery. In case of periumbilical adhesions, the camera trocar access can be achieved by a modified Hasson technique in the region of the Lee-Huang point. On principle, the differences between traditional and robotic-assisted laparoscopic port placement are illustrated in Fig. 20.1.

If an SLN biopsy is planned, the intracervical injection of patent blue or indocyanine green (ICG) at 3, 6, 9, and 12 o'clock is applied at this point of the procedure (bearing in mind that the SLN mapping shall be performed within 15–60 minutes after the ICG injection). With the required equipment for ICG fluorescence imaging of the SLN (e.g., daVinci-FireFly™ system for robotics and Stryker Novadaq™ system for traditional laparoscopy, see Figs. 20.2 and 20.3), this technique is easily applicable and capable of being integrated to the surgical procedure.

We prefer to use the VCare® uterine manipulator for its easy handling (the general use and handling of uterine manipulators in oncologic surgery especially in terms of safety precautions and tumor biological considerations will be discussed in future not only for cervical cancer surgery but also in EC surgery because a potential risk of tumor cell dissemination has to be assumed as well) and place a urinary catheter. The four robotic and the assistant ports are inserted in the

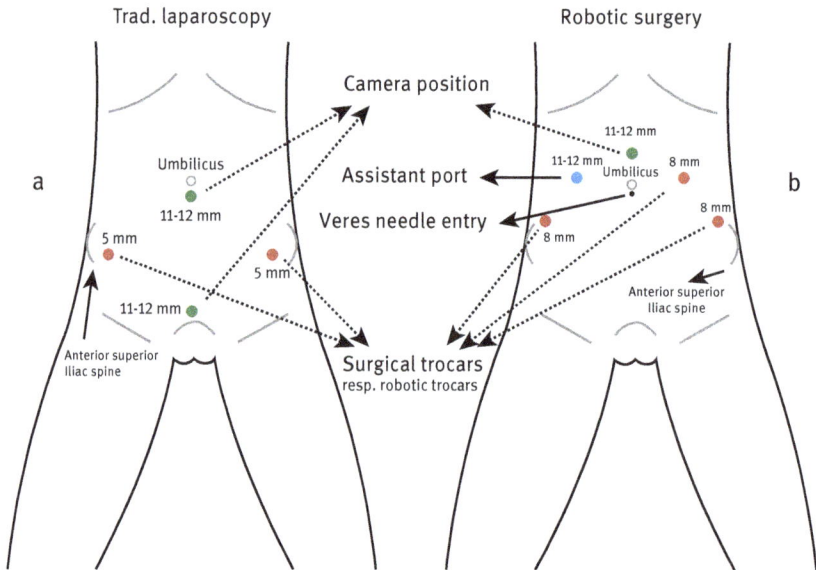

Fig. 20.1: Standard trocar placement for surgical staging of endometrial cancer: (a) traditional and (b) robotic surgery (daVinci™ S and SI system and the daVinci™ Xi system permits a more variable trocar placement); in traditional laparoscopy, the subumbilical camera trocar is used for the pelvic part of the procedure, and for para-aortic LND, the suprapubic camera position is utilized. In robotic surgery, a more cranial position of the camera is necessary (5–7 cm supraumbilical), thus using a region nearby the Lee-Huang point; in expected major peritoneal adhesions, a modified Hasson technique can be performed in this location, as well.

so-called "sunrise distribution" (see Figs. 20.1 and 20.4); however, any reasonable placement to optimize visualization shall be favored. For traditional laparoscopy, we use the conventional technique for peritoneal access at the umbilicus and insert the working trocars as illustrated in Fig. 20.1.

We start the procedure with a panoramic view of the abdominal cavity in a 360-degree manner, followed by the collection of the peritoneal cytology. The patient is then maneuvered into a steep Trendelenburg position, and the robotic system is docked on from the patients' legs or in the side-docking technique. Docking with the daVinci Xi™ system is much more sophisticated due to the modified patient side cart, which is the most important innovation in the generation of daVinci™ systems.

For dissection and coagulation, we use the monopolar scissors and a bipolar forceps. In our opinion, the Maryland forceps is too delicate for tissue rigidity. For retraction, we utilize a grasping forceps. For suturing, we use the Mega Suture Cut™ needle driver. In the conventional procedure, a sealing instrument is inevitable apart from the graspers and different scissors, especially the Metzenbaum scissors.

The Fallopian tubes are sealed proximal to the uterus to prevent the dissemination of cancerous cells. First, we typically start the surgical staging procedure for early-stage EC (1A, B, G1-3) with the radical hysterectomy (type B according to

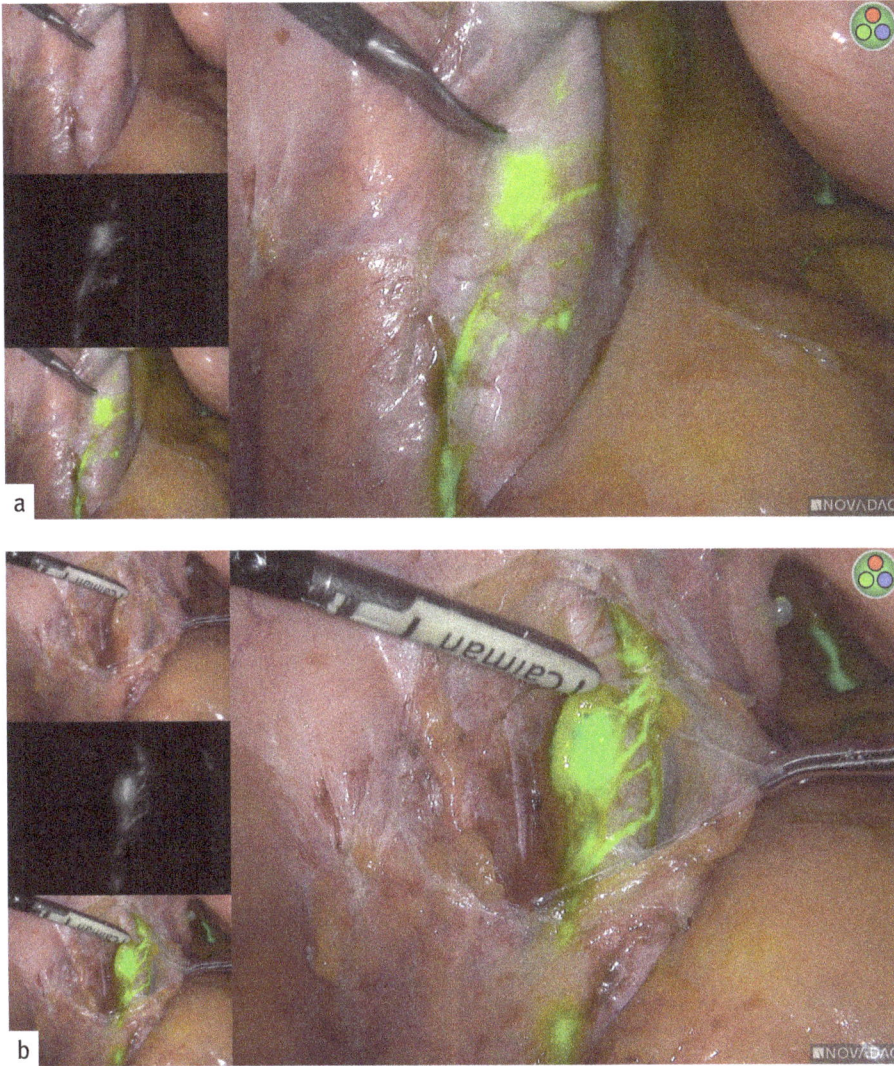

Fig. 20.2: Sentinel node biopsy in traditional laparoscopic endometrial cancer staging using fluorescence imaging with indocyanine green (Novadaq™ system by Stryker Inc., ICG: Verdye®, 25 mg/50 mg powder, Diagnostic Green, Germany). (a) Transperitoneal visualization of an SLN on the left external iliac artery; (b) dissection of the SLN (amazing presentation of the lymphatic vessels).

Querleu-Morrow classification corresponding to the type 2 Piver hysterectomy, also known as the TeLinde modification, or type C/Piver 3 in case of suspected stage 2 EC, respecting the principles of nerve-sparing hysterectomy and the concept of mesometrial structures), in order to send the specimen to the frozen section as early as possible. In robotics, arm 3 retracts the medial third of the round ligament to medially elevating the IP ligament with the ureter. Then, visualization of the latter is done.

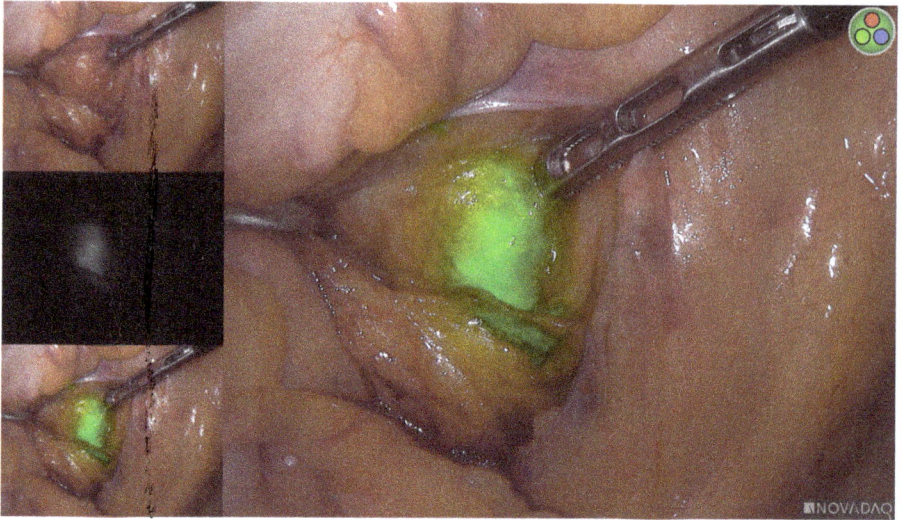

Fig. 20.3: Sentinel node biopsy in traditional laparoscopic endometrial cancer staging using fluorescence imaging with indocyanine green (Novadaq™ system by Stryker Inc., ICG: Verdye®, 25 mg/50 mg powder, Diagnostic Green, Germany). Detection of an SLN below the aortic bifurcation (frequent SLN location in endometrial and cervical cancer).

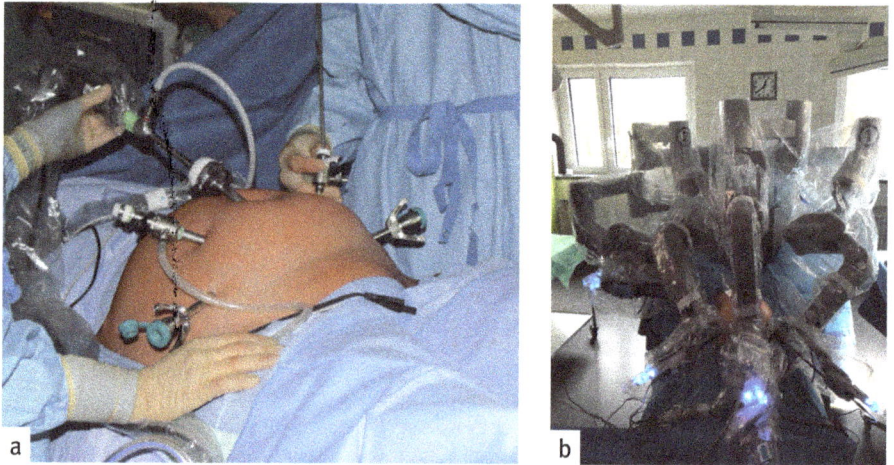

Fig. 20.4: (a) Arrangement of trocars in the so-called sunrise position. (b) Robotic procedure for endometrial cancer staging (between legs docked patient side cart, daVinci S™ system).

Arm 2 grasps the lateral peritoneum opposite of arm 3 for countertraction, so arm 1 can transect the peritoneum laterally and parallel to the IP ligament. Arm 3 grabs the uterus and retracts it to cephalad while arm 2 grasps the lateral pedicle of the round ligament for countertraction, so arm 1 can transect the round ligament and extend the transection into the anterior leaf of the broad ligament, continuing along the line of the vesicouterine reflection to meet the anterior midline of the pelvic peritoneum. Arm 3 grabs the medial stump of the round ligament, and arm 2 stays at the lateral stump of the round ligament, so arm 1 can develop the perivesical (Latzko's fossa) and pararectal spaces. The uterine vessels are transected at their origin from the internal iliac vessels, the medial part of the parametrium is dissected, and the ureter is mobilized from the peritoneum (Okabayashi space) and exposed to the point of its insertion into the bladder. The vesicouterine ligament is then transected laterally to mobilize the bladder further inferiorly so sufficient vaginal margins can be maintained. The filling of the bladder with 100–200 ml of saline solution facilitates the identification of the vesical wall. Arm 3 then grabs the uterus and anteverts, and arm 2 tractions the inferior part of the posterior visceral peritoneum so arm 1 can dissect it horizontally to expose the rectovaginal space. The uterosacral ligaments are divided between the mid and posterior section of the ligament.

For colpotomy, arm 3 retroverts and tractions the uterus toward the cephalad, arm 2 holds the bladder flap, and arm 1 colpotomizes. Uterine manipulation with the inserted device crucially simplifies all these surgical steps, including the identification of the vaginal border of the dissection area. It is performed by the first surgical assistant or, if available, of a second assistant. In traditional laparoscopy, the surgical steps of hysterectomy correspond to the described robotic steps but are managed by less holding features, thus resulting in a higher physical strain for the surgeon. The specimen is delivered through the vagina in toto. A balloon catheter is inserted into the vagina and filled up with water as needed to maintain the capnoperitoneum.

For para-aortic lymph node dissection, the retroperitoneum is accessed by arm 3 elevating the peritoneum overlying the distal aorta and arm 2 lifting the third portion of the duodenum to enable dissection up to the left renal vein. Before performing the LNE, the inferior mesenteric artery and the left ureter have to be identified. Remarkably, on the left side of the aorta, a high amount of lymph nodes can be retrieved. Then, arm 1 transects the peritoneum vertically to enter the retroperitoneum. Arm 1 starts the dissection, while arm 3 exposes the retroperitoneum by retracting the left leaf of the peritoneum and arm 2 lifts the peri- and inter-aorto-caval lymphatic tissue. For the dissection of the right area of the vena cava, arm 3 or the assistant pulls the right ureter and right leaf of the peritoneum to the right side. As arm 2 lifts the lymphatic tissue, arm 3 dissects it. In traditional laparoscopy, the camera position is changed to the suprapubic trocar for para-aortic LNE and the screen is positioned above the head of the patient. For the retraction of the peritoneal leaves, we insert two to three special laparoscopic retractor disposables (e.g., TPEA lifter®, Brenner Medical). The lymph node specimens are collected in marked endobags and delivered vaginally, later on. Hemostatic agents can be applied if required.

For pelvic lymph node dissection, we expose the previously opened retroperitoneal space by retracting the lateral stump of the round ligament anteriorly with arm 3 while arm 1 incises the posterior leaf of the broad ligament toward cephalad, parallel to the external and common iliac vessels. The bedside assistant takes over the traction on the lateral peritoneum for pelvic LNE on the right side and on the sigmoid medially for the pelvic LNE on the left side. The latter step requires sufficient mobilization of the sigmoid colon along the physiological adhesion beforehand. As the fatty tissue under the IP ligament is well exposed, arm 2 can then lift it, and the dissection of the external iliac lymphatic nodes up to the common iliac vessels is accomplished by arm 1. The ureter is tracked medially with arm 3 or laterally depending on the side of the pelvic LNE and with progression of the LNE along the external and common iliac vessels toward the cephalad.

The obturator lymph node dissection is performed easiest in the caudo-cranial direction, starting at the inferior edge of the superior ramus of pubis in order to identify the obturator nerve most safely and straightforward. Arm 3 still retracts the peritoneum anteriorly while arms 1 and 2 perform the LNE.

For pelvic and para-aortic LNE in traditional laparoscopy, the basic surgical steps are identical, however, again a physical challenge for the surgeon and assistant. In addition, anatomical exposure can be more intricate or requires additional placements of trocars.

The lymph node specimens are collected in marked endobags and delivered vaginally. Lastly, as for the omentum, an omental biopsy or a full omentectomy can be performed according to the uterine risk factors. For a complete omentectomy, it is advisable to perform this as the last procedure because the robotic system shall be redocked at the patients' right or left shoulder and the Trendelenburg position shall be reversed. The sunrise distribution can be maintained. For an infracolic omentectomy, we start with the central third of the transverse colon. Arm 3 retracts the omentum at the distal end while arm 2 lifts the transverse colon for countertraction and arm 1 dissects the omentum. It is delivered per vaginam.

In conventional laparoscopy, infragastric or infracolic omentectomy can be performed with less expenditure regarding the technical equipment, either subsequent to the para-aortic LNE or followed after the pelvic LNE when the camera position has been changed.

The horizontal closure of the vaginal vault is done by vertical stitches in a figure-of-8 fashion, commencing with one on both lateral margins: Arm 3 lifts up the bladder flap, arm 2 grasps the anterior then posterior lip of the vagina, and arm 1 (having changed to a needle holder) secures the sutures. We favor figure-of-8-stitches over running sutures to prevent vaginal cuff dehiscence as a typical complication of MIS procedures in general. For this reason we also use late absorbable suture material (such as polydioxanone) for vaginal closure, both in robotics and conventional laparoscopic procedures.

The robotic system is then undocked.

Finally, one drain is inserted into the left lower abdominal port site. The pneumoperitoneum and ports are removed and incision closure is performed, including fascia closure in trocar sites of > 1 cm.

References

[1] Ferlay J, Shin HR, Bray F, Forman D, Mathers C, Parkin DM. GLOBOCAN 2008. Cancer incidence and mortality worldwide. IARC CancerBase No. 10 [Internet]. Lyon, France: International Agency for Research on Cancer; 2010; Vol. Available at: http://globocan.iarc.fr.

[2] Ferlay J, Soerjomataram I, Ervik M, et al. GLOBOCAN 2012 v1.1, Cancer Incidence and Mortality Worldwide: IARC CancerBase No. 11 [Internet]. Lyon, France: International Agency for Research on Cancer 2014: http://globocan.iarc.fr.

[3] Humphrey MM, Apte SM. The use of minimally invasive surgery for endometrial cancer. Cancer Control J Moffitt Cancer Center 2009;16(1):30–7.

[4] Creasman WT, Odicino F, Mausinneuve P, et al. Carcinoma of the corpus uteri. (26th Annual Report on the Results of Treatment in Gynecological Cancer). Int J Gynecol Obstet 2006;95(Suppl 1):105–43.

[5] Hecht JL, Mutter GL. Molecular and pathologic aspects of endometrial carcinogenesis. J Clin Oncol 2006;24:4783–91.

[6] Sherman ME. Theories of endometrial carcinogenesis: a multidisciplinary approach. Mod Pathol 2000;13:295–308.

[7] Felix AS, Weissfeld JL, Stone RA, et al. Factors associated with type I and type II endometrial cancer. Cancer Causes Control 2010;21:1851–6.

[8] Lax SF. Dualistic model of molecular pathogenesis in endometrial carcinoma. Zentralblatt fuer Gynaekol Jan 2002;124(1):10–6.

[9] Shapiro S, Kelly JP, Rosenberg L, et al. Risk of localized and widespread endometrial cancer in relation to recent and discontinued use of conjugated estrogens. N Engl J Med 1985;313(16):969–72.

[10] Pike MC, Peters RK, Cozen W, et al. Estrogen-progestin replacement therapy and endometrial cancer. J Natl Cancer Inst 1997;89(15):1110–6.

[11] Fisher B, Costantino JP, Redmond CK, et al. Endometrial cancer in tamoxifen-treated breast cancer patients: findings from the National Surgical Adjuvant Breast and Bowel Project (NSABP) B-14. J Natl Cancer Inst 1994;86(7):527–37.

[12] Berton-Rigaud D, Devouassoux-Shisheboran M, Ledermann JA, et al. Gynecologic Cancer Inter-Group (GCIC): consensus review for uterine and ovarian carcinosarcoma. Int J Gynecol Cancer 2014;24(9 Suppl 3):S55–60.

[13] Bishop EA, Java JJ, Moore KN, et al. Surgical outcomes among elderly women with endometrial cancer treated by laparoscopic hysterectomy: a NRG/Gynecologic Oncology Group study. Am J Obstet Gynecol 2018 Jan;218(1):109.e1–11.

[14] Kashima H, Shiozawa T, Miyamoto T, et al. Autocrine stimulation of IGF1 in estrogen-induced growth of endometrial carcinoma cells: involvement of the mitogen-activated protein kinase path way followed by up-regulation of cyclin D1 and cyclin E. Endocr Relat Cancer 2009 Mar;16(1):113–22.

[15] Mills KT, Bellows CF, Hoffman AE, Kelly TN, Gagliardi G. Diabetes mellitus and colorectal cancer prognosis: a meta-analysis. Dis Colon Rectum 2013 Nov;56(11):1304–19.

[16] Kleeff J, Costello E, Jackson R, et al. The impact of diabetes mellitus on survival following resection and adjuvant chemotherapy for pancreatic cancer. Br J Cancer 2016;115:887–94.

[17] Lindemann K, Cvancarova M, Eskild A. Body mass index, diabetes and survival after diagnosis of endometrial cancer: a report from the HUNT-survey. Gynecol Oncol 2015;139:476–80.

[18] Nagle CM, Crosbie EJ, Brand A, et al. The association between diabetes, comorbidities, body mass index and all-cause and cause-specific mortality among women with endometrial cancer. Gynecol Oncol 2018 Jul;150(1):99–105.

[19] Binder PS, Peipert JF, Kallogjeri D, et al. Adult comorbidity evaluation 27 score as a predictor of survival in endometrial cancer patients. Am J Obstet Gynecol 2016;215(766):766.e1–9.

[20] Robbins JR, Gayar OH, Zaki M, Mahan M, Buekers T, Elshaikh MA. Impact of age-adjusted Charlson comorbidity score on outcomes for patients with early-stage endometrial cancer. Gynecol Oncol 2013;131:593–597.

[21] Bats AS, Rossi L, Le Frere-Belda MA, et al. Lynch syndrome and endometrial cancer. Bull Cancer 2017 Dec;104(12):1013–102.

[22] Beiner ME, Finch A, Rosen B, et al. The risk of endometrial cancer in women with BRCA1 and BRCA2 mutations. A prospective study. Gynecol Oncol 2007 Jan;104(1):7–10.

[23] Zhou B, Yang L, Sun Q, et al. Cigarette smoking and the risk of endometrial cancer: a meta-analysis. Am J Med 2008;121(6):501–8.

[24] Lee DO, Jung MH, Kim HY. Prospective comparison of biopsy results from curettage and hysteroscopy in postmenopausal uterine bleeding. J Obstet Gynaecol Res 2011 Oct;37(10):1423–6.

[25] Burke WM, Orr J, Leitao M, et al. Endometrial cancer: a review and current management strategies: part I. Gynecologic Oncology 2014;134:385–92.

[26] Savelli L, Ceccarini M, Ludovisi M, et al. Preoperative local staging of endometrial cancer: transvaginal sonography vs. magnetic resonance imaging. Ultrasound Obstet Gynecol 2008;31(5):560–6.

[27] Olawaiye AB, Rauh-Hain JA, Withiam-Leitch M, Rueda B, Goodman A, del Carmen MG. Utility of pre-operative serum CA-125 in the management of uterine papillary serous carcinoma. Gynecol Oncol 2008;110(3):293–8.

[28] Antonsen SL, Høgdall E, Christensen IJ, et al. HE4 and CA125 levels in the preoperative assessment of endometrial cancer patients: a prospective multicenter study (ENDOMET). Acta Obstet Gynecol Scand 2013 Nov;92(11):1313–22.

[29] Juhasz-Böss I, Haggag H, Baum S, Kerl S, Rody A, Solomayer E. Laparoscopic and laparotomic approaches for endometrial cancer treatment: a comprehensive review. Arch Gynecol Obstet 2012;286(1):167–72.

[30] SGO Clinical Practice Endometrial Cancer Working Group, Burke WM, Orr J, Leitao M, et al. Endometrial cancer: a review and current management strategies: Part II. Gynecol Oncol 2014;134:393–402.

[31] Leblanc E, Samouelian V, Boulanger L, Narducci F. Are there still contraindications to laparoscopic treatment of endometrial carcinoma? Gynécol Obstét Fertil 2010;38:119–25.

[32] Berretta R, Merisio C, Melpignano M, et al. Vaginal versus abdominal hysterectomy in endometrial cancer: a retrospective study in a selective population. Int J Gynecol Cancer 2008 Jul–Aug;18(4):797–802.

[33] Creasman WT, Morrow CP, Bundy BN, Homesley HD, Graham JE, Heller PB. Surgical pathologic spread patterns of endometrial cancer: a Gynecologic Oncology Group study. Cancer 1987;60(Suppl)(8):2035–41.

[34] Mariani A, Dowdy SC, Cliby WA, et al. Prospective assessment of lymphatic dissemination in endometrial cancer: a paradigm shift in surgical staging. Gynecol Oncol 2008 Apr;109(1):11–18.

[35] Todo Y, Kato H, Kaneuchi M, Watari H, Takeda M, Sakuragi N. Survival effect of para-aortic lymphadenectomy in endometrial cancer (SEPAL study): a retrospective cohort analysis. Lancet 2010 Apr 3;375(9721):1165–72.

[36] Chan JK, Cheung MK, Huh WK, et al. Therapeutic role of lymph node resection in endometrioid corpus cancer: a study of 12,333 patients. Cancer 2006;107:1823–30.

[37] Lee CL, Kusunoki S, Huang KG, Wu KY, Huang CY, Yen CF. Long-term survival outcomes of laparoscopic staging surgery in treating endometrial cancer: 20 years of follow-up. Taiwan J Obstet Gynecol 2016 Aug;55(4):545–51.

[38] ASTEC study Group, Kitchener H, Swart AM, Qian Q, Amos C, Parmar MK. Efficacy of systematic pelvic lymphadenectomy in endometrial cancer (MRC ASTEC trial): a randomised study. Lancet 2009 Jan 10;373(9658):125–36. doi: 10.1016/S0140-6736(08)61766-3.

[39] ASTEC/EN.5 Study Group: Blake P, Swart AM, Orton J, et al. Adjuvant external beam radiotherapy in the treatment of endometrial cancer (MRC ASTEC and NCIC CTG EN.5 randomised trials): pooled trial results, systematic review, and meta-analysis. Lancet 2009 Jan 10;373(9658):137–46.

[40] Ballester M, Dubernard G, Lécuru F, et al. Detection rate and diagnostic accuracy of sentinel-node biopsy in early stage endometrial cancer: a prospective multicentre study (SENTI-ENDO). Lancet Oncol 2011;12(5):469–76.

[41] Togami S, Kawamura T, Fukuda M, Yanazume S, Kamio M, Kobayashi H. Prospective study of sentinel lymph node mapping for endometrial cancer. Int J Gynaecol Obstet [Epub ahead of print August 20, 2018].

[42] Bourgin C, Lambaudie E, Houvenaeghel G, Foucher F, Levêque J, Lavoué V. Impact of age on surgical staging and approaches (laparotomy, laparoscopy and robotic surgery) in endometrial cancer management. Eur J Surg Oncol 2017 Apr;43(4):703–9.

[43] Nout RA, Smit VT, Putter H, et al. Vaginal brachytherapy versus pelvic external beam radiotherapy for patients with endometrial cancer of high-intermediate risk (PORTEC-2): an open-label, non-inferiority, randomised trial. Lancet 2010 Mar 6;375(9717):816–23.

[44] Lambrou NC, Gómez-Marín O, Mirhashemi R, et al. Optimal surgical cytoreduction in patients with stage III and stage IV endometrial carcinoma: a study of morbidity and survival. Gynecol Oncol 2004 Jun;93(3):653–8.

[45] Reich H, DeCaprio J, McGlynn F. Laparoscopic hysterectomy. J Gynecol Surg 1989;5:213–6.

[46] Dargent D, Salvat J. L'envahissement ganglionnaire pelvien. Paris: Medsi-McGraw Hill; 1989.

[47] Childers JM, Hatch KD, Tran AN, Surwit E. Laparoscopic para-aortic lymphadenectomy in gynecologic malignancies. Obstet Gynecol 1993;82:741–7.

[48] Childers JM, Brzechffa PR, Hatch KD, Surwit EA. Laparoscopically assisted surgical staging (LASS) of endometrial cancer. Gynecol Oncol 1993;51(1):33–8.

[49] Reich H, McFlynn F. Total laparoscopic hysterectomy. Gynaecol Endosc 1993;2:59–63.

[50] Keys HM, Roberts JA, Brunetto VL, et al. A phase III trial of surgery with or without adjunctive external pelvic radiation therapy in intermediate risk endometrial adenocarcinoma: a Gynecologic Oncology Group study. Gynecol Oncol 2004 Mar;92(3):744–51.

[51] Walker JL, Piedmonte MR, Spirtos NM, et al. Laparoscopy compared with laparotomy for comprehensive surgical staging of uterine cancer: Gynecologic Oncology Group Study LAP2. J Clin Oncol 2009 Nov 10;27(32):5331–6.

[52] AAGL position statement: route of hysterectomy to treat benign uterine disease. J Minim Invasive Gynecol 2011;18:1–3.

[53] Galaal K, Bryant A, Fisher AD, Al-Khaduri M, Kew F, Lopes AD. Laparoscopy versus laparotomy for the management of early stage endometrial cancer. Cochrane Database Syst Rev 2012 Sep 12;(9);Art. No. CD006655.

[54] Acholonu UC Jr, Chang-Jackson SC, Radjabi AR, et al. Laparoscopy for the management of early-stage endometrial cancer: from experimental to standard of care. J Minim Invasive Gynecol 2012 Jul–Aug;19(4):434–42.

[55] Lu Q, Liu H, Liu C, et al. Comparison of laparoscopy and laparotomy for management of endometrial carcinoma: a prospective randomized study with 11-year experience. J Cancer Res Clin Oncol 2013 Nov;139(11):1853–9.

[56] de la Orden SG, Reza MM, Blasco JA, Andradas E, Callejo D, Pérez T. Laparoscopic hysterectomy in the treatment of endometrial cancer: a systematic review. J Minim Invasive Gynecol 2008 Jul–Aug;15(4):395–401.

[57] Fader AN, Java J, Tenney M, et al. Impact of histology and surgical approach on survival among women with early-stage, high-grade uterine cancer: an NRG Oncology/Gynecologic Oncology Group ancillary analysis. Gynecol Oncol 2016 Dec;143(3):460–5.

[58] Fader AN, Seamon LG, Escobar PF, et al. Minimally invasive surgery versus laparotomy in women with high grade endometrial cancer: a multi-site study performed at high volume cancer centers. Gynecol Oncol 2012 Aug;126(2):180–5.

[59] Corrado G, Cutillo G, Pomati G, et al. Surgical and oncological outcome of robotic surgery compared to laparoscopic and abdominal surgery in the management of endometrial cancer. Eur J Surg Oncol 2015 Aug;41(8):1074–81.

[60] Seamon LG, Cohn DE, Henretta MS, et al. Minimally invasive comprehensive surgical staging for endometrial cancer: robotics or laparoscopy? Gynecol Oncol 2009 Apr;113(1):36–41.

[61] Lim PC, Kang E, Park DH. Learning curve and surgical outcome for robotic-assisted hysterectomy with lymphadenectomy: case-matched controlled comparison with laparoscopy and laparotomy for treatment of endometrial cancer. J Minim Invasive Gynecol 2010 Nov–Dec;17(6):739–48.

[62] Park DA, Lee DH, Kim SW, Lee SH. Comparative safety and effectiveness of robot-assisted laparoscopic hysterectomy versus conventional laparoscopy and laparotomy for endometrial cancer: a systematic review and meta-analysis. Eur J Surg Oncol 2016 Sep;42(9):1303–14.

[63] Guy MS, Sheeder J, Behbakht K, Wright JD, Guntupalli SR. Comparative outcomes in older and younger women undergoing laparotomy or robotic surgical staging for endometrial cancer. Am J Obstet Gynecol 2016 Mar;214(3):350.e1–10.

[64] Lim PC, Kang E, Park DH. Learning curve and surgical outcome for robotic-assisted hysterectomy with lymphadenectomy: case-matched controlled comparison with laparoscopy and laparotomy for treatment of endometrial cancer. J Minim Invasive Gynecol 2010 Nov–Dec;17(6):739–48.

[65] O'Malley DM, Smith B, Fowler JM. The role of robotic surgery in endometrial cancer. J Surg Oncol 2015 Dec;112(7):761–8.

[66] Wright JD, Ananth CV, Tergas AI, et al. An economic analysis of robotically assisted hysterectomy. Obstet Gynecol 2014 May;123(5):1038–48.

[67] Herling SF. Robotic-assisted laparoscopic hysterectomy for women with endometrial cancer—complications, women's experiences, quality of life and a health economic evaluation. Dan Med J 2016 Jul;63(7).

[68] Chan JK, Gardner AB, Taylor K, et al. Robotic versus laparoscopic versus open surgery in morbidly obese endometrial cancer patients—a comparative analysis of total charges and complication rates. Gynecol Oncol 2015 Nov;139(2):300–5.

[69] Eltabbakh GH, Shamonki MI, Moody JM, Garafano LL. Hysterectomy for obese women with endometrial cancer: laparoscopy or laparotomy? Gynecol Oncol 2000 Sep;78(3 Pt 1):329–35.

[70] Stephan JM, Goodheart MJ, McDonald M, et al. Robotic surgery in supermorbidly obese patients with endometrial cancer. Am J Obstet Gynecol 2015 Jul;213(1):49.e1–8.

[71] Uccella S, Bonzini M, Palomba S, et al. Impact of obesity on surgical treatment for endometrial cancer: a multicenter study comparing laparoscopy vs open surgery, with propensity-matched analysis. J Minim Invasive Gynecol 2016 Jan;23(1):53–61.

[72] Iavazzo C, Gkegkes ID. Robotic assisted hysterectomy in obese patients: a systematic review. Arch Gynecol Obstet 2016 Jun;293(6):1169–83.

[73] Corrado G, Chiantera V, Fanfani F, et al. Robotic hysterectomy in severely obese patients with endometrial cancer: a multicenter study. J Minim Invasive Gynecol 2016 Jan;23(1):94–100.

[74] Backes FJ, Rosen M, Liang M, et al. Robotic hysterectomy for endometrial cancer in obese patients with comorbidities: evaluating postoperative complications. Int J Gynecol Cancer 2015 Sep;25(7):1271–6.

[75] Fontaine KR, Redden DT, Wang C, Westfall AO, Allison DB. Years of life lost due to obesity. JAMA 2003 Jan 8;289(2):187–93.

[76] Alektiar KM, Venkatraman E, Abu-Rustum N, Barakat RR. Is endometrial carcinoma intrinsically more aggressive in elderly patients? Cancer 2003 Dec 1;98(11):2368–77.

[77] Jolly S, Vargas CE, Kumar T, et al. The impact of age on long-term outcome in patients with endometrial cancer treated with postoperative radiation. Gynecol Oncol 2006 Oct;103(1):87–93.

[78] De Marzi P, Ottolina J, Mangili G, et al. Surgical treatment of elderly patients with endometrial cancer (≥ 65 years). J Geriatr Oncol 2013 Oct;4(4):368–73.

[79] Lachance JA, Everett EN, Greer B, et al. The effect of age on clinical/pathologic features, surgical morbidity, and outcome in patients with endometrial cancer. Gynecol Oncol 2006 Jun;101(3):470–5.

[80] Siesto G, Uccella S, Ghezzi F, et al. Surgical and survival outcomes in older women with endometrial cancer treated by laparoscopy. Menopause 2010 May–Jun;17(3):539–44.

[81] Fleming ND, Lentz SE, Cass I, Li AJ, Karlan BY, Walsh CS. Is older age a poor prognostic factor in stage I and II endometrioid endometrial adenocarcinoma? Gynecol Oncol 2011 Feb;120(2):189–92.

[82] Zeng XZ, Lavoue V, Lau S, et al. Outcome of robotic surgery for endometrial cancer as a function of patient age. Int J Gynecol Cancer 2015 May;25(4):637–44.

[83] Le diagnostic [Internet]. Fondation ARC pour la recherche sur le cancer. [cité 14 fevr 2015]. Available at: http://www.fondation-arc.org/Le-cancer-chez-la-personne-agee/oncogeriatrie-le-diagnostic.html.

[84] Wright JD, Lewin SN, Barrena Medel NI, et al. Morbidity and mortality of surgery for endometrial cancer in the oldest old. Am J Obstet Gynecol 2011 Jul;205(1):66.e1–8.

[85] Backes FJ, ElNaggar AC, Farrell MR, et al. Perioperative outcomes for laparotomy compared to robotic surgical staging of endometrial cancer in the elderly: a retrospective cohort. Int J Gynecol Cancer 2016 Nov;26(9):1717–21.

[86] Doo DW, Guntupalli SR, Corr BR, et al. Comparative surgical outcomes for endometrial cancer patients 65 years old or older staged with robotics or laparotomy. Ann Surg Oncol 2015 Oct;22(11):3687–94.

[87] Lavoue V, Zeng X, Lau S, et al. Impact of robotics on the outcome of elderly patients with endometrial cancer. Gynecol Oncol 2014 Jun;133(3):556–62.

[88] Vaknin Z, Perri T, Lau S, et al. Outcome and quality of life in a prospective cohort of the first 100 robotic surgeries for endometrial cancer, with focus on elderly patients. Int J Gynecol Cancer 2010 Nov;20(8):1367–73.

[89] Vaknin Z, Ben-Ami I, Schneider D, Pansky M, Halperin R. A comparison of perioperative morbidity, perioperative mortality, and disease-specific survival in elderly women (> or =70 years) versus younger women (<70 years) with endometrioid endometrial cancer. Int J Gynecol Cancer 2009 Jul;19(5):879–83.

[90] Monson K, Litvak DA, Bold RJ. Surgery in the aged population: surgical oncology. Arch Surg 2003 Oct;138(10):1061–7.

[91] Turrentine FE, Wang H, Simpson VB, Jones RS. Surgical risk factors, morbidity, and mortality in elderly patients. J Am Coll Surg 2006 Dec;203(6):865–77.

[92] Nordin AJ, Chinn DJ, Moloney I, Naik R, de Barros Lopes A, Monaghan JM. Do elderly cancer patients care about cure? Attitudes to radical gynecologic oncology surgery in the elderly. Gynecol Oncol 2001 Jun;81(3):447–55.

[93] Bourgin C, Saidani M, Poupon C, et al. Endometrial cancer in elderly women: Which disease, which surgical management? A systematic review of the literature. EJSO 2016;42:166–75.

[94] Fried LP, Tangen CM, Walston J, et al. Cardiovascular Health Study Collaborative Research Group. Frailty in older adults: evidence for a phenotype. J Gerontol A Biol Sci Med Sci 2001 Mar;56(3):M146–56.

[95] Makary MA, Segev DL, Pronovost PJ, et al. Frailty as a predictor of surgical outcomes in older patients. J Am Coll Surg 2010 Jun;210(6):901–8.

[96] Revenig LM, Canter DJ, Taylor MD, et al. Too frail for surgery? Initial results of a large multidisciplinary prospective study examining preoperative variables predictive of poor surgical outcomes. J Am Coll Surg 2013 Oct;217(4):665–70.e1.

[97] Common perioperative Complications in Older Patients [Internet]. [cité 28 mars 2014]. Available at: http://www.springer.com/cda/content/document/cda_download document/9781441969989-c29. pdf?SGWID.0-0-45-1152939-p174128180.

[98] Shih KK, Yun E, Gardner GJ, Barakat RR, Chi DS, Leitao MM Jr. Surgical cytoreduction in stage IV endometrioid endometrial carcinoma. Gynecol Oncol 2011;122(3):608–11.

[99] Lambrou NC, Gómez-Marín O, Mirhashemi R, et al. Optimal surgical cytoreduction in patients with stage III and stage IV endometrial carcinoma: a study of morbidity and survival. Gynecol Oncol 2004;93(3):653–8.

Lucas Minig, Vanna Zanagnolo and Javier Magrina

21 Minimally invasive surgery (MIS) for epithelial ovarian cancer (EOC)

21.1 Introduction

Early-stage epithelial ovarian cancer (EOC) is defined as a tumor confined to one or both ovaries without evidence of local or distant spread. The recommended treatment by the International Federation of Gynecology and Obstetrics (FIGO) consists of surgical staging based on hysterectomy, bilateral salpingo-oophorectomy, omentectomy, pelvic and aortic lymphadenectomy, multiple peritoneal biopsies, and appendectomy (for mucinous histology) through midline incision [1], With this type of treatment and with the addition of platinum-based chemotherapy in selected group of patients, the 5-year survival ranges over 90% [2].

In the last 30 years, minimally invasive laparoscopic surgery has become increasingly integrated as a surgical approach for the treatment of endometrial and cervical cancer. However, the acceptance and wide application of laparoscopy for women with EOC are limited [3]. Long surgeons' learning curve, long operative time, and the paucity of data regarding the long-term oncological outcomes constitute some of the main obstacles. The clinical evidence to help quantify the risks and benefits of laparoscopy for the management of early-stage EOC as routine clinical practice is based on case series [4–13] or a few comparative studies with laparotomy [3, 14–22]. Recent evidence suggests a role of laparoscopy to evaluate tumor resectability in women with AEOC [23]. Limited evidence suggests a role of minimally invasive surgery (MIS) for cytoreduction in selected women undergoing primary, interval, or secondary debulking [24]. Therefore, the current chapter will describe the current role of laparoscopy in the management of women with EOC.

21.2 Surgical staging of women with apparently early-stage ovarian cancer

Early-stage EOC is defined as a tumor confined to one or both ovaries without visible or microscopic evidence of local or distant spread. The surgical removal of organs and tissues that may be potentially affected by microscopic disease seems to be the best alternative to determine the true extension of the disease due to the limitations of current diagnostic methods such as positron emission tomography–computed tomography (CT) or nuclear magnetic resonance imaging [25].

https://doi.org/10.1515/9783110535204-021

21.2.1 Surgical technique

Surgical staging of apparently early-stage EOC requires a well-trained surgical team, an adequate preparation of the patient, as well as appropriate surgical instruments and equipment. Furthermore, the patient needs to be in a semilithotomy position over an antisliding device to prevent sliding when in the Trendelenburg position.

21.2.1.1 Intraoperative diagnosis of apparently early-stage ovarian cancer with immediate staging

This procedure is a two-step surgery: pelvic and abdominal approach. The first trocar (11 mm) is placed at the umbilicus by using the Veress or open technique. Three 5-mm trocars are introduced in the pelvis as shown in Fig. 21.1.

Surgical staging should start with the aspiration of free fluid or pelvic washing for cytological analysis of tumor cells. The next step is a thorough inspection of the parietal and visceral peritoneal surfaces of the entire peritoneal surfaces of the pelvis, middle, and upper abdomen. Any suspicious lesions are excised if the inspection is negative, and random peritoneal biopsies along the natural flow path of peritoneal fluid should be done. This begins in the Douglas pouch and extends through the paracolic spaces to the hemi-diaphragms. Biopsies should be large (4–5 cm^2) and 5 to 10 in number [26].

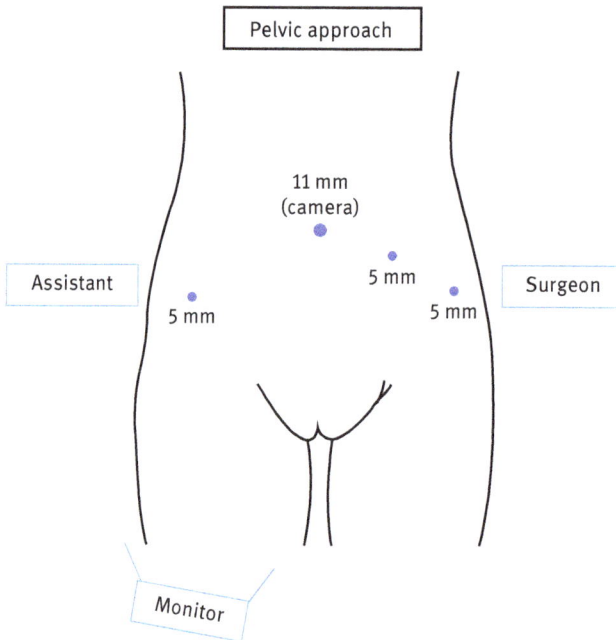

Fig. 21.1: Trocars' distribution for pelvic approach.

With a preoperative diagnosis of a suspicious adnexal mass, the tumor should be amenable to place in an endobag for removal and without apparent gross metastatic disease limited. During the initial surgical inspection, the affected ovary should be ideally free of dense adhesions and without any evidence of an ovarian surface tumor [26]. In the absence of extra-tumor disease, the adnexal dissection and its subsequent removal must be carefully performed to avoid cyst rupture, potentially affecting the needs for adjuvant therapies and prognosis of the disease [27, 28]. Thus, tumor size must be small enough to enter fully into an endoscopic bag to be removed intact [29, 30]. If the frozen section reveals an invasive epithelial ovarian carcinoma, full surgical staging, as previously described, needs to be performed [31]. At this point, total simple hysterectomy Bilateral Salpingo-oophorectomy(BSO), omentectomy, biopsies, and pelvic and aortic lymph node dissection are performed. All specimens are removed through the open the vagina before closure.

Despite the fact that some port sites are used for the second part of the surgery, additional incisions are required, as Fig. 21.2 shows.

The abdominal part of the operation includes infracolic omentectomy, appendectomy (for mucinous histology), and aortic transperitoneal lymphadenectomy. The left infrarenal node dissection is the most complicated procedure for staging early-stage EOC patients. It is estimated that nodal invasion is present in approximately 10% of these patients, and the most common location is in the left infrarenal group [32]. In addition to prognostic information, identifying patients with nodal involvement will select a small group of women who will require adjuvant chemotherapy only because of positive nodes [33].

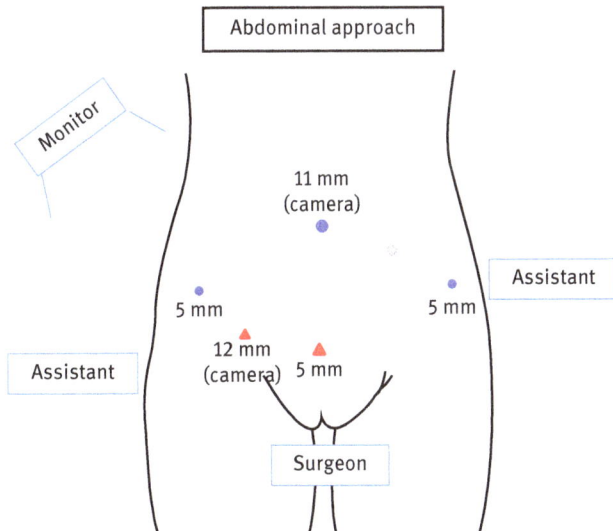

Fig. 21.2: Trocars' distribution for the abdominal approach. Trocars in the triangle represent the additional access.

21.2.1.2 Surgical restaging of an apparently early-stage ovarian cancer

In some instances, patients undergo delayed surgical staging after an incidental diagnosis of an apparently early-stage EOC. In this case, the surgical restaging can start by performing an extraperitoneal para-aortic lymphadenectomy [34]. For some authors, this approach may be safer and easier, especially in obese women or in patients with multiple intraabdominal adhesions [34, 35]. In these cases, surgical staging begins with a transumbilical diagnostic laparoscopy to assess the peritoneal cavity. In the absence of intraperitoneal disease, an extraperitoneal para-aortic lymphadenectomy is performed via a left-sided approach. A 10-mm incision is made 3 cm medial to the anterosuperior iliac spine. The extraperitoneal space is developed using finger dissection of the peritoneum over the psoas muscle and the left flank. CO_2 is insufflated and the space is created. Two additional 5-mm trocars are then introduced in the midaxillary line in the preperitoneal space under laparoscopic guidance. One trocar is located just above the iliac crest and the other one 1–2 cm below the left inferior costal margin. An additional 5-mm laparoscopic trocar can be inserted between the camera and the trocar above the iliac crest to obtain better exposure of the surgical field. After finishing this procedure, the surgery can proceed by performing the pelvic approach as previously mentioned once the robotic column is undocked and redocked (Fig. 21.1).

Therefore, performing laparoscopic MIS staging should be considered only in carefully selected patients.

21.2.2 Clinical evidence

The feasibility of laparoscopic staging requires the evaluation of several aspects, including the frequency of complications, the rate of conversion to laparotomy, and the risk of recurrence. Laparoscopic surgical staging in early-stage EOC should be performed only in cases where the surgeon and the surgical team can meet the same quality indicators of safety and oncologic radicality with procedures performed by laparotomy. Thus, referral to a surgeon with a sufficient level of surgical preparation is the recommended strategy [36]. In this regard, several studies have shown that about 30% of patients with apparently early-stage disease operated on by general gynecologists or general surgeons are upstaged by gynecologic oncologists because of findings of disease in retroperitoneal lymph nodes, peritoneal biopsies, or omentum [36].

To date, a total of 11 retrospective studies comparing laparotomy with laparoscopy are published in the literature [3, 14–22]. The studies included 3065 patients, of whom 1450 underwent laparoscopy and 1615 underwent surgical staging for apparent early-stage EOC by laparotomy. In a meta-analysis recently published [37], laparoscopy was associated with a significantly lower estimated blood loss (Weighted Mean However it generally known WMD: –156.5 ml; 95% confidence interval [CI]: –216.4, –96.5) and shorter length of hospital stay (WMD: –3.7 days; 95% CI: –5.2, –2.1). Transfusion rate was higher in laparotomy patients (odds ratio [OR]: 0.21; 95% CI: 0.10, 0.43). On the other hand, operative time and intraoperative complications were similar between both surgical approaches.

Even though postoperative complications were lower in the laparoscopy group (OR: 0.48; 95% CI: 0.29, 0.81), grade 3 or worse complication rates were similar between the two approaches (OR: 0.83; 95% CI: 0.24, 2.92). Upstaging rate (OR: 0.81; 95% CI: 0.55, 1.20) as well as cysts' rupture rate (OR: 1.32; 95% CI: 0.52, 3.38) were similar between both groups. The numbers of pelvic (WMD: –1.09; 95% CI: –5.70, 3.51) and para-aortic (WMD: 1.92; 95% CI: –0.80, 4.65) nodes was similar. Laparotomy was associated with a longer time to chemotherapy than laparoscopy was (WMD: –5.16 days; 95% CI: –8.68, –1.64). Recurrence rate (OR: 0.75; 95% CI: 0.47, 1.20) and survival (OR: 0.76; 95% CI: 0.55, 1.05) was similar between both surgical approaches. The limited evidence published indicates that laparoscopy is feasible and safe for the staging of early EOC.

21.2.3 Sentinel node mapping with indocyanine green

Laparoscopic sentinel lymph node (SLN) detection by using indocyanine green (ICG) is currently under investigation [38]. A recent multicenter Italian study reported 10 cases of apparent stage I EOC schedule for a laparoscopic surgical staging. A total of 0.5 to 1 ml of ICG solution was injected close to the ovary, into the dorsal and ventral side of the proper ovarian parenchyma, and in the suspensory ligament with a 22-gauge needle. Subsequently, by using the real-time fluorescent infrared light of the SPIES camera, the entire retroperitoneal area was explored to find the fluorescent tracer in the lymphatic channels and to identify the anatomical location of the SLNs.

At least one sentinel node was detected in 9/10 patients (90%). The median number of lymph nodes removed per patient was 2 (range 0–2). All the detected SLNs were identified ipsilateral to the site of injection. In 3/10 (30%) patients, a common iliac SLN was found, and two of those cases were associated with an aortic SLN, whereas in one case, only one SLN was discovered. All the 15 SLNs removed were negative for metastasis upon final pathology. In the absence of positive nodes, the sensitivity cannot be calculated. Specificity and negative predictive value were 100%. Even though this technique appears to be safe and promising, aiming to reduce the morbidity and complications associated with a full lymphadenectomy in this setting of patients, more studies are needed before its implementation into clinical practice [38].

21.3 Laparoscopy for abdominal evaluation of tumor distribution in advanced stage (Fagotti criteria)

In advanced-stage ovarian cancer, the role of laparoscopy has been described as a tool to triage for resectability and second-look evaluations, with limited studies on its role in cytoreductive procedures [23]. The number of patients with advanced EOC (AEOC) who undergo an optimal cytoreductive procedure widely varies in the literature,

depending on either surgeon's training/clinical setting and patient's characteristics. Therefore, a certain number of women still undergo explorative laparotomy only, followed by neoadjuvant chemotherapy (NACT). Several approaches, including assessment of CA-125 serum levels and CT scan, have been attempted to identify preoperatively those patients who will achieve optimal cytoreduction (residual tumor less than 1 cm), thus avoiding unnecessary laparotomies. The accuracy of these approaches has been limited by several factors, such as the number of patients, retrospective nature of the studies, and the significant difference of optimal cytoreduction rate among the centers [23]. The possible advantages for a laparoscopic evaluation before cytoreductive surgery include the following:
- The assessment of intraperitoneal disease.
- The reduction of unnecessary laparotomy resulting in suboptimal cytoreduction, and therefore, patients who are not candidates for cytoreduction may start immediately NACT.
- Collection of tissue for definitive diagnosis and molecular analysis [23].

In 1998, Vergote et al. [39] published the first study evaluating the role of laparoscopy prior to upfront surgery in a retrospective analysis of 285 patients with advanced ovarian carcinoma. Later, two Italian studies were published, in 2005 and 2006 [40, 41], suggesting a role for laparoscopy in identifying patients with AEOC who are candidates for NACT versus primary debulking surgery (PDS).

Fagotti et al. first suggested that laparoscopy is able to provide the same information as standard laparotomy regarding intraperitoneal diffusion of AEOC and consequently to accurately assess the chances of optimal cytoreduction in these patients [23]. The characteristics required for the definition for each laparoscopic feature are as follows: massive peritoneal involvement and/or a miliary pattern of distribution for peritoneal carcinomatosis (score 2); widespread infiltrating carcinomatosis and/or confluent nodules to the most part of the diaphragmatic surface (score 2); large infiltrating nodules and/or involvement of the root of the mesentery supposed on the basis of limited movements of the various intestinal segments (score 2); tumor diffusion along the omentum up to the large stomach curvature (score 2); possible large/small bowel resection (excluding recto-sigmoid resection) and/or extended carcinomatosis on the ansae (score 2); obvious neoplastic involvement of the gastric wall (score 2); and liver surface lesions larger than 2 cm (score 2). Afterward, by summing the scores relative to all parameters, they set up a laparoscopy-based quantitative predictive model (predictive index value [PIV]), which, since it reflects a continuum of progressive tumor diffusion, provides an objective score related to intraabdominal disease diffusion and predicts the likelihood of optimal cytoreduction. The performance of this model was validated in a larger prospective cohort of AEOC patients [42]. The overall accuracy rate of the laparoscopic procedure ranged between 77.3% and 100%. At a PIV >8, the probability of optimally resecting the disease at laparotomy was equal to 0, and the rate of unnecessary exploratory laparotomy was 40.5%. Therefore, the authors concluded that the proposed laparoscopic model appears a reliable and flexible tool to predict optimal cytoreduction in advanced ovarian cancer.

In 2013, Fagotti *et al.* published the results of a prospective multicentric trial Olympia-MITO 13 designed to report the accuracy of laparoscopy to describe intraabdominal diffusion of AEOC and to verify the reproducibility of the scoring system in the description of tumor spread. The most difficult feature to assess was mesenteric retraction; however, an accuracy rate of 80% or greater was reached in three of the four satellite centers. The authors' conclusion was that laparoscopy allows an accurate and reliable assessment of intraperitoneal diffusion of disease in AEOC patients in trained gynecological oncology centers [43].

More recently [44], the same authors published an updated laparoscopy-based model to predict incomplete cytoreduction (residual disease = 0) in AEOC, after the introduction of upper abdominal surgery. A total of 234 women with newly diagnosed AEOC underwent laparotomy PDS after staging laparoscopy (S-LPS). In the new model, laparoscopic assessments of mesenteral retraction and miliary carcinomatosis on the serosa of the small bowel were considered as absolute criteria of unresectability, and therefore, these two parameters had been excluded from the updated version of the model, whereas the following laparoscopic parameters were included: (1) massive peritoneal involvement and/or a miliary pattern of distribution for parietal peritoneal carcinomatosis; (2) wide spread infiltrating carcinomatosis and/or confluent nodules to the most part of the diaphragmatic surface; (3) tumor diffusion along the omentum up to the large stomach curvature; (4) possible large/small bowel resection (excluding recto-sigmoid involvement); (5) obvious neoplastic involvement of the stomach and/or lesser omentum and/or spleen; and (6) liver surface lesions larger than 2 cm [42, 43]. Based on the presented results, LPS is confirmed as an accurate tool in the prediction of complete PDS in women with AEOC. The updated LPS-PIV showed improved discriminating performance, with a lower rate of inappropriate laparotomy explorations at the established cutoff value of 10.

Other studies have confirmed the feasibility of complete cytoreductive surgery assessed by laparoscopy [45, 46].

Two RCTs were undertaken to investigate this issue. The first, from the Netherlands [45], a multicenter, randomized controlled trial, evaluated the role of laparoscopy before PDS leaving residual tumor (RT) of <1 cm in women with AEOC. Participating patients were randomly assigned to either laparoscopy or PDS. Laparoscopy was used to guide the selection of primary treatment: either primary surgery or NACT followed by interval surgery. The primary outcome was futile laparotomy, defined as a PDS with residual disease of >1 cm. Futile laparotomy occurred in 10 (10%) of 102 patients in the laparoscopy group versus 39 (39%) of 99 patients in the primary surgery group (*p* < .001). In advanced ovarian cancer patients, these data suggest that performance of diagnostic laparoscopy prior to PDS is reasonable with the aim, if cytoreduction to <1 cm of residual disease seems feasible, to proceed with upfront surgery.

The second study, from Italy, is the SCORPION trial [47], which compared surgical complications and progression-free survival from primary surgery versus interval debulking surgery (IDS). After confirmation of histology and assessment of PI score at S-LPS, patients were assigned to treatment arms. The results of this study demonstrate that NACT/IDS may be preferable to PDS in patients with a very high tumor load in the abdomen in terms of perioperative moderate/severe morbidity, whereas quality of life measurements show no differences at the end of treatment between the two arms.

In conclusion, existing studies suggest a valuable role for laparoscopy in objectively assessing the chances for optimal PDS in patients with AEOC (FIGO stages III and IV).

21.4 MIS for advanced ovarian cancer

Most patients with EOC are diagnosed with stage IIIC and IV, and most of them have extensive peritoneal metastases. If the disease can be removed to no visible tumor, i.e., complete tumor resection, primary surgery can be performed via laparotomy [48] in most patients or by MIS—laparoscopy or robotics—in a smaller proportion of patients [49]. When the metastases cannot be completely removed with primary chemo-cytoreduction, NACT with the goal to completely remove the residual tumor burden at interval debulking is recommended. Either via laparotomy or MIS, most patients will recur, in which case a secondary debulking via laparotomy or MIS will be carried out depending on the extent of the disease [24]. Whether it is primary, secondary, or interval debulking, patient selection for MIS follows the same principles outlined in another section of this chapter. A careful patient selection is mandatory for a successful tumor resection by MIS, due to the limitations of this approach in EOC.

Unfortunately, an MIS approach has not found much support among gynecologic oncologists due to the fear of leaving disease, or inadequate surgeon's expertise, or the lack of standardization of the MIS techniques. It is not surprising that, due to the advantages of robotics over laparoscopy, most studies relate to robotics [24].

Laparoscopy provides immediate access to all four abdominal quadrants, while the da Vinci S and Si (Intuitive Surgical Inc., Sunnyvale, CA, USA) systems require rotation of the operating table to access lower and upper abdomen. Others preferred a hybrid procedure laparoscopy-robotics: a portion of the operation is performed via robotics while laparoscopy is used to remove other disease not reachable by robotics, therefore avoiding table rotation [50, 51]. The problem with the S and Si models was solved with the development of the da Vinci Xi system (Intuitive Surgical Inc., Sunnyvale, CA, USA), which allows rotation of the robotic arms for removal of disease in any of the quadrants [50], and the introduction of the camera at any of the port sites. However, additional trocars may be required to access all disease sites. Hand-assisted robotic surgery [52] was reported to facilitate resection in areas difficult to access and where palpation can be helpful.

The evidence regarding MIS in advanced or recurrent EOC is limited, although positive to the use of that approach in selected patients [24, 50, 51, 53–56]. The most important requirement for a successful MIS debulking, whether for primary, interval, or secondary disease, is careful patient selection, as indicated above. This requires appropriate preoperative evaluation, detailed laparoscopic exploration prior to debulking, and surgeon's expertise. Laparoscopic exploration is mandatory to select patients with localized disease to areas amenable to resection, and with absent peritoneal nodular metastases.

21.4.1 MIS for primary debulking

A comparison of robotics, laparoscopy, and laparotomy for AEOC was reported in 2011 [53]. A total of 76 patients with advanced stage were operated by robotics ($n = 15$), laparoscopy ($n = 20$), and laparotomy. Patients in each surgical approach were divided into three subgroups according to the number of major surgical procedures performed—one, two, or three or more—such as bowel resection, full thickness diaphragmatic resection, partial liver resection, and splenectomy. The study showed a significant reduction in blood loss and hospital stay for women who underwent robotic and/or laparoscopic approach compared to laparotomy. Intraoperative and postoperative complications were similar among the three different surgical groups.

Robotic patients undergoing two or more major surgical procedures had a longer operating time than did those who underwent laparoscopy or laparotomy. There were no differences in overall survival among the three groups, but there was a higher progression-free survival for the robotic group, most likely related to initial extent of disease.

Another study [56] compared 63 robotic and 26 laparotomy patients with EOC. This is the only study with significant improvement in overall survival for robotic patients, due to a substantial heterogeneity regarding inclusion criteria and different surgical procedures between both groups. Surgical staging for early stage disease was performed in 40% of robotic patients as compared to 27% of laparotomy patients. No patients underwent bowel resection in the robotic group, while it was performed in 38% of laparotomy patients.

In 2014, Nezhat et al. [51] reported the results of women with advanced stage/recurrent EOC that underwent robotics (10 patients), laparoscopy (29 patients), and laparotomy (8 patients). In case of diffuse abdominal implants, laparotomy was the surgical approach of choice. A significantly higher blood loss and longer hospital stay were noted in laparotomy patients, while there were no differences relative to operating time and intraoperative and postoperative complications among the three groups. It was concluded that MIS seems to be an acceptable approach in selected patients since laparoscopic and robotic perioperative outcomes were comparable and not inferior to laparotomy.

MIS is an adequate approach in highly selected patients with AEOC with localized disease amenable to complete resection. In patients with of diffuse disease, large omental cake, or requiring three or more major surgical procedures, laparotomy or NACT is preferred.

21.4.2 MIS for interval debulking

The feasibility and safety of MIS for interval debulking are well documented in the literature. Alletti *et al.* [57] demonstrated its feasibility in a multicenter trial in patients with complete clinical response to NACT. Comparison studies of MIS with laparotomy for interval debulking have also shown benefits for the MIS approach. As with primary and secondary debulking, it is obvious that the only candidates for MIS are highly selected patients with localized disease amenable to complete resection, which is a small proportion of patients with AEOC, even after NACT.

As compared to laparotomy, interval debulking patients operated by MIS had similar or longer operating times [58, 59], reduced blood loss [58–60], shorter hospital stay [58–60], similar complications rate [58–60], similar rates of tumor resection [58–60], similar operative mortality [58], shorter interval to chemotherapy [59], similar readmission rates [58], similar recurrence rate, and similar survival [58–60]. More importantly, a meta-analysis showed that MIS was not inferior to laparotomy for interval debulking [61].

As is the case with primary and secondary debulking, MIS can also be used for interval debulking following similar criteria for patient selection as for primary and secondary debulking and with similar patient benefits.

21.4.3 MIS for secondary debulking

MIS is feasible and safe for patients requiring a secondary cytoreduction [51, 54, 55, 62]. As with primary debulking, careful patient selection is mandatory for a successful complete tumor resection via MIS.

A comparison study of robotics (10 patients), laparoscopy (9 patients), and laparotomy (33 patients) for secondary debulking concluded that MIS was preferable due to lower blood loss and shorter hospital stay. Again, careful patient selection and surgeon's expertise were mandatory requirements for a successful debulking [54].

A multi-institutional study was performed in 48 women with localized recurrent EOC and absent peritoneal nodular implants who underwent secondary robotic cytoreduction. An optimal debulking was achieved in 36 (82%) patients, with an acceptable complication rate of 13.6% (6 patients). It was concluded that selected patients with recurrent EOC are candidates for secondary surgical cytoreduction via MIS, in this study via robotics. Surgical and oncological outcomes appear to be favorable as compared to previous reports of laparotomy debulking for recurrent EOC [55].

21.4.4 Port-site metastasis

Port-site metastasis is an important concern when performing MIS in patients with AEOC. The highest risk for port-site metastasis is the presence of carcinomatosis and ascites [63]. There is a 17–47% incidence of subclinical implantation of malignant cells at trocar sites [63, 64], but clinical manifestation is present in only 5% of them [64] and, as already indicated, is related to carcinomatosis and ascites [63, 64]. Microscopic tumor implantation at trocar sites does not appear to be related to the interval period between laparoscopy and definitive surgery or chemotherapy and has no impact on survival [63, 64]. One study recommended proceeding with immediate surgical resection at time of laparoscopy or to NACT within 7 days later. Clinical port-site metastasis in patients undergoing primary or secondary debulking via MIS was not observed [53, 54].

21.5 Conclusion

Laparoscopy has become the standard approach for the evaluation of optimal debulking prior to laparotomy in patients with AEOC. MIS staging is preferable for patients with apparent early-stage ovarian cancer. There is a clear role of MIS for highly selected patients with localized disease amenable to complete resection undergoing primary, interval, or secondary debulking. This constitutes a small proportion of patients with advanced ovarian cancer.

References

[1] Berek J, Crum C, Friedlander M. FIGO CANCER REPORT 2012. Cancer of the ovary, fallopian tube, and peritoneum. Int J Gynaecol Obstet 119S2;S118–29.
[2] Jemal A, Siegel R, Xu J, Ward E. Cancer statistics, 2010. CA Cancer J Clin 2012;60:277–300.
[3] Bogani G, Cromi A, Serati M, et al. Laparoscopic and open abdominal staging for early-stage ovarian cancer: our experience, systematic review, and meta-analysis of comparative studies. Int J Gynecol Cancer 2014 Sep;24(7):1241–9.
[4] Leblanc E, Querleu D, Narducci F. Laparoscopic restaging of early stage invasive adnexal tumors: a 10-year experience. Gynecol Oncol 2004;94:624–9.
[5] Tozzi R, Köhler C, Ferrara A, Schneider A. Laparoscopic treatment of early ovarian cancer: surgical and survival outcomes. Gynecol Oncol 2004;93:199–203.
[6] Spirtos NM, Eisekop SM, Boike G, Schlaerth JB, Cappellari JO. Laparoscopic staging in patients with incompletely staged cancers of the uterus, ovary, fallopian tube, and primary peritoneum: a Gynecologic Oncology Group (GOG) study. Am J Obstet Gynecol 2005;193:1645–9.
[7] Colomer AT, Jiménez AM, Bover Barceló MI. Laparoscopic treatment and staging of early ovarian cancer. J Minim Invasive Gynecol 2008;15:414–9.
[8] Jung US, Lee JH, Kyung MS, et al. Feasibility and efficacy of laparoscopic management of ovarian cancer. J Obstet Gynaecol Res 2009;35:113–8.
[9] Nezhat FR, Ezzati M, Chuang L, et al. Laparoscopic management of early ovarian and fallopian tube cancers: surgical and survival outcome. Am J Obstet Gynecol 2009;200:83.e1–6.

[10] Schreuder HW, Pattij TO, Zweemer RP, van Baal MW, Verheijen RH. Increasing experience in laparoscopic staging of early ovarian cancer. Gynecol Surg 2012;9:89–96.

[11] Brockbank EC, Harry V, Kolomainen D, et al. Laparoscopic staging for apparent early stage ovarian or fallopian tube cancer. First case series from a UK cancer centre and systematic literature review. Eur J Surg Oncol 2013;39:912–7.

[12] Montanari G, Di Donato N, Del Forno S, et al. Laparoscopic management of early stage ovarian cancer: is it feasible, safe, and adequate? A retrospective study. Eur J Gynaecol Oncol 2013;34(5):415–8.

[13] Gallotta V, Ghezzi F, Vizza E, et al. Laparoscopic staging of apparent early stage ovarian cancer: Results of a large, retrospective, multi-institutional series. Gynecol Oncol 2014;135(3):428–34.

[14] Chi DS, Abu-Rustum NR, Sonoda Y, et al. The safety and efficacy of laparoscopic surgical staging of apparent stage I ovarian and fallopian tube cancers. Am J Obstet Gynecol 2005;192:1614–9.

[15] Park JY, Kim DY, Suh DS, et al. Comparison of laparoscopy and laparotomy in surgical staging of early-stage ovarian and fallopian tubal cancer. Ann Surg Oncol 2008;15:2012–9.

[16] Park JY, Bae J, Lim MC, et al. Laparoscopic and laparotomic staging in stage I epithelial ovarian cancer: a comparison of feasibility and safety. Int J Gynecol Cancer 2008;18:1202–9.

[17] Lee M, Kim SW, Paek J, et al. Comparisons of surgical outcomes, complications, and costs between laparotomy and laparoscopy in early-stage ovarian cancer. Int J Gynecol Cancer 2011 Feb;21(2):251–6.

[18] Koo YJ, Kim JE, Kim YH, et al. Comparison of laparoscopy and laparotomy for the management of early-stage ovarian cancer: surgical and oncological outcomes. J Gynecol Oncol 2014 Apr;25(2):111–7.

[19] Liu M, Li L, He Y, et al. Comparison of laparoscopy and laparotomy in the surgical management of early-stage ovarian cancer. Int J Gynecol Cancer 2014;24:352–7.

[20] Minig L, Saadi J, Patrono MG, Giavedoni ME, Cárdenas-Rebollo JM, Perrotta M. Laparoscopic surgical staging in women with early stage epithelial ovarian cancer performed by recently certified gynecologic oncologists. Eur J Obstet Gynecol Reprod Biol 2016 Jun;201:94–100.

[21] Lu Q, Qu H, Liu C, Wang S, Zhang Z, Zhang Z. Comparison of laparoscopy and laparotomy in surgical staging of apparent early ovarian cancer: 13-year experience. Medicine (Baltimore) 2016 May;95(20):e3655.

[22] Ditto A, Bogani G, Martinelli F, et al. Minimally invasive surgical staging for ovarian carcinoma: a propensity-matched comparison with traditional open surgery. J Minim Invasive Gynecol 2017 Jan 1;24(1):98–102.

[23] Fagotti A, Vizzielli G, Fanfani F, et al. Introduction of staging laparoscopy in the management of advanced epithelial ovarian, tubal and peritoneal cancer: impact on prognosis in a single institution experience. Gynecol Oncol 2013 Nov;131(2):341–6.

[24] Minig L, Padilla Iserte P, Zorrero C, Zanagnolo V. Robotic surgery in women with ovarian cancer: surgical technique and evidence of clinical outcomes. J Minim Invasive Gynecol 2016 Mar–Apr;23(3):309–16.

[25] Drieskens O, Stroobants S, Gysen M, Vandenbosch G, Mortelmans L, Vergote I. Positron emission tomography with FDG in the detection of peritoneal and retroperitoneal metastases of ovarian cancer. Gynecol Obstet Invest 2003;55:130–4.

[26] Leblanc E, Sonoda Y, Narducci F, Ferron G, Querleu D. Laparoscopic staging of early ovarian carcinoma. Curr Opin Obstet Gynecol 2006 Aug;18(4):407–12.

[27] Vergote I, De Brabanter J, Fyles A, et al. Prognostic importance of degree of differentiation and cyst rupture in stage I invasive epithelial ovarian carcinoma. Lancet 2001;357:176–82.

[28] Bakkum-Gamez JN, Richardson DL, Seamon LG, et al. Influence of intraoperative capsule rupture on outcomes in stage I epithelial ovarian cancer. Obstet Gynecol 2009 Jan;113(1):11–7.

[29] Ramirez PT, Frumovitz M, Wolf JK, Levenback C. Laparoscopic port-site metastases in patients with gynecological malignancies. Int J Gynecol Cancer 2004;14:1070 –7.

[30] Tozzi R, Schneider A. Laparoscopic treatment of early ovarian cancer. Curr Opin Obstet Gynecol 2005 Aug;17(4):354–8.

[31] Benedet JL, Bender H, Jones III H, Ngan HY, Pecorelli S. FIGO staging classifications and clinical practice guidelines in the management of gynecologic cancers; FIGO committee on gynecologic oncology. Int J Gynaecol Obstet 2000;70:209–62.

[32] Bachmann C, Krämer B, Brucker SY, et al. Relevance of pelvic and para-aortic node metastases in early-stage ovarian cancer. Anticancer Res 2014 Nov;34(11):6735–8.

[33] Skirnisdottir I, Sorbe B. Lymph node sampling is of prognostic value in early stage epithelial ovarian carcinoma. Eur J Gynaecol Oncol 2005;26:181–5.

[34] Díaz-Feijoo B, Gil-Ibáñez B, Pérez-Benavente A, et al. Comparison of robotic-assisted vs conventional laparoscopy for extraperitoneal paraaortic lymphadenectomy. Gynecol Oncol 2014 Jan;132(1):98–101.

[35] Pakish J, Soliman PT, Frumovitz M, et al. A comparison of extraperitoneal versus transperitoneal laparoscopic or robotic para-aortic lymphadenectomy for staging of endometrial carcinoma. Gynecol Oncol 2014 Feb;132(2):366–71.

[36] Vernooij F, Heintz AP, Witteveen PO, van der Heiden-van der Loo M, Coebergh JW, van der Graaf Y. Specialized care and survival of ovarian cancer patients in the Netherlands: nationwide cohort study. J Natl Cancer Inst 2008;100(6):399–406.

[37] Bogani G, Borghi C, Leone Roberti Maggiore U, et al. Minimally invasive surgical staging in early-stage ovarian carcinoma: a systematic review and meta-analysis. J Minim Invasive Gynecol 2017 May–Jun;24(4):552–62.

[38] Buda A, Bussi B, Di Martino G, et al. Sentinel lymph node mapping with near-infrared fluorescent imaging using indocyanine green: a new tool for laparoscopic platform in patients with endometrial and cervical cancer. J Minim Invasive Gynecol 2016 Feb 1;23(2):265–9.

[39] Vergote I, De Wever I, Tjalma W, Van Gramberen M, Decloedt J, van Dam P. Neoadjuvant chemotherapy or primary debulking surgery in advanced ovarian carcinoma: a retrospective analysis of 285 patients. Gynecol Oncol 1998 Dec;71(3):431–6.

[40] Angioli R, Palaia I, Zullo MA, et al. Diagnostic open laparoscopy in the management of advanced ovarian cancer. Gynecol Oncol 2006;100(3):455–61.

[41] Fagotti A, Fanfani F, Ludovisi M, et al. Role of laparoscopy to assess the chance of optimal cytoreductive surgery in advanced ovarian cancer: a pilot study. Gynecol Oncol 2005;96:729–35.

[42] Fagotti A, Ferrandina G, Fanfani F, et al. Prospective validation of a laparoscopic predictive model for optimal cytoreduction in advanced ovarian carcinoma. Am J Obstet Gynecol 2008 Dec;199(6):642.e1–6.

[43] Fagotti A, Vizzielli G, De Iaco P, et al. A multicentric trial (Olympia-MITO 13) on the accuracy of laparoscopy to assess peritoneal spread in ovarian cancer. Am J Obstet Gynecol 2013 Nov;209(5):462.e1–11.

[44] Petrillo M, Vizzielli G, Fanfani F, et al. Definition of a dynamic laparoscopic model for the prediction of incomplete cytoreduction in advanced epithelial ovarian cancer: proof of a concept. Gynecol Oncol 2015 Oct;139(1):5–9.

[45] Rutten MJ, Gaarenstroom KN, Van Gorp T, et al. Laparoscopy to predict the result of primary cytoreductive surgery in advanced ovarian cancer patients (LapOvCa-trial): a multicentre randomized controlled study. BMC Cancer 2012 Jan 20;12:31. doi: 10.1186/1471-2407-12-31.

[46] Chesnais M, Lecuru F, Mimouni M, Ngo C, Fauconnier A, Huchon C. A pre-operative predictive score to evaluate the feasibility of complete cytoreductive surgery in patients with epithelial ovarian cancer. PLoS One 2017 Nov 8;12(11):e0187245.

[47] Fagotti A, Ferrandina G, Vizzielli G, et al. Phase III randomised clinical trial comparing primary surgery versus neoadjuvant chemotherapy in advanced epithelial ovarian cancer with high tumour load (SCORPION trial): final analysis of peri-operative outcome. Eur J Cancer 2016 May;59:22–33.

[48] Stuart GC, Kitchener H, Bacon M, et al; participants of 4th Ovarian Cancer Consensus Conference (OCCC); Gynecologic Cancer Intergroup. 2010 Gynecologic Cancer InterGroup (GCIG) consensus statement on clinical trials in ovarian cancer: report from the Fourth Ovarian Cancer Consensus Conference. Int J Gynecol Cancer 2011 May;21(4):750–5.

[49] Magrina JF, Zanagnolo V, Noble BN, Kho RM, Magtibay P. Robotic approach for ovarian cancer: perioperative and survival results and comparison with laparoscopy and laparotomy. Gynecol Oncol 2011 Apr;121(1):100–5.

[50] Chen CH, Chiu LH, Chen HH, Chan C, Liu WM. Comparison of robotic approach, laparoscopic approach and laparotomy in treating epithelial ovarian cancer. Int J Med Robot 2016 Jun;12(2):268–75.

[51] Nezhat FR, Finger TN, Vetere P, et al. Comparison of perioperative outcomes and complication rates between conventional versus robotic-assisted laparoscopy in the evaluation and management of early, advanced, and recurrent stage ovarian, fallopian tube, and primary peritoneal cancer. Int J Gynecol Cancer 2014;24(3):600–7.

[52] Fornalik H, Brooks H, Moore ES, Flanders NL, Callahan MJ, Sutton GP. Hand-assisted robotic surgery for staging of ovarian cancer and uterine cancers with high risk of peritoneal spread: a retrospective cohort study. Int J Gynecol Cancer 2015 Oct;25(8):1488–93.

[53] Magrina JF, Zanagnolo V, Noble BN, Kho RM, Magtibay P. Robotic approach for ovarian cancer: perioperative and survival results and comparison with laparoscopy and laparotomy. Gynecol Oncol 2011;121(1):100–5.

[54] Magrina JF, Cetta RL, Chang YH, Guevara G, Magtibay PM. Analysis of secondary cytoreduction for recurrent ovarian cancer by robotics, laparoscopy and laparotomy. Gynecol Oncol 2013;129(2):336–40.

[55] Escobar PF, Levinson KL, Magrina J, et al. Feasibility and perioperative outcomes of robotic-assisted surgery in the management of recurrent ovarian cancer: a multi-institutional study. Gynecol Oncol 2014;134(2):253–6.

[56] Feuer GA, Lakhi N, Barker J, Salmieri S, Burrell M. Perioperative and clinical outcomes in the management of epithelial ovarian cancer using a robotic or abdominal approach. Gynecol Oncol 2013;131(3):520–4.

[57] Alletti G, Bottoni C, Fanfani F, et al. Minimally invasive interval debulking surgery in ovarian neoplasm (MISSION trial-NCT02324595): a feasibility study. Am J Obstet Gynecol 2016 Apr;214(4):503.e1–6.

[58] Melamed A, Nitecki R, Boruta DM, et al. Laparoscopy compared with laparotomy for debulking ovarian cancer after neoadjuvant chemotherapy. Obstet Gynecol 2017 May;129(5):861–9.

[59] Alletti G, Petrillo M, Vizzielli G, et al. Minimally invasive versus standard laparotomic interval debulking surgery in ovarian neoplasm: A single-institution retrospective case-control study. Gynecol Oncol 2016 Dec;143(3):516–20.

[60] Corrado G, Mancini E, Cutillo G, et al. Laparoscopic debulking surgery in the management of advanced ovarian cancer after neoadjuvant chemotherapy. Int J Gynecol Cancer 2015;25(7):1253–7.

[61] Qin M, Jin Y, Ma L, Zhang YY, Pan LY. The role of neoadjuvant chemotherapy followed by interval debulking surgery in advanced ovarian cancer: a systematic review and meta-analysis of randomized controlled trials and observational studies. Oncotarget 2017 Dec 27;9(9):8614–28.

[62] Eriksson AGZ, Graul A, Yu MC, et al. Minimal access surgery compared to laparotomy for secondary surgical cytoreduction in patients with recurrent ovarian carcinoma: perioperative and oncologic outcomes. Gynecol Oncol 2017 Aug;146(2):263–7.

[63] Heitz F, Ognjenovic D, Harter P, et al. Abdominal wall metastases in patients with ovarian cancer after laparoscopic surgery: incidence, risk factors, and complications. Int J Gynecol Cancer 2010;20(1):41–6.

[64] Vergote I, Marquette S, Amant F, Berteloot P, Neven P. Port-site metastases after open laparoscopy: a study in 173 patients with advanced ovarian carcinoma. Int J Gynecol Cancer 2005 Sep–Oct;15(5):776–9.

Marc Possover

22 Neuropelveology—the medicine of the pathologies of the pelvic nerves and plexuses

The pelvis contains major somatic and autonomic nerves and plexuses, which are responsible for the transportation of all afferent and efferent information in the lower half of the human body. Efferent fibers are involved in pelvic organ functions, principally those of sexuality, voiding and storage in the pelvic organs, and equilibrium when standing or walking. Afferent fibers transport all sensitive information generated in the lower limbs and pelvis to the central nervous system. Pelvic nerve pathologies therefore lead to a combination of sensory dysfunctions with pelvic and low extremity visceral and/or somatic pain syndrome and motor dysfunctions with pelvic organ dysfunctions and difficulties with walking, balance, and coordination of the lower extremities.

22.1 The neuropelveological approach in the diagnosis and treatment of "chronic pelvic pain"

Chronic pelvic pain (CPP) is a condition with many faces—it is defined as nonmalignant pain perceived in structures related to the pelvis and accompanied by symptoms as consequences of a well-defined pathology, e.g., infection, endometriosis, hemorrhoids, anal fissure, pudendal neuropathy, sacral spinal cord pathology, vascular and cutaneous disease, or psychiatric conditions [1, 2]. CPP has been estimated to have a prevalence of between 4% and 15% [3, 4]. If identifiable disease conditions are excluded, idiopathic pain conditions and CPP syndromes (CPPSs) can be defined. The International Continence Society has defined CPPS as constant or recurrent pain in the pelvis of nonmalignant origin that is present for at least 6 months [5]. In CPPS, the pain is often accompanied by symptoms related to organs in the pelvis, without a proven infection or other obvious pathology, e.g., lower urinary tract symptoms or sexual, bowel, pelvic floor, or gynecological problems [5]. These symptoms are often accompanied by negative cognitive, behavioral, sexual, or emotional consequences with an important impact on the quality of life [6]. CPPS is often combined with chronic low lumbar pain (LLP), which has a high prevalence in the general population (6–45%) [7]. Because of the stigma and social isolation of these patients, it is not surprising that other associated problems may coexist, such as depression, anxiety, and drug addiction. CPP/CPPS and LLP present a major challenge to healthcare providers because of their unclear etiology, complex natural history, and poor response to therapy. These patients often approach several new physicians with a combination of unrealistic hopes for a cure and suspicion related to past diagnosis and treatment failures. The goal of treatment is then often to reduce pain and other

https://doi.org/10.1515/9783110535204-022

symptoms without a real search for a potential etiologic treatment. These patients are all too often sidelined and are offered no alternative other than to accept medical pain management and antidepressants, with their known side effects and the dangers of dependence for the rest of their lives.

Pathology of the pelvic nerves and plexuses may explain such "unknown pain conditions" and associated pelvic organ dysfunctions. Pathologies of the pelvic somatic nerves may produce neuropathic pain in the lower back, the genito-anal areas, and the lower extremities, but also pelvic organ dysfunction as in CPPS [8]. Considering the number of pelvic pathologies and invasive procedures in proximity to the pelvic nerves that could potentially induce neuronal compression, entrapment, or damage, reports in the literature are rare. The incidence of pelvic nerve pathologies seems widely underestimated, mainly because of the lack of awareness that such lesions may exist, lack of diagnosis and acceptance, as well as the declaration and reporting of such lesions. Neurosurgical procedure techniques are well established in nerve lesions of the upper limbs, but surgical exploration of the pelvic retroperitoneal area and the pelvic nerves is still unusual for neurosurgeons. The only nerve that has been truly investigated in pelvic nerve pathology is pudendal neuralgia (Alcock's canal syndrome) because the nerve is easily accessible for neurophysiological explorations, infiltrations, and surgical decompression. In contrast, endopelvic nerves are difficult to access and have been much less investigated in the past. Nevertheless, pathologies of the pelvic nerves may explain many cases of CPP/CPPS [9]. Management of pelvic nerve pathologies requires good integration and knowledge of all pelvic organ systems, neuro-functional pelvic anatomy, and the musculoskeletal, neurologic, and psychiatric aspects, and no current specialty seems to be devoted to this field. The concept of "neuropelveology," the first medical practice focused on the pathologies of the pelvic nervous system was introduced more than 10 years ago [10]. Neuropelveology combines the knowledge required for a proper neurologic diagnosis for intractable CPP/CPPS and LLP. Because of growing interest from the medical community, the International Society of Neuropelveology (ISoN) (www.theison.org) was founded in 2014 with one major objective: to provide universal access to education in neuropelveology. The neuropelveological approach to pelvic neuropathies may not only explain many cases of CPPS but also enable new therapeutic options from noninvasive treatments to laparoscopic neurofunctional procedures. Advances in video endoscopy and microsurgical instruments enable good access to all areas in the retroperitoneal pelvic space [11], providing the necessary visibility with magnification of the structures and the possibility to work with appropriate instruments for adequate neurofunctional procedures such as nerve decompression and neurolysis [12–15]. Laparoscopy is also the only technique that enables selective placement of electrodes to all pelvic nerves and plexuses. This technique of *laparoscopic implantation of neuroprothesis*, also called the "LION procedure," enables the selective placement of electrodes in direct contact with the nerves under direct visualization [10].

Laparoscopic neuropelveological procedures may be reserved for experienced surgeons in laparoscopic retroperitoneal pelvic surgery, but diagnosis of pelvic nerve pathologies is accessible for all physicians [16]. It is essential to adopt a "neurological way of thinking." Standard medical training imparts the concept that the location of the pain and its etiology correspond to the same area. In pathologies of the pelvic nerves, however, the location of the patient's pain (dermatomes) and the sensomotor dysfunctions of the pelvic organs and the lower extremities reveal which nerves are involved in the pain process, whereas the etiology is mostly located on the path from the dermatome to the brain. A neuropelveological workup aims to determine which nerves, at which level, are involved in pain generation and always follows five steps in the following subsections:

1. Determination whether the pain is visceral or somatic
2. Determination of the nerve pathways involved in the relay of pain information to the brain
3. Evaluation of the neurological level of pain (central vs. pelvic vs. peripheral)
4. Establishment of a potential etiology
5. Confirmation of and therapy for a potential etiology.

Steps 1 to 3 are achieved by referencing the patient's history, while the neurological examination with the direct transvaginal/rectal digital palpation of the pelvic somatic nerves may confirm the diagnosis. Modern imaging and/or laparoscopic visualization may offer an effective etiologic diagnosis and, in most patients, the corresponding etiologic treatment.

Because neuropelveology is now accessible for all physicians, it is no longer acceptable to ignore the pathologies of the pelvic nerves as a potential etiology for CPP/CPPS and LLP, and it seems reasonable to advise all "pelvic physicians" on the need for proper knowledge of neuropelveology, at least for the recognition of neuropelveological conditions [17]. The ISoN proposes an E-learning program accessible to all physicians for the acquisition of such knowledge (www.theison.org).

22.2 The neuropelveological approach to pelvic organ dysfunction

22.2.1 Pelvic organ dysfunctions

Urinary incontinence, bladder overactivity, sexual dysfunction, and other pelvic floor disorders are common problems affecting millions of people of all ages, gender, and race. Overactive bladder (OAB) is a condition that affects millions of citizens worldwide.

The US Department of Health and Human Services estimates that approximately 13 million Americans suffer from urinary incontinence. Urinary incontinence is an underreported problem that increases with age, affecting 50–84% of the elderly in long-term care facilities. Moreover, 10% to 30% of American women/girls aged 15–64 years are thought to suffer from it, compared to between 1.5% and 5% of men. Over half of all nursing home residents are thought to be affected by urinary incontinence. It is estimated that 20% of all women over the age of 40 are affected by urinary incontinence.

Recent international population and nonpopulation studies reported OAB in 10–17% of the adult population, depending on sex. In the US, a population-based study reported that 16.0% of men and 16.9% of women experienced OAB, which corresponds to approximately 33 million people [18]. Also, sexual dissatisfaction and/or trouble with penis/clitoris erection affects both women and men. Up to 30 million American men are affected by erectile dysfunction (ED). Women's sexual health, like men's, is important to overall emotional and physical well-being. The three most common sexual dysfunctions in males are decreased libido, ED, and ejaculatory dysfunction. ED is a common problem in primary care and currently affects more than 150 million men worldwide, with a projected prevalence increase to 322 million men by the year 2025. The safety and efficacy of phosphodiesterase 5 (PDE5) inhibitors has been well documented. First-line therapy for the treatment of ED is medication with a PDE5 inhibitor. A contraindication for the use of PDE5 inhibitors is the intake of nitrates, and patients with severe cardiovascular comorbidities should not use a PDE5 inhibitor. Up to 50% of patients suffering from ED present a suboptimal answer to the PDE5 inhibitors. During recent years, downsizing of catheter material has facilitated endovascular revascularization of small-caliber erection-related arteries. In a study known as the ZEN study [19], procedural success was 100%, with no major adverse events during follow-up. About 60% of patients undergoing stent placement showed functional improvement subsequent to endovascular revascularization. However, the restenosis rate was reported to be as high as 34% in these small-caliber arteries after 6 months of follow-up.

22.2.2 Electrical stimulation of the pelvic nerves as an attractive treatment

Electrical stimulation of pelvic nerves in the pelvic floor may provide an effective therapy for a variety of disorders. Electrical stimulation has emerged as an alternative and attractive treatment for refractory cases of bladder overactivity, urinary incontinence, and also bladder retention (incapacity of bladder emptying). Also the stimulation may be effective in restoring sexual function or alleviating pelvic floor or genital pain. Continuous or intermittent electrical nerve stimulation strategies are used to treat lower urinary tract dysfunction. Neuromodulation is used to treat both overactivity and underactivity, but it is currently also used to treat bladder pain. Electrical stimulation is performed at different sites in the human body and therefore targets different nerves.

Sacral Nerve Stimulator (SNS) has proven efficacy in both refractory OAB, neurogenic bladder disease, bladder retention, and fecal incontinence [20]. Sacral nerve stimulation enables stimulation of pudendal fibers—the key player of the functions of the pelvic organs, including the genital organs—contained in the sacral nerve root and also activates other fibers that are present in the sacral nerve root. This in turn produces some patient discomfort, such as feeling of electricity in the leg. In an attempt to target the pudendal nerve more specifically, Spinelli *et al.* described a surgical procedure that places an electronic lead into Alcock's canal via either a perineal approach or a posterior approach [21]. Groen *et al.* investigated the applicability of a mini-neurostimulator called the Bion® that was placed near the pudendal nerve in Alcock's canal [22]. Despite these positive outcomes, no follow-up study of this device has been done since. Peters *et al.* investigated whether isolated pudendal nerve stimulation (PNS) was superior to SNS with a cross-over study in 30 patients. Results were remarkably in favor for PNS, which was chosen as the superior lead in 79.2%, with an average reduction of symptoms of 63% compared to 46% for the SNS group [23]. Transcutaneous electrical nerve stimulation is still in evaluation and seems inferior to other OAB treatments like SNS and PNS but is noninvasive and applicable for ambulant therapy. The percutaneous dorsal genital nerve stimulation is still an experimental neuromodulation technique to treat neurogenic bladder and OAB disease and is not applied in routine clinical practice [24]. The nerve is a direct branch of the pudendal nerve and could therefore, in theory, be more closely related to the main nerves that control lower urinary tract function compared to, for instance, the posterior tibial nerve. Because part of the distal pudendal nerve lies superficially to the skin outside the pelvis, this nerve can be stimulated using surface electrodes attached to the overlying skin. This application is also limited due to intolerance of the required high stimulation amplitude. In patients with intact sensitivity, this leads to stimulation amplitudes that are less effective or too low to be effective, which subsequently results in incontinence. Surface electrodes have additional limitations such as difficulties in daily proper placement and hygiene. Implanted electrodes are more suitable, but implanted electrodes in the penis or near the clitoris have to endure mechanical stress of penile erections and external pressure, with risk for cable/electrode breakage and dislocation. A technique for percutaneous implantation of an electrode near the origin of the DNP, close to the Alcock's canal, has also been developed. Because such a technique lacks direct vision to the nerve during implantation, X-ray screening and neurophysiological monitoring of the nerve are usually mandatory. The technique is not easy and also exposes patients to electrode migration and failure since the lead is not fixed to any anatomical structure and patients are sitting on the lead.

22.2.3 Genital nerves stimulation—an attractive alternative for gynecologists

Because the laparoscopic approach to the pelvic nerves enables selective exposure of all pelvic nerves and plexuses, the technique of laparoscopic implantation of lead electrodes to different nerves has been developed—the LION procedure [25, 26]. These procedures present significant advantages compared to all percutaneous techniques of implantation but still present some surgical difficulties and are not reproducible by every laparoscopic surgeon. However, gynecologists are untrained not only in the LION procedures but also in classical percutaneous techniques of implantation. This is, in fact, a pity because most patients suffering from OAB and incontinences are women. As a consequence, all our efforts over the last few years have been focused on the development of a surgical technique for the implantation of neuroprothesis to the pelvic nerves, straightforward enough to be reproduced by most laparoscopic surgeons and urogynecologists. Because gynecologists are usually trained in both the laparoscopic Burch procedure (dissection of the space of Retzius) and Tention free vaginal tape (TVT) procedure, the GNS procedure—genital nerves stimulation—is a new technique for implantation that may be easily accessible for every gynecologist. The technique combines a percutaneous approach from below, similar to the TVT procedure, with a primary endoscopic dissection of the Retzius space as in the Burch procedure. The procedure starts with the laparoscopic trans- or retroperotineal dissection of the Retzius space with exposure of the pubic arch. Then the patients are placed lying on their back with their legs in a position of 30 degrees abduction and 30 degrees flexion of the hips and the procedure is carried out on as per a TVT procedure. A sagittal incision about 1–2 mm is made approximately 1 cm below the external urethral meatus in a female (infrapubic parapenile incision in a male). A curve needle driver is inserted into the incision. The tip is oriented at an angle of 5–10 degrees from the midline, toward the symphysis. The inserter tip will be approximately in the 11 o'clock position (or 1 o'clock position on the right side). The inserter is advanced, contacting the inferior edge of the pubic ramus. While maintaining contact with the bone, further advance is made into the Retzius space, previously dissected by laparoscopy. During the insertion, the surgeon controls the position of the inserters by palpation, as per standard surgery, but also by endoscopic view to avoid injury to the pelvic organs, vessels, or nerves. The spear of the curve driver needle is removed by laparoscopy and the electrode lead is introduced retrograde into the shaft of the curve driver needle. By retraction of the curve needle driver, the electrode lead is left in the right position under the pubic bone, transfixing the urogenital diaphragm down to the genital organ, in contact to the cavernous (from the pelvic splanchnic nerves) and dorsal nerves of the penis/clitoris (ventral branch of the pudendal nerve). This technique provides a selective and distal stimulation of key nerves involved in controlling the functions of the pelvic organs, including:

- overactivity of the bladder, urge incontinence, and bladder retention [27];
- idiopathic fecal incontinence, frequency, and retention [28]; and
- ED in males, and sexual dysfunction in females.

However, it is evident beyond any doubt that large cohort studies are necessary to determine the applicability of the GNS by gynecologists and urogynecologists but also by general surgeons and urologists.

The LION procedure to the pelvic somatic nerves further allows for control of neurogenic pain syndromes [29] and may also represent a potent alternative to current methods for neuromodulation in the treatment of visceral pain mediated by the autonomic nerve system [30]. Recent studies have demonstrated that pelvic nerve stimulation might also induce changes that affect the central nervous system to engage residual spinal and peripheral pathways for the recovery of voluntary motion of the legs in chronic paraplegics [31, 32].

This evolution in the management of pathologies and dysfunctions of the pelvic nerves and plexuses requires more interdisciplinary exchange of knowledge between clinical physicians and basic researchers and should encourage young physicians to devote time and energy to the field of clinical and experimental pelvic nerve medicine, *neuropelveology* [33]. This new field of medicine not only offers diagnostic and therapeutic options for many intractable conditions but also opens the door wide for physicians, revealing the mystery of the pelvic nerves and plexuses with further new fields of application that are simply ready and waiting to be discovered by future generations.

References

[1] Fall M, Baranowski AP, Elneil S, et al. EAU guidelines on chronic pelvic pain. Eur Urol 2010;57:35–48.

[2] Engeler D, Baranowski AP, Elneil S, et al. Guidelines on chronic pelvic pain. Eur Assoc Urol 2012;7:869–910.

[3] Howard FM. Chronic pelvic pain. Obstet Gynecol 2003;101:594–611.

[4] Daniels JP, Khan KS. Chronic pelvic pain in women. BMJ (Clinical Research Ed) 2010;341:c4834.

[5] Abrams P, Cardozo L, Fall M, et al. The standardisation of terminology of lower urinary tract function: report from the Standardisation Sub-committee of the International Continence Society. Am J Obstet Gynecol 2002;187:116–26.

[6] Engeler DS, Baranowski AP, Dinis-Oliveira P, et al. The 2013 EAU guidelines on chronic pelvic pain: is management of chronic pelvic pain a habit, a philosophy, or a science? 10 years of development. Eur Urol 2013;64:431–9.

[7] Allegri M, Montella S, Salici F, et al. Mechanisms of low back pain: a guide for diagnosis and therapy. F1000Research 2016;5.

[8] Gebhart GF, Bielefeldt K. Physiology of visceral pain. Compr Physiol 2016;6:1609–33.

[9] Possover M. Intractable neural pelvic pain. In: Gomel V, Brill AI, eds. Reconstructive and Reproductive Surgery in Gynecology. London: Informa Health Care; 2010:200–10.

[10] Possover M, Baekelandt J, Chiantera V. The laparoscopic implantation of neuroprothesis (LION) procedure to control intractable abdomino-pelvic neuralgia. Neuromodulation 2007;10:18–23.

[11] Zanatta A, Rosin MM, Machado RL, Cava L, Possover M. Laparoscopic dissection and anatomy of sacral nerve roots and pelvic splanchnic nerves. J Minim Invasive Gynecol 2014;21:982–3.

[12] Possover M, Schneider T, Henle KP. Laparoscopic therapy for endometriosis and vascular entrapment of sacral plexus. Fertil Steril 2011;95:756–8.

[13] Lemos N, Possover M. Laparoscopic approach to intrapelvic nerve entrapments. J Hip Preserv Surg 2015;2:92–8.

[14] Possover M, Forman A. Pelvic neuralgias by neuro-vascular entrapment: anatomical findings in a series of 97 consecutive patients treated by laparoscopic nerve decompression. Pain Physician 2015;18:E1139–43.

[15] Possover M, Kostov P. Laparoscopic management of sacral nerve root schwannoma with intractable vulvococcygodynia: report of three cases and review of literature. J Minim Invasive Gynecol 2013;20:394–7.

[16] Quaghebeur J, Wyndaele JJ. Chronic pelvic pain syndrome: role of a thorough clinical assessment. Scand J Urol 2015;49:81–9.

[17] Possover M, Andersson KE, Forman A. Neuropelveology: an emerging discipline for the management of chronic pelvic pain. Int Neurourol J 2017;21:243–6.

[18] Stewart WF, Van Rooyen JB, Cundiff GW, et al. Prevalence and burden of overactive bladder in the United States. World J Urol 2003;20:327–36.

[19] Rogers JH, Goldstein I, Kandzari DE, et al. Zotarolimus-eluting peripheral stents for the treatment of erectile dysfunction in subjects with suboptimal response to phosphodiesterase-5 inhibitors. J Am Coll Cardiol 2012;60:2618–27.

[20] van Kerrebroeck PE, van Voskuilen AC, Heesakkers JP, et al. Results of sacral neuromodulation therapy for urinary voiding dysfunction: outcomes of a prospective, worldwide clinical study. J Urol 2007;178:2029–34.

[21] Spinelli M, Malaguti S, Giardiello G, Lazzeri M, Tarantola J, Van Den Hombergh U. A new minimally invasive procedure for pudendal nerve stimulation to treat neurogenic bladder: description of the method and preliminary data. Neurourol Urodyn 2005;24:305–9.

[22] Groen J, Amiel C, Bosch JL. Chronic pudendal nerve neuromodulation in women with idiopathic refractory detrusor overactivity incontinence: results of a pilot study with a novel minimally invasive implantable mini-stimulator. Neurourol Urodyn 2005;24:226–30.

[23] Peters KM, Feber KM, Bennett RC. Sacral versus pudendal nerve stimulation for voiding dysfunction: a prospective, single-blinded, randomized, crossover trial. Neurourol Urodyn 2005;24:643–7.

[24] Martens FM, Heesakkers JP, Rijkhoff NJ. Surgical access for electrical stimulation of the pudendal and dorsal genital nerves in the overactive bladder: a review. J Urol 2011;186:798–804.

[25] Possover M. The laparoscopic implantation of neuroprothesis to the sacral plexus for therapy of neurogenic bladder dysfunctions after failure of percutaneous sacral nerve stimulation. Neuromodulation 2010;13:141–4.

[26] Possover M. A novel implantation technique for pudendal nerve stimulation for treatment of overactive bladder and urgency incontinence. J Minim Invasive Gynecol 2014;21:888–92.

[27] Farag FF, Martens FM, Rijkhoff NJ, Heesakkers JP. Dorsal genital nerve stimulation in patients with detrusor overactivity: a systematic review. Curr Urol Rep 2012;13:385–8.

[28] Worsoe J, Fynne L, Laurberg S, Krogh K, Rijkhoff NJ. Electrical stimulation of the dorsal clitoral nerve reduces incontinence episodes in idiopathic faecal incontinent patients: a pilot study. Colorectal Dis 2012;14:349–55.

[29] Possover M, Baekelandt J, Chiantera V. The laparoscopic approach to control intractable pelvic neuralgia: from laparoscopic pelvic neurosurgery to the LION procedure. Clin J Pain 2007;23:821–5.

[30] Gupta P, Ehlert MJ, Sirls LT, Peters KM. Percutaneous tibial nerve stimulation and sacral neuromodulation: an update. Curr Urol Rep 2015;16:4.

[31] Possover M. The LION procedure to the pelvic nerves for recovery of locomotion in 18 spinal cord injured peoples—a case series. Surg Technol Int 2016;29:19–25.

[32] Possover M, Forman A. Recovery of supraspinal control of leg movement in a chronic complete flaccid paraplegic man after continuous low-frequency pelvic nerve stimulation and FES-assisted training. Spinal Cord Series Cases 2017;3:16034.

[33] Possover M, Forman A, Rabischong B, Lemos N, Chiantera V. Neuropelveology: new groundbreaking discipline in medicine. J Minim Invasive Gynecol 2015;22:1140–1.

Sven Becker and Morva Tahmasbi-Rad

23 Complications of laparoscopic surgery and their management

23.1 Introduction

Complications are the limiting factor of all surgery. More than performing the actual surgery, learning how to avoid complications before, during, and after surgery is the most important task of every surgeon. Severe complications can destroy the lives of those patients that we intend to cure. Complications such as uretero-vaginal fistulas, which might be the result of less than 2 seconds of inattentive preparation, can lead to years of hardship, suffering, accusations, and litigation. Excellent surgery is about performing the right surgery for the right patient without any complications. Minimally invasive surgery is technically challenging. This chapter will go through the major causes of complications in laparoscopy both for simple and for advanced gynecologic patients and present strategies for prevention, early detection, and intra- and postoperative management.

23.2 Incidence of and literature about complications—general considerations

Traditionally, intraoperative complications in regular and advanced laparoscopic and minimally invasive surgery are thought to be no more common than in open surgery, while post-operative complications, mostly involving the abdominal wall, are much rarer [1]. There is additional evidence indicating that for specific advanced indications, the rate of severe intraoperative complications might actually be lower for laparoscopic surgery than for either abdominal or vagina surgery [2].

23.3 Is laparoscopy different from open or vaginal surgery?

Laparoscopic surgery is mentally and physically more demanding on the surgeon and tends to have a longer learning curve than open surgery. This is mostly due to the more difficult management of intraoperative bleeding.

Where in open surgery, pressure can be applied to control (excessive) bleeding, often allowing for a short break and a moment of relaxation in surgery, laparoscopic surgery becomes more difficult with every additional amount of blood obscuring the surgical field. The generally low rates of laparo-conversion observed in the literature reflects mostly on the fact that surgeons attempting laparoscopic advanced surgery

https://doi.org/10.1515/9783110535204-023

tend to be experienced surgeons using additional caution when facing a new and challenging situation [3].

Laparoscopic surgery requires a completely different mindset than open or vaginal surgery. Most surgery requires a refined technique, but laparoscopy requires a refined approach that is not immediately obvious—and even more true in oncology cases.

23.4 Complications of indication

Laparoscopy has been well established for treatment of most gynecologic pathologies and has become standard treatment for many of them.

Complications of indication often have little do to with laparoscopy. The decision to operate on a cervical cancer extending all the way to the pelvic sidewall will lead to complicated surgery, no matter what the approach is. If the indication is wrong, the technique cannot improve on that.

"Indication is science, operation is art"—the proper indication for laparoscopic interventions is no different than for open surgery. However, not everything that is possible laparoscopically should be done laparoscopically. Patients with multiple midline laparotomies can always be assessed laparoscopically through a Palmer's point incision, but the length of time required for a laparoscopic adhesiolysis and the likelihood of its success need to be balanced against the overall time available and the willingness of the surgical team to go through with this approach.

Classical complications of indication in laparoscopic surgery for gynecologic disease that will increase complication rates are as follows:
1. Concurrent medical comorbidities preventing Trendelenburg positioning
2. Complication of wrong approach
3. Giant uterus, requiring hours of morcellation
4. Laparoscopic radical hysterectomy in stage III cervical cancer
5. Laparoscopic approach to stage II ovarian cancer
6. Complication of improper oncologic approach (laparotomy better than laparoscopy)

23.5 Intraoperative complications

The best approach to complications is to avoid them altogether. The following 20 "Frankfurt" points summarize the key issues that must be addressed in the laparoscopic surgical theater to allow for an atmosphere of zero tolerance against laparoscopic complications. Such surgical "advice" always has a strong subjective component and consequently should not be viewed as rules, but rather as recommendations.

Experienced surgeons have fewer complications than inexperienced surgeons do. Everyone assumes that this is true—and it probably is [4]. One could easily devise a randomized trial proving that, but what patients would willingly accept to participate in such a study? Unwillingly, they participate every day.

Again, the following points are teaching points that are the result of experience combined with an extensive research of the existing literature. They are not to be taken dogmatically. Ultimately, in every surgical theater there is only one person holding all the responsibility: the surgeon. He or she must decide, case by case, which advice to accept and which way is the best.

Twenty Frankfurt points to reduce complications:
1. Check the setup yourself.
2. Make sure the patient cannot slide cephalad.
3. Use a manipulator.
4. Place the manipulator yourself.
5. Use the same access approach every time. Different options exist.
6. Use the CO_2 pressure-guided approach.
7. Use 20 mmHg whenever possible intraoperatively.
8. Position lateral additional trocars high and lateral.
9. Position the main working median trocar midway *between* the symphysis and navel.
10. Always take down sigma attachments to the left lateral psoas space/pelvic sidewall.
11. Always have the uterus pushed in at maximum.
12. Check uterine manipulation frequently.
13. Avoid bleeding always.
14. Make it look beautiful.
15. Always take down bladder anteriorly before coagulating uterine vessels.
16. Desvascularize on both sides before cutting to minimize retrograde bleeding.
17. Use monopolar energy with extreme caution.
18. Total hysterectomy—colpotomy: make sure you have dissected the whole cap.
19. Total hysterectomy—colpotomy: start opening the vagina posteriorly.
20. Take advantage of new technologies (harmonic scalpel, three-dimensional laparoscopy).

23.6 Intraoperative complications specific to laparoscopy and how to avoid them

a. Entry-related complications
Laparoscopic entry can potentially lead to catastrophic vascular or bowel injury, even though the overall incidence is very low. This is true for both benign as

well as oncology cases. The incidence of entry-injury is highly dependent on the surgeon's experience and the attention that is being paid to this seemingly routine moment of the surgery.

The most recent Cochrane review of the subject did not find different rates of complications with either the open laparoscopy or the direct Verres-needle approach [5].

Entry-related complications can involve the bowel. These can be easily repaired if properly recognized. If a bowel injury is suspected, every effort must be made to detect it. While the bowel injury by itself is not fatal, a protracted peritonitis followed by sepsis due to an unrecognized bowel injury can be.

The most feared complication of entry is a vascular injury. Particularly injuries to the large arteries have the potential to be fatal. The blood loss from even a small lesion to the aorta or the iliac vessels is such that only minutes remain, before the circulation of the patient collapses—often with fatal consequences. Different factors increase the likelihood of vascular entry injury: lack of experience, very thin patients, failed attempts, small changes from the usual positioning, inadvertent veering off the central midline, and, most importantly, inattention. Often, the initial injury does not lead to directly visible hemorrhage but to retroperitoneal hematoma. Management of big vessel injuries can be summed up with two strategies: immediate midline laparotomy to apply immediate pressure while calling in a vascular surgeon to perform the actual repair. Any delay in diagnosis can be fatal. Transverse laparotomy is contraindicated. The sooner a vascular surgeon is called, the better.

b. Bowel injuries

Bowel injuries in laparoscopy are most often due to inadvertent thermic lesions to the bowel. These lesions, if not properly diagnosed, can lead to delayed necrosis and perforation, leading to the typical clinical course of unrecognized bowel lesions: normal course during the first 24 hours after surgery, followed by a slow deterioration with CRP (C-reactive protein) increase, ileus, fever, and a general deterioration often apparent by day 3. Clinical course can be insidious, leading to the general rule of postoperative laparoscopy management: if the patient does not improve along the usual timeframe, never hesitate to perform a diagnostic repeat laparoscopy. To avoid thermic and, thus, delayed injuries, meticulous preparation is mandatory. However, simple preventive measures include removing all small bowel out of the space of Douglas (Trendelenburg) and using thermic instruments only where they are clearly visible at all times, as well as avoiding electric instruments for manipulation.

c. Ureteral injuries

While postoperative hemorrhage usually occurs during the first 24 hours after surgery and bowel injuries become apparent on day 3, ureteral injuries can become symptomatic almost at any time after surgery. Many uretero-vaginal fistulas do not declare themselves until 5–6 weeks postoperatively. How can we prevent such lesions? The number 1 rule is to visualize the ureter, for which accessing the pelvic sidewall is the paramount step. Dissecting down the bladder during hysterectomies is another way to prevent such lesions. Using uterine manipulation and pushing in the uterus to maximally distance the ureters from the uterine artery is another important strategy.

d. Positioning injuries

It remains unclear whether positioning injuries are more common in laparoscopic surgery, as general opinion will have it. Padding and dry positioning are as important for laparoscopy as for any other surgery. There has been speculation whether Trendelenburg positioning combined with the use of leg rests could increase the number of compartment syndromes. While occasional compartment syndromes have been described with laparoscopy, there appears to be no overall increase.

e. Conversion to laparotomy

Conversion to laparotomy should not be considered a complication as it only replaces one possible legitimate approach with another. In fact, not performing laparotomy when it should be done can lead to unnecessary complications. Laparotomy should not be considered either a complication or a failure [6].

23.7 Postoperative complications

"The surgery is only over 8 weeks after surgery." The postoperative course is clearly determined by the quality of the intraoperative surgery provided, but not entirely so. As every surgeon knows, often the most disastrous complications occur completely unexpectedly.

The first 24 hours after surgery know mostly one complication: hemorrhage. Hemorrhage must be avoided during surgery—for better visualization and reduction of intraoperative complications. Because intraoperative hemostasis is essential, postoperative hemorrhage after laparoscopy is rare. Three different sources of postoperative hemorrhage are common: (1) bleeding from an insufficiently coagulated ovary after ovarian cystectomy, (2) arterial bleeding from the pelvic sidewall after hysterectomy or radical hysterectomy (insufficiently coagulated uterine artery, arterial bleeders from the vaginal cuff), and (3) bleeding from an unrecognized venous laceration. As postoperative bleeding occurs mostly unexpected, there can be only one strategy to deal with this complication: extreme vigilance in postoperative surveillance, frequent control of hemoglobin, an attentive eye for changes in vital signs, and, as advocated by some, abdominal bleeding monitoring through 24-hour drainage. Most importantly, in cases of doubt, the strategy has to be "reoperation" to clarify the situation.

Around day 2 to day 4, unrecognized bowel injuries, either sharp or thermic, tend to become obvious. During that time, postsurgical recovery should accelerate. In the context of an "early" peritonitis and ileus secondary to bowel injury, the clinical course is different. Initially, unspecific symptoms dominate: slight nausea, no bowel movements, diminished bowel sounds, and increasing abdominal discomfort. At the same time, the patient might develop a low-level fever, tachycardia. Laboratory changes are usually obvious at this stage: leukocytosis and increasing C-reactive protein. The initial diagnostic step should be a computed tomography scan. Abdominal X-ray is often nondiagnostic, as air is always present intraabdominally after surgery [7].

There are no tricks to prevent bowel surgery. In our opinion, restricting the cutting or coagulating instrument to the median working trocar creates maximal visibility of the most "dangerous" object in the abdomen. The simultaneous use of two electrical instruments should be reserved to the experienced surgeon only. Most bowel injury in laparoscopy is thermic.

Bladder and/or ureter injures can become symptomatic almost at any time after surgery, either through infection and peritonitis or through urinoma formation, kidney symptoms secondary to distention of the renal pelvis, urinary tract infections, and, in case of fistula formation, uncontrollable and continuous loss of urine [8]. The most feared complication is uretero-vaginal fistula, in which most cases probably are the result of necrosis of some part of the ureter becoming involved with the healing area of the vaginal suture line. As such, uretero-vaginal fistulas are the postoperative manifestation of an intraoperative but inapparent injury. With benign hysterectomy, the incidence of bladder injury is quoted at 1%, and ureteral injury, about 0.3% [9].

To prevent bladder injuries, there are some strategies to be kept in mind: (1) use a uterine manipulator, (2) dissect the bladder down always, (3) if in doubt, fill the bladder with saline, and (4) do not hesitate to perform a cystoscopy at the end of the procedure, if only to document that all was done to ensure maximal safety for the patient.

Wound infection is extremely rare in laparoscopy as opposed to laparotomy and need not be discussed.

A complication that appears to be slightly more frequent after laparoscopic hysterectomy than after abdominal hysterectomy is vaginal cuff dehiscence. Even though most data come from hysterectomies for benign indications, it is likely that these numbers equally apply to laparoscopic hysterectomy for oncology cases. The overall incidence of this complication that can cause peritonitis usually requires repeat surgery and potentially delays subsequent treatments such as radiation is low (<1%). Retrospective data show that continuous suture might reduce the incidence of this complication while few other factors have shown to alter its rate [10].

With regard to long-term complications, adhesion formation leading to long-term problems such as ileus and difficult reoperation is of particular importance for oncologic patients with an increased inherent risk for repeat surgery in the case of recurrence.

There exists ample evidence that laparoscopy strongly decreases the incidence of postoperative adhesion formation, creating a major advantage for laparoscopic oncologic surgery [11].

23.8 Managing complications—treating the patient and the surgeon

Complications need to be recognized, treated, and endured both by the patient and by the physician. Often, their management can be time-consuming and it can be very hard not just for the patient but also for the surgeon, who tends to see any complication as a personal failure. The patient needs to be managed medically—by reoperation if necessary—but also psychologically. Openness about the situation is usually the best approach. Patients are always aware that something went wrong and the only way to maintain their trust is an honest approach. A lot of time listening and explaining must be spent with the patient and the family, but every hour spent in the immediate postcomplication period can save years of litigation and bitterness. At the same time, the complication needs to be "put aside" by the surgeon. The next surgery requires, as always, the same basic confidence as the previous one. There are no good insecure surgeons. Complication do injury not only to our patients, but also to ourselves as surgeons.

23.9 How to improve and how to train surgeons

Even though the association is rarely made, talking about complications really means talking about training. Well-trained surgeons have fewer complications than poorly trained surgeons do [12]. The critical phase is the early part of the much quoted learning curve. In this context, an article about minimally invasive surgery would not be complete without the discussion of robotic vs. conventional laparoscopy. While overall complications rates between these two different approaches have been very similar, robotic minimally invasive surgery seems to have a faster learning curve [13, 14].

Surgery is a noble craft as much as a science. Advances in both technical and medical aspects have made it an incredibly safe part of modern medicine. This is particularly true for laparoscopy [15, 16]. The most important risk factor for complications aside from the patient is the surgeon.

Because of that, training future surgeons well has the potential to reduce complications more than anything else. Hippocrates must have known something about this when he made training almost the centerpiece of his famous oath.

Whatever we know about surgery, we must pass it on, slowly, diligently, patiently, and painfully, to future generations to make sure that our children, too, can go to the operating theater confident that "everything will be alright."

23.10 Conclusion and outlook

In minimally invasive gynecologic practice, most classically open surgical procedures can now be performed laparoscopically. Laparoscopic surgery has many advantages, as shown by a large body of literature. Intraoperative complications are similar or less when compared to open surgery. Postoperative complications are less frequent. The proper approach to complication-free laparoscopy requires a different mindset from open surgery. Technology has the potential to create an ever safer surgical environment. Particularly, improvements of visualization such as three-dimensional imaging systems have the potential to further reduce already the low complication rates in advanced laparoscopy cases.

List of typical complications in complex surgery:
- Hemorrhage (vessel injury)
- Bowel injury
- Bladder injury
- Ureteral injury
- Neuronal injury

List of specifically laparoscopic injuries:
- Entry injuries (retroperitoneal hematoma)
- CO_2 intoxication
- Cardiac problems due to positioning
- Neuronal problems due to positioning
- Emphysema due to CO_2 insufflation
- Hematoma due to trocar placement

References

[1] De Gouveia De Sa M, Claydon LS Whitlow B. Laparoscopic versus open sacrocolpopexy for treatment of prolapse of the apical segment of the vagina: a systematic review and meta-analysis. Int Urogynecol J 2016;27(1):3–17.
[2] Beck T, Morse C, Gray, H, Goff B, Urban R, Liao J. Route of hysterectomy and surgical outcomes from a state-wide gynecologic oncology population: is there a role for vaginal hysterectomy? Am J Obstet Gynecol 2016;214(3):348.e1–9.
[3] Chopin N, Malaret JM, Lafay-Pillet MC, et al. Total laparoscopic hysterectomy for benign uterine pathologies: obesity does not increase the risk of complications. Hum Reprod 2009;24(12):3057–62.
[4] Lönnerfors C, Reynisson P, Geppert B, Persson J. The effect of increased experience on complications in robotic hysterectomy for malignant and benign gynecological disease. J Robot Surg 2015 Dec;9(4):321–30.
[5] Ahmad G, Gent D, Henderson D, O'Flynn H, Phillips K, Watson A. Laparoscopic entry techniques (Cochrane—review). Cochrane Database Syst Rev 2015;31:8.
[6] Sandberg EB, Cohen SL, Jansen FW, Einarsson JI. Analysis of risk factors for intraoperative conversion of laparoscopic myomectomy. J Minim Invasive Gynecol 2015;22(6S):S62.
[7] Llarena NC, Shah AB, Milad MP. Bowel injury in gynecologic laparoscopy: a systematic review. Obstet Gynecol 2015;125(6):1407–17.
[8] Bige O, Demir A, Saatli B, et al. Laparoscopy versus laparotomy for the management of endometrial carcinoma in morbidly obese patients: a prospective study. J Turk Ger Gynecol Assoc 2015;16:164–9.

[9] Wattiez A, Soriano D, Cohen SB. The learning curve of total laparoscopic hysterectomy: comparative analysis of 1647 cases. J Am Assoc Gynecol Laparosc 2002;9:339–45.

[10] Weizman NF, Manoucheri E, Vitonis AF, Hicks GJ, Einarsson JI, Cohen SL. Vaginal cuff dehiscence: risk factors and associated morbidities. J Surg Educ 2015;72(2):212–9.

[11] Kavic SM, Kavic SM. Adhesions and adhesiolysis: the role of laparoscopy. JSLS 2002;6(2):99–109.

[12] Bjerrum F, Sorensen JL, Konge L, et al. Procedural specificity in laparoscopic simulator training: protocol for a randomised educational superiority trial. BMC Med Educ 2014;14:215.

[13] Chandra V, Nehra D, Parent R, et al. A comparison of laparoscopic and robotic assisted suturing performance by experts and novices. Surgery 2010;147:830–9.

[14] Moore LJ, Wilson MR, Waine E, et al. Robotic technology results in faster and more robust surgical skill acquisition than traditional laparoscopy. J Robotic Surg 2015;9:67–73.

[15] Ciccione A, Autorino R, Breda A, et al. Three dimensional vs standard laparoscopic: comparative assessment using a validated program for laparoscopic urologic skills. Urology 2013;82:1444–50.

[16] Romero-Loera S, Cardenas-Lailson LE, Concha Bermejillo F, et al. Comparacion de destrezas en simulador de laparoscopia: imagen en 2D vs. 3D. Cirugia y Cirujanos 2016;84(1):37–44.

Ayesha Mahmud and Justin Clark

24 Hysteroscopy: instrumentation for diagnostic and operative hysteroscopy, distension media, and office hysteroscopy

24.1 Introduction

Hysteroscopy is the cornerstone of modern-day endoscopy in gynecology. In recent years, technological developments have greatly expanded the utility of hysteroscopy procedures in gynecology. It is now possible to perform a comprehensive hysteroscopic examination of the uterine cavity without the need for cervical dilation or routine use of anesthesia [1]. Consequently, diagnostic and operative hysteroscopy is now routinely performed worldwide in both office (outpatient) and inpatient settings.

Office hysteroscopy provides quick access and safe and cost-effective service as compared to inpatient hysteroscopy, avoiding the risks of anesthesia and prolonged recovery. On balance, the choice of setting for hysteroscopy is mainly influenced by the patient's preference, the complexity of the case, and the inclination of the surgeon. Irrespective of the chosen setting, the success of hysteroscopy hinges on the expertise of the clinician, the availability of endoscopic and ancillary equipment, and the setting for hysteroscopy. This chapter will provide a brief overview of the instruments used for diagnostic and operative hysteroscopy, the role of distension media, and office hysteroscopy.

24.2 Instruments for diagnostic and operative hysteroscopy

A typical "hysteroscope" usually consists of the following components, i.e., a light source for illumination, an inflow and outflow channel for distension media, an operating channel with a sheath (for instrumentation in operative hysteroscopy), and the use of a lens-telescope system for visual control and imaging. Studies suggest that the hysteroscope size considerably impacts the acceptability and success of ambulatory hysteroscopy [2]. Randomized controlled trials comparing different hysteroscope sizes have shown that hysteroscope sizes with an outer-sheath diameter of 3–3.5 mm are associated with far less intraoperative pain when compared with 5-mm hysteroscopes [3–5]. Other studies have concluded that hysteroscope size did not influence the procedural success rate [4, 6]. This suggests that operator skills and training impact patient acceptability. At present, a variety of hysteroscopes (operative and diagnostic) are available, which include rigid, flexible, and miniature semirigid/rigid

https://doi.org/10.1515/9783110535204-024

hysteroscopes. The choice of hysteroscope should be guided by its features, intended function (operative or diagnostic), and patient acceptability.

24.2.1 Light source

The technical quality and specifications of the light source impact image quality for hysteroscopy. A high-quality cold light source (175 watts or 300 watts) with a Xenon lamp is preferable for good quality images (Fig. 24.1). The primary concern with light sources is the thermal dissipation of energy, which increases with increasing operative time. Insulated fiber-optic or fluid light cables measuring between 3.5–5 mm and 180–30 cm in length are used for light transmission [1].

24.2.2 Imaging systems

A variety of imaging systems are available with add-on or built-in video recording and image printing technology. The quality of the imagining system depends on the video camera resolution, sensitivity, signal-to-noise ratio, and quality of video imaging. Newer high-definition cameras provide superior image quality and resolution (Fig. 24.2).

24.2.3 Endoscopes

Generally, the use of *flexible fiberscopes* is limited by their associated costs, lack of durability, and suitability for autoclaving [1]. In contrast, *rigid telescopes* are preferred

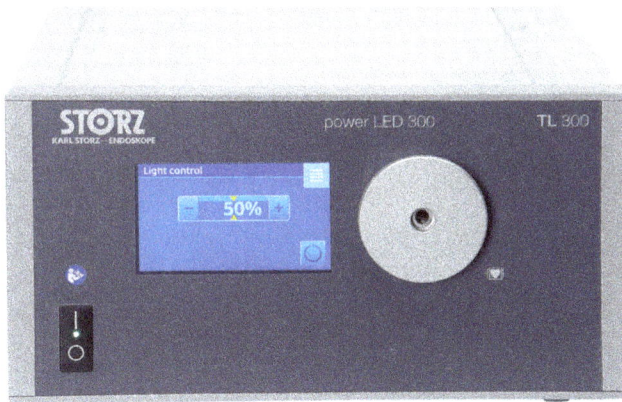

Fig. 24.1: LED cold light source. (Photo courtesy of Karl Storz.)

and available with different viewing angles, e.g., 0, 12, or 30 degrees, allowing for better visualization of the uterine cavity when adjusted correctly to the endocervical canal (Fig. 24.3).

Zero-degree telescopes allow visualization along the natural view orientation but require more side-to-side movement associated with procedural pain, whereas, 12 degrees or 30 degrees is preferred for operative procedures because instruments can be seen at higher magnification and a wider field of view is obtained such that the operating instrument can be kept in view at all times. The wider field of view afforded by 30-degree telescopes are preferred for diagnostic hysteroscopy as they allow better visualization of the uterine cavity and the tubal ostia with minimal rotational movement, less cervical irritation, and better patient tolerance and comfort.

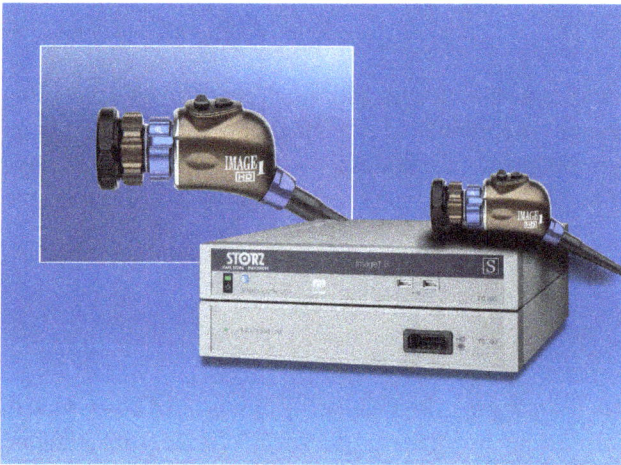

Fig. 24.2: High-definition video endoscopy system. (Photo courtesy of Karl Storz.)

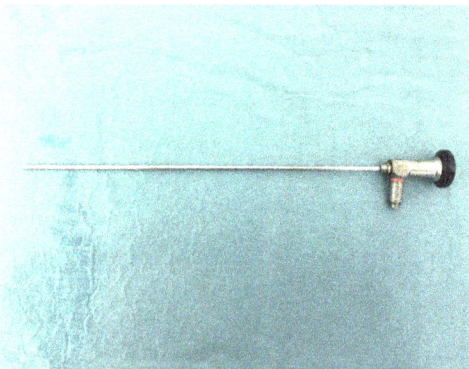

Fig. 24.3: A 30-degree rigid hysteroscope.

24.2.4 Diagnostic hysteroscopes

By design, diagnostic hysteroscopes are ergonomic miniature endoscopes. Most ambulatory units use hysteroscopes with an outer diameter of 3 mm for diagnostic purposes, e.g., the BETTOCCHI® hysteroscope. The use of smaller-diameter hysteroscopes renders the procedures less invasive and more tolerable for patients. The BETTOCCHI® Integrated Office Hysteroscope (B.I.O.H™) or the Alphascope™ are examples of more recent modification of conventional hysteroscope design. They allow the operator to maintain optimal visualization through suction, irrigation, and simultaneous instrumentation through operating sheaths for operative treatments. Versapoint™ is another example of a miniature bipolar electrosurgical system that allows easy removal of polyps without the need for large-diameter hysteroscopes (Fig. 24.4).

24.2.5 Operative hysteroscopes

Operative hysteroscopes by design include a larger-diameter (between 3.2 and 5.3 mm) sheath to accommodate operative instruments and the flow of fluid distention media.

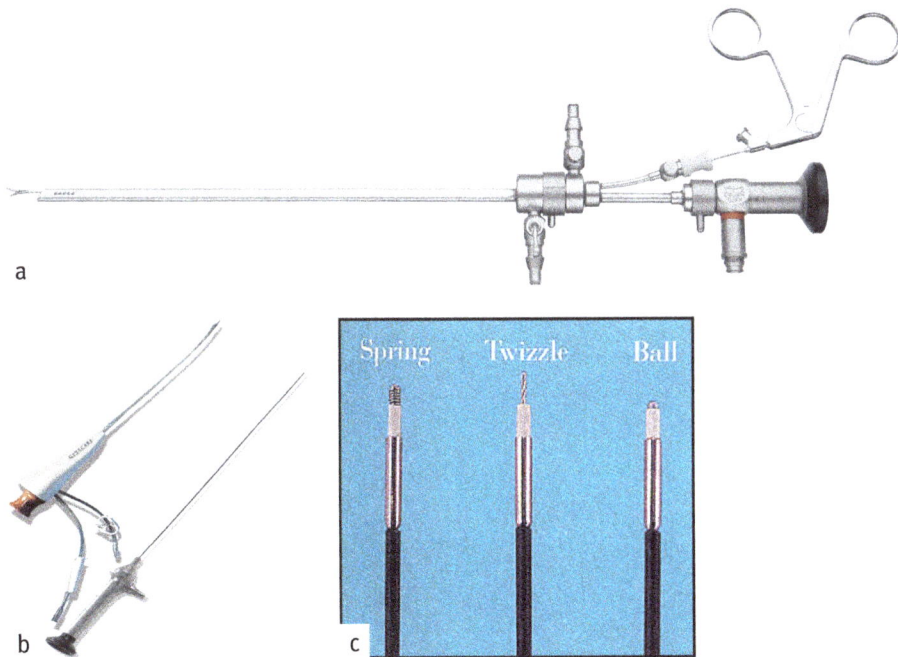

Fig. 24.4: (a) BETTOCHI® hysteroscope. (Photo courtesy of Karl Storz.) (b) Alphascope™. (Photo courtesy of Johnson & Johnson.) (c) Versapoint™ electrodes. (Photo courtesy of Johnson & Johnson.)

Operative instruments are mostly semirigid in design and much smaller in diameter (5 Fr or 1.67 mm). These include scissors, probes, monopolar and bipolar electrodes, along with a variety of biopsy forceps. Procedures such as adhesiolysis for minor adhesions, polypectomy, or directed biopsy can be performed effectively with these instruments [7–9] (Fig. 24.5).

More complicated procedures such as removal of a submucosal fibroid or excision of the endometrium require the use of larger-diameter electrosurgical devices such as the resectoscope (Fig. 24.6).

Resectoscope telescopes have viewing angles of 12 or 30 degrees, with an outer sheath diameter of 7.3 or 8.7 mm for continuous-flow irrigation (of distension media) [10]. A cutting loop is the primary operative instrument used with monopolar or

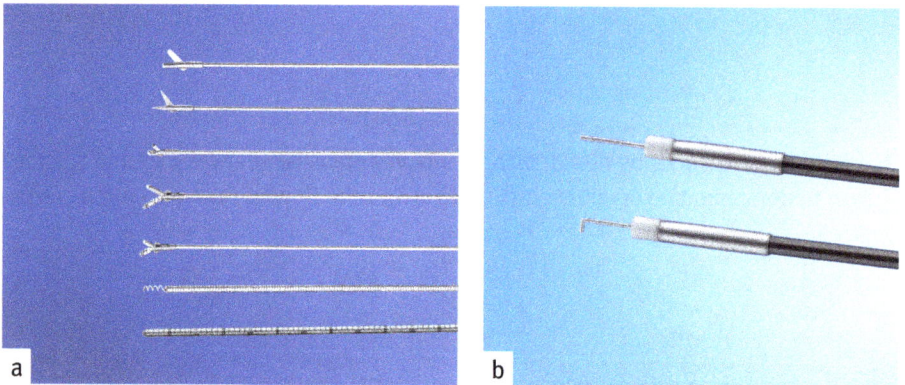

Fig. 24.5: (a) 5-Fr mechanical instruments. (b) 5-Fr bipolar electrodes. (Photos courtesy of Karl Storz.)

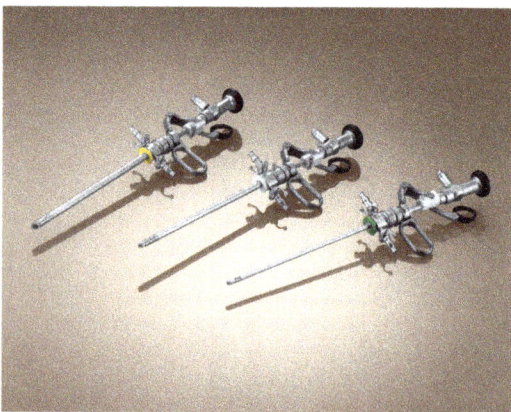

Fig. 24.6: 26-Fr bipolar resectoscope. (Photo courtesy of Karl Storz.)

bipolar electricity circuits. Also, tools such as micro-knives and coagulating electrodes can also be used with the resectoscope. Monopolar resectoscope requires the
use of nonconductive media due to the associated risk of thermal injury. In comparison, bipolar resectoscope is generally safer than monopolar as the thermal loop limits
the spread of heat to surrounding tissue lowering the risk of thermal injury and can be
safely used with a conductive media such as normal saline. High-frequency electrosurgical systems are used with resectoscopes for power supply control.

More recently, hysteroscopic morcellators, now called hysteroscopic tissue
removal systems (HTRS), that maintain visualization through simultaneous tissue
cutting and removal has become increasingly popular [11]. HTRS are electricity driven mechanical devices comprising a 0-degree telescope with a specialized operating channel that allows the use of disposable cutting instruments and
is connected to an external suction system. Examples of these systems include
TRUCLEAR™, Myosure™, Integrated Bigatti Shaver (IBS), and the SYMPHION™
(Fig. 24.7). These HTRS come in a variety of sizes so that some are suitable and
indicated for office removal of polyps and fibroids, whereas others are designed
for removal of larger fibroids and chronic retained products of conception under
regional or general anesthesia. Trials have shown that tissue removal systems have a
quicker learning curve, are faster to complete, less painful, more tolerable, and allow
better surgical excision of polyps compared to electrosurgical devices such as the
resectoscope [11, 12].

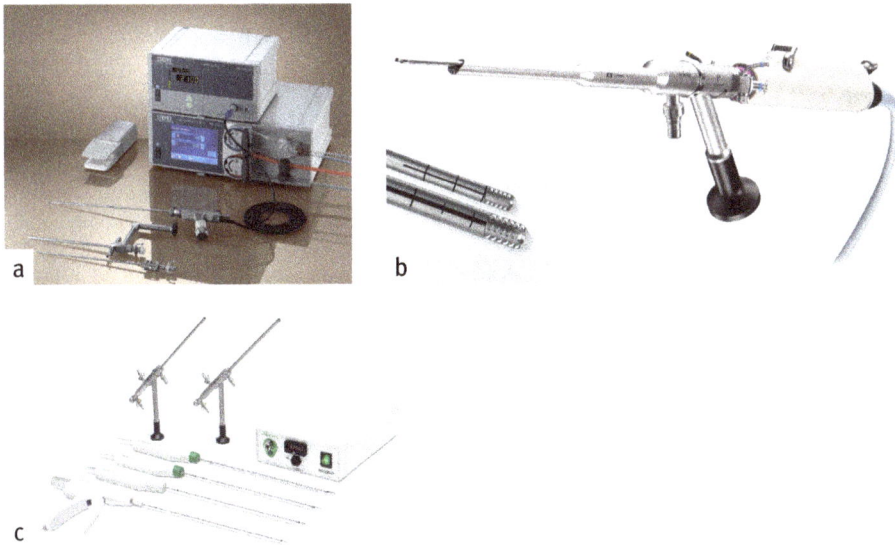

Fig. 24.7: (a) Integrated Bigatti Shaver™. (Photo courtesy of Karl Storz.) (b) Truclear™. (Photo courtesy
of Medtronic.) (c) Myosure™. (Photo courtesy of Hologic.)

24.3 Distension media

Optimal visualization of the uterine cavity requires the use of distension media that can accommodate both diagnostic and operative hysteroscopy. Fluid (i.e., glycine, dextran, water, sorbitol, and normal saline) and gaseous distention media (i.e., carbon dioxide) have both been described in the literature. Generally, fluid distention media are preferred in comparison to gaseous ones, i.e., carbon dioxide, which require special insufflation equipment and whose use is limited to diagnostic purposes. In contrast, fluid-based media allow for simultaneous removal of blood and debris, adjusting for optimal visualization for both diagnostic and operative hysteroscopy. Carbon dioxide use is also associated with a small risk of air embolism, and for this reason, the use of an electronic hystero-insufflator (to monitor intrauterine pressure and gas insufflation) is advisable. Hence, it is not surprising that much of the newer operative hysteroscopic systems are built to accommodate for fluid distension media with automated fluid management systems (Fig. 24.8).

The preference for "a particular" type of fluid distention media depends on the safety profile of the selected fluid, the type of operative system (mechanical or electrosurgical technology), and the purpose of the hysteroscopy. As such, isotonic normal saline is the preferred fluid distension media for operative hysteroscopy as its "normal physiologically compatible" nature allows for less risk of severe osmotic imbalance in the event of inadvertent fluid overload (hypovolemic hyponatremia) [13]. This advantage makes it a safe choice for mechanical operative

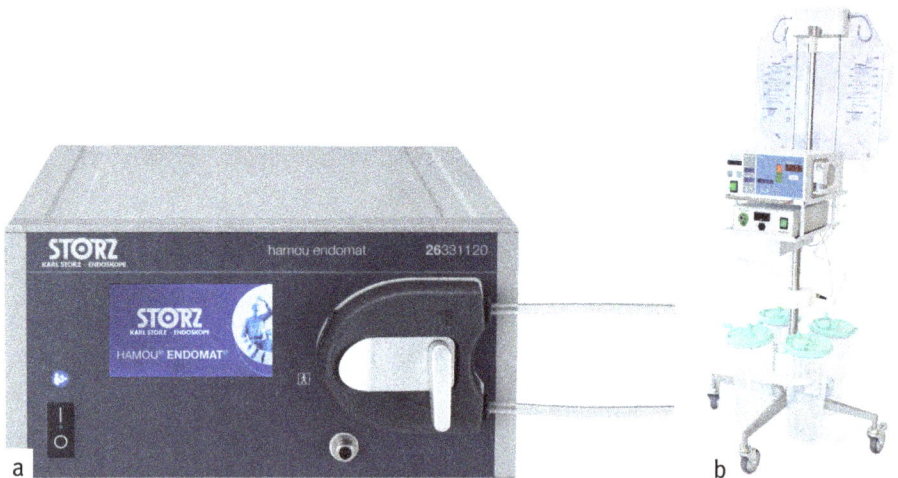

Fig. 24.8: (a) Hamou Endomat™. (Photo courtesy of Karl Storz.) (b) Aquilex™ fluid control system. (Photo courtesy of Hologic.)

procedures (e.g., polypectomy). Although regarding pain and visualization, normal saline is no different from carbon dioxide, the procedural completion time with normal saline has been found to be much quicker [14]. Similarly, operative technology using different electrical circuits, i.e., monopolar or bipolar instruments, also impacts the choice of fluid distension media. Monopolar instruments require the use of nonconductive, nonionic, hypo-osmolar solutions (e.g., sorbitol or glycine), whereas bipolar instruments require the use of conductive, ionic solutions (e.g., normal saline or Ringer's lactate). Tab. 24.1 provides a summary of the types of distension media and their clinical application [15]. Irrespective of which fluid is used, the risk of fluid overload with or without electrolyte imbalance remains a major concern.

Fluid overload can complicate up to 5% of operative hysteroscopy procedures [15]. Fluid overload occurs from intravascular absorption of excess fluid into the body's circulation, with a resultant expansion of the extracellular fluid volume. This can lead to serious, life-threatening complications such as pulmonary edema, hypertension, neurological impairment, seizures, and cardiac failure [16]. The joint British Society For Gynaecological Endoscopy/European Society for Gynaecological Endoscopy (BSGE/ESGE) guidance suggests that "A fluid deficit of more than 1000 ml should be used as a threshold to define fluid overload when using hypotonic solutions in healthy women of reproductive age" [15]. The guidance also recommends using a fluid deficit threshold of 2500 ml when using isotonic fluid media for the same group of women [15]. Generally, the newer generation bipolar systems are considered safe as they do not impact serum osmolality or sodium levels. However, given the risks of fluid overload, a precautionary approach is warranted.

Several operative factors contribute to an increased risk of fluid overload, including prolonged procedures requiring large diameter endoscopes with concurrent fluid irrigation (increase exposure and absorption of larger fluid volumes); endometrial resection for pathology or treatment (risk of increased fluid absorption by exposure of myometrium blood vessels); increased intrauterine pressure; low mean arterial pressure; use of hypotonic electrolyte free fluids (e.g., glycine), and a

Tab. 24.1: Types of distension media and clinical applications.

Type of fluid distension media	Osmolality (mOsm/l)	Type of electrolyte solution	Type of hysteroscopy
Normal saline	285 (iso-osmolar)	Electrolyte-containing	Diagnostic and operative
Ringer's lactate	279 (iso-osmolar)	Electrolyte-containing	Operative
Glycine 1.5%	200 (hypo-osmolar)	Electrolyte-free	Operative
Dextrose 5% (in water)	256 (hypo-osmolar)	Electrolyte-free	Operative
Sorbitol 3%	165 (hypo-osmolar)	Electrolyte-free	Operative

larger uterine cavity [17–21], For example, transcervical resection of fibroids (TCRF) requires the use of a large-diameter scope (resectoscope) with concurrent irrigation for clear visualization and removal of fibroid fragments, which can take much longer than a simple polypectomy procedure. Premenopausal women and those with known cardiac or renal disease are more at risk of serious complications [15]. Therefore, it is advisable to correctly measure the fluid input and output during the procedure to recognize and manage any fluid deficits.

The joint BSGE/ESGE guidance advocates the use of a structured fluid management in liaison with the anesthetist throughout the procedure [15]. The use of closed systems, fluid reservoir containing drapes, and automated fluid measurement systems can help facilitate this process. Additional measures such as the use of preoperative GnRH agonists before TCRF and use of intracervical diluted vasopressin have been advocated to lower the risk of prolonged operative hysteroscopy [15]. Moreover, where possible, the use of local anesthesia with sedation can reduce the risk of fluid overload. Therefore, clinicians can significantly lower the risk of fluid overload by following current BSGE/ESGE guidance for liquid distention media in operative hysteroscopy.

24.4 Office hysteroscopy

Office hysteroscopy is now a permanent fixture in ambulatory gynecology. It also remains the gold standard for assessment and treatment of uterine cavity pathology. Initially, the scope of office hysteroscopy was limited to diagnosis only. However, with advances in medical technology and miniaturization of instruments, a variety of minor operative procedures can now be completed in outpatient settings [22–24]. This includes endometrial polypectomy, resection of fibroids, localization of intrauterine contraceptive devices, minor adhesiolysis and endometrial ablation, etc. Moreover, office hysteroscopy is a well-accepted, accessible, cost-effective, and safe alternative to inpatient hysteroscopy [25, 26]. Using evidence-based best practice guidance can help minimize complications and optimize the patient experience of office hysteroscopy [27].

References

[1] Mencaglia L, Cavalcanti De Albuquerque Neto L, and Arias Alvarez RA. Manual of Hysteroscopy Diagnostic, Operative and Office Hysteroscopy. Tuttlingen: Endo-Press; 2013.
[2] Romani F, Guido M, Morciano A, et al. The use of different size-hysteroscope in office hysteroscopy: our experience. Arch Gynecol Obstet 2013;288(6):1355e9.
[3] Campo R, Molinas CR, Rombauts L, et al. Prospective multicentre randomized controlled trial to evaluate factors influencing the success rate of office diagnostic hysteroscopy. Hum Reprod 2005;20(1):258e63.

[4] Giorda G, Scarabelli C, Franceschi S, et al. Feasibility and pain control in outpatient hysteroscopy in postmenopausal women: a randomized trial. Acta Obstet Gynecol Scand 2000;79(7):593e7.

[5] De Angelis C, Santoro G, Re ME, et al. Office hysteroscopy and compliance: mini-hysteroscopy versus traditional hysteroscopy in a randomized trial. Hum Reprod 2003;18(11):2441e5.

[6] Rullo S, Sorrenti G, Marziali M, et al. Office hysteroscopy: comparison of 2.7- and 4-mm hysteroscopes for acceptability, feasibility and diagnostic accuracy. J Reprod Med 2005;50(1):45e8.

[7] Bettocchi S, Ceci O, Nappi L, et al. Operative office hysteroscopy without anesthesia: analysis of 4863 cases performed with mechanical instruments. J Am Assoc Gynecol Laparosc 2004;11:59–61.

[8] Nathani F, Clark TJ. Uterine polypectomy in the management of abnormal uterine bleeding: a systematic review. J Minim Invasive Gynecol 2006;13:260–8.

[9] Timmermans A, Veersema S. Ambulatory transcervical resection of polyps with the Duckbill polyp snare: a modality for treatment of endometrial polyps. J Minim Invasive Gynecol 2005;12:37–9.

[10] Di Spiezio Sardo A, Mazzon I, Bramante S, et al. *Hysteroscopic myomectomy: a comprehensive review of surgical techniques.* Hum Reprod Update 2008;14.2: 101–19. Web.

[11] van Dongen H, Emanuel MH, Wolterbeek R, Trimbos J, Jansen FW. Hysteroscopic morcellator for removal of intrauterine polyps and myomas: a randomized controlled pilot study among residents in training. J Minim Invasive Gynecol 2008;15:466–71.

[12] Smith PP, Malick S, Clark TJ. Bipolar radiofrequency compared with thermal balloon ablation in the office: a randomized controlled trial. Obstet Gynecol 2014;124:219–25.

[13] Berg A, Sandvik L, Langebrekke A, Istre O. A randomized trial comparing monopolar electrodes using glycine 1.5% with two different types of bipolar electrodes (TCRis, Versapoint) using saline, in hysteroscopic surgery. Fertil Steril 2009;91:1273–8.

[14] Cooper NAM, Smith P, Khan KS, Clark TJ. A systematic 1798 review of the effect of the distension medium on pain during outpatient hysteroscopy. Fertil Steril 2011;95:264–71.

[15] Umranikar S, Clark TJ, Saridogan E, et al. BSGE/ESGE guideline on management of fluid distension media in operative hysteroscopy. Gynecol Surg 2016;13(4):289–303.

[16] Istre O, Bjoennes J, Naess R, Hornbaek K, Forman A. Postoperative cerebral oedema after transcervical endometrial resection and uterine irrigation with 1.5% glycine. Lancet 1994;344:1187–9.

[17] Varol N, Maher P, Vancaillie T, et al. A literature review and update on the prevention and management of fluid overload in endometrial resection and hysteroscopic surgery. Gynaecol Endosc 2002;11(1):19–26.

[18] Garry R, Hasham F, Kokri MS, Mooney P. The effect of pressure on fluid absorption during endometrial ablation. J Gynecol Surg 1992;8(1):1–10.

[19] Hasham F, Garry R, Kokri MS, Mooney P. Fluid Absorption during laser ablation of the endometrium in the treatment of menorrhagia. Br J Anaesth 1992;68:151–4.

[20] Bennett K, Ohrmundt C, Maloni J. Preventing intravasation in women undergoing hysteroscopic procedures. AORN J 1996;64(5):792–9.

[21] Paschopoulos M, Polyzos NP, Lavasidis LG, Vrekoussis T, Dalkalitsis N, Paraskevaidis E. Safety issues of hysteroscopic surgery. Ann N Y Acad Sci 2006;1092:229–34.

[22] Clark TJ, Gupta JK. Handbook of Outpatient Hysteroscopy: A Complete Guide to Diagnosis and Therapy. CRC Press; 2005.

[23] Clark TJ, Godwin J, Khan KS, Gupta JK. Ambulatory endoscopic treatment of symptomatic benign endometrial polyps: feasibility study. Gynaecol Endosc 2002;11:91–7.

[24] Kremer C, Duffy S, Moroney M. Patient satisfaction with outpatient hysteroscopy versus day case hysteroscopy: randomised controlled trial. BMJ 2000;320:279–82.

[25] Wortman M, Daggett A, Ball C. Operative hysteroscopy in an office-based surgical setting: review of patient safety and satisfaction in 414 cases. JMIG 2013;20:56–63.

[26] Moawad NS, Santamaria E, Johnson M, Shuster J. Cost effectiveness of office hysteroscopy for abnormal uterine bleeding. JSLS 2014;18.

[27] Best practice in outpatient hysteroscopy. RCOG, Green-top Guideline No. 59, March 2011.

Mark Hans Emanuel

25 Hysteroscopic surgery for submucosal fibroids

25.1 Diagnosis and preoperative evaluation

To address the absence of consensus about the nomenclature of causes for abnormal uterine bleeding, the Fédération Internationale de Gynécologie et d'Obstétrique has designed the PALM-COEIN (polyp, adenomyosis, leiomyoma, malignancy and hyperplasia, coagulopathy, ovulatory disorders, endometrial disorders, iatrogenic causes, and not classified) PALM-COEIN classification system [1]. This classification system categorizes the submucosal variant of fibroids according to our publication in 1993 [2]: intracavitary myomas that are attached to the endometrium by a narrow stalk are classified as type 0; types 1 and 2 myomas require that a portion of the lesion is intramural, with type 1 being 50% or less and type 2 more than 50%. In most cases, fibroids with deeper intramural extension have a larger volume. During their growth, it takes longer for a type 2 fibroid to reach the uterine cavity and start being symptomatic than it takes for a type 0 fibroid; the last variant tends to be smaller. Type 3 myomas are completely extracavitary but abut the endometrium. Type 4 lesions are intramural myomas that are entirely within the myometrium, with no extension to the endometrial surface.

During the last two decades, transvaginal ultrasonography of the uterus has become a routine procedure in the diagnostic work-up of several gynecological problems. It has been demonstrated that a normal sonographic finding is very accurate for the exclusion of clinically significant intracavitary abnormalities [3]. However, in the presence of uterine pathology, diagnostic accuracy and reproducibility decline. To improve the image in these cases, sonographic examination using artificial uterine cavity distension was first described at our department [4]. Saline infusion sonohysterography (SIS) and gel instillation sonohysterography (GIS) are extensively described in the literature [5–10]. It is accepted that SIS/GIS improves the diagnostic accuracy of transvaginal ultrasonography in case of abnormal or inconclusive findings and that SIS/GIS is an effective early diagnostic step in the evaluation of patients with pre- and postmenopausal abnormal uterine bleeding. For an adequate preoperative evaluation of a submucous myoma, it has been proven that a concomitant three-dimensional contrast ultrasonographical examination has a low inter- and intraobserver variability with a good reproducibility of measuring the protrusion of the fibroid into the cavity [11]. Apart from properly classifying the intramural extension of the myoma, especially the evaluation of the thickness of the myometrium between the intramural portion of the myoma and the serosa is important to prevent perforation during hysteroscopic treatment. There are no generally accepted limits of this thickness, although a minimal of 5 mm is often mentioned. The surgeon should

https://doi.org/10.1515/9783110535204-025

always be aware of this thickness and extreme caution should be employed while addressing the deepest intramurally located part of the fibroid.

25.2 Preoperative preparation

Although a thin endometrium improves visualization of the borders of a myoma during hysteroscopic procedures, endometrial preparation was never subject of a randomized controlled trials (RCTs) related to hysteroscopic myomectomy. The same counts for the use of medication that is known to reduce the size of the myoma. One would expect that preoperative use could result in more complete removals; however, this was never proven for gonadotrophin-releasing hormone analogs (GnRHa). The use of GnRHa for 3 to 4 months prior to fibroid surgery reduces both uterine volume and fibroid size. They are beneficial in the correction of preoperative iron deficiency anemia, if present [12]. The preoperative use of ulipristal acetate, a selective progesteron receptor modulator (SPRM), showed similar results [13], amenorrhea and fibroid size reduction, but advantages during hysteroscopic surgery were never studied. In a meta-analysis of 11 randomized controlled trials involving 780 women with symptomatic uterine fibroids, it was demonstrated that mifepristone (another SPRM) could also effectively reduce uterine and fibroid volume and alleviate symptoms, including hypermenorrhea. Again, no effects on surgical outcome were described [14].

25.3 Hysteroscopic surgery

Only very small fibroids (<1 cm) can be treated with conventional instruments with a diameter of 3–7 French. During diagnostic preoperative hysteroscopic procedures, a myoma can possibly be incised around its border at the transition to the normal myometrium in order to promote the expulsion of the myoma toward the uterine cavity, eventually resulting in less intramural extension [15]. Some authors state that hysteroscopic myomectomy with conventional (nonelectrosurgical) use of instruments (cold loop resection) is a safe and effective procedure of notable importance for fertility patients [16].

The first use of a resectoscope for the removal of a submucous myoma was described in 1978 by Neuwirth [17].

Tissue that has been cut must be removed from the uterine cavity by taking out the hysteroscope after grasping the loose tissue elements with a forceps or the loop-electrode in case of the resectoscope. Although the removal of tissue under visual control, instead of using a curette, is the most effective way, it takes a large number of steps, which can be tiring in the long run, inconvenient to perform, and consequently found hard to learn. For these reasons, operative hysteroscopy has a rather long learning curve and the number of gynecologists who perform operative hysteroscopy is still low.

Hysteroscopic morcellation could resolve some of the above-mentioned difficulties. The first tissue removal system TRUCLEAR™ (Medtronic, Minneapolis, MN, USA) was invented by the author. Its action is based on mechanical cutting and aspiration [18]. The system uses no electrocoagulation and there is no lateral thermal or electrical energy spread. Hemostasis occurs by spontaneous myometrial contraction. The removed tissue is discharged through the device, is collected in a tissue-trap, and is available for pathological analysis.

A new development in hysteroscopic morcellation is the recent availability of a smaller outer diameter TRUCLEAR™ system with a 2.9-mm cutting blade and a 5.0-mm hysteroscope for office or ambulatory use with no or local anesthesia. The very similar morcellator system Myosure™ was introduced a few years later by Hologic (Bedford, MA, USA). Other companies that recently came with alternative tissue removal systems are Storz (Tutlingen, Germany) and Boston Scientific (Marlborough, MA, USA).

During hysteroscopic surgery of fibroids, the intravasation of distension fluid is strongly related to surgery time and to the location of the fibroid. Especially, resection of fibroids with deeper intramural extension cause more intravasation [19]. Apart from a longer surgery time, this can also be explained by the vascular architecture of the myometrium; deeper in the myometrium, the number of vessels decrease, but their size in diameter increases [20].

Distention and visualization are improving with higher intrauterine pressure and flow; however, the lowest pressure and flow in which distention and visualization are acceptable are advised. This is to prevent fluid loss as much as possible, and the intramural part of the fibroid is expelled to the cavity easier and better.

Uterine vascularity may be enhanced by myomas or other pathology. A low pressure and a high flow usually create better visualization than high pressure and low flow. However, intraoperative bleeding is generally not a significant problem because a rapid liquid flow will clean the image and after the procedure, uterine contractions will diminish bleeding rapidly.

25.4 Operative procedures

Hysteroscopic surgery of fibroids is not generally implemented in daily practice; still, many cases are referred to centers with more expertise. Besides, surgical trainees and gynecologists perform less surgery than in the past because of limited work hours. In a study, we examined the case volume of surgeons by looking at the number of hysteroscopic myomectomies performed across the years [21]. High-volume surgeons (performing approximately 20 hysteroscopic myomectomies annually) resected more tissue and a higher amount of tissue per time than low-volume surgeons did (performing approximately four procedures annually). There was no significant difference in complications.

Since hysteroscopic removal of fibroids means the removal of a certain volume of tissue, it is of utmost importance to know amount of tissue that has to be removed.

One should realize that with increasing diameter (2R), the volume ($4/3\pi R^3$) increases much faster (to the third power) (Tab. 25.1). It is obvious that this is of great influence on the ultimate surgery time that is necessary for the complete removal a myoma by hysteroscopical techniques (Fig. 25.1).

The basic strategy to remove a fibroid hysteroscopically, irrespective of the technology used, is to start at the periphery and remove tissue further toward the center of the fibroid. One should never cut the stalk in case of a type 0 fibroid. In case of a type 1–2 fibroid, the intracavitary part is first removed and then the intramural part for which the visual overview of the capsular area (the compressed normal myometrium surrounding the fibroid) is mandatory for a complete removal and to prevent perforation.

In case of an incomplete removal, mostly caused by a premature cessation of the procedure because of excessive intravastion, possibly persistent symptoms dictate further management. If abnormal bleeding is sufficiently treated by an incomplete myoma removal, a wait-and-see policy is an option. In many cases, the residual fibroid tissue is damaged by devascularization and coagulation in a way that spontaneous resorption of the fibroid remnant tissue can be expected further, although this

Tab. 25.1: The relation between the diameter (2R) and the volume ($4/3\pi R^3$) of a sphere.

Diameter in cm	Volume in cm³ (ml)
0.2	0.004
0.4	0.03
0.6	0.11
0.8	0.27
1.0	0.52
1.2	0.90
1.4	1.43
1.6	2.14
1.8	3.04
2.0	4.18
2.2	5.56
2.4	7.22
2.6	9.18
2.8	11.49
3.0	14.14
3.2	17.16
3.4	20.58
3.6	24.43
3.8	28.73
4.0	33.51
4.2	38.79
4.4	44.60
4.6	50.97
4.8	57.91
5.0	65.45

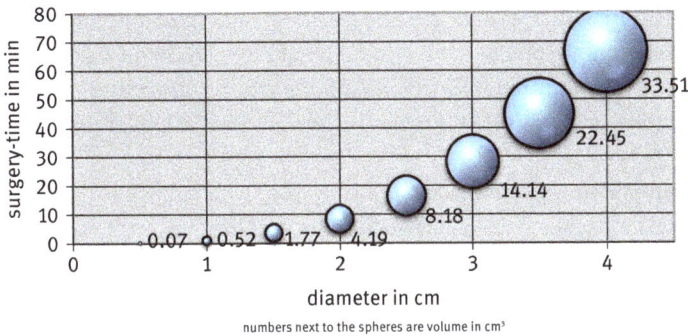

Fig. 25.1: Diameter versus surgery time (tissue removal rate 0.5 cm³/min).

can take months when observed by repeated ultrasonographical examination [22, 23]. Such a policy seems not very adequate in case of subfertility because of the long time passing by.

When surgical techniques are performed in a proper state-of-the-art way, there is no need for standard measures to prevent adhesions. However, when the endometrial lining is damaged unintentionally, it is not evident whatever measure should be taken, but it seems logical to perform a second look hysteroscopy after a few weeks. Furthermore, it is advised not to resect opposite submucous myomas in one session. In such cases, adhesion formation can be easily prevented by removing such multiple myomas in two settings (one for the anterior wall and one for the posterior wall).

25.5 Postoperative care

The patient may immediately resume normal activities; she should be driven home and refrain from strenuous activities and those requiring mental alertness. She should contact the surgeon if she develops fever, foul discharge, heavy bleeding, or persistent pain.

Later imaging studies (ultrasound and/or second look hysteroscopy) can be used to determine whether the surgery was successful, especially when there was doubt about the completeness of the fibroid removal. The appropriate timing for postoperative evaluation should be individualized and is based upon the difficulty of the procedure, the recurrence of symptoms, and the needs of the patient.

There are no RCTs supporting any specific postoperative measures.

25.6 Outcome and recurrence

Although there seems to be international consensus in many guidelines about the need for hysteroscopic removal of submucous myomas, in case of heavy menstrual bleeding or subfertility, no RCTs have been performed to date. A published "study" that promised to be the first RCT evaluating the effect of hysteroscopic myomectomy appeared to be an example of blatant scientific plagiarism [24]. The article was retracted at the request of the editors of *Fertility and Sterility* as it duplicates a paper by other authors reporting about an RCT concerning subfertility and hysteroscopic polypectomy [25].

In a recent Cochrane review, it is stated that hysteroscopic myomectomy at least might increase the odds of clinical pregnancy, but the evidence is at present not conclusive [26]. More randomized studies are needed to substantiate the effectiveness of the hysteroscopic removal of suspected submucous fibroids in women with unexplained subfertility or prior to assisted reproductive techniques.

A recurrence can be defined as the need for further surgery. We analyzed a group of 258 women who were treated with transcervical resection of submucous myomas without endometrial ablation [27]. In case of incomplete resection, a repeat procedure was offered. Long-term follow-up was obtained. An independent prognostic value of uterine size and number of submucous myomas for recurrence was noted. The surgery-free percentage of 165 patients with normal sized uteri and not more than two myomas was 94.3% at 2 years and 90.3% at 5 years. Similar results were published by others [28, 29].

References

[1] Munro MG, Critchley HO, Broder MS, Fraser IS; FIGO Working Group on Menstrual Disorders. FIGO classification system (PALM-COEIN) for causes of abnormal uterine bleeding in nongravid women of reproductive age. Int J Gynaecol Obstet 2011 Apr;113(1):3–13.

[2] Wamsteker K, Emanuel MH, de Kruif JH. Transcervical hysteroscopic resection of submucous fibroids for abnormal uterine bleeding: results regarding the degree of intramural extension. Obstet Gynecol 1993 Nov;82(5):736–40.

[3] Emanuel MH, Verdel MJC, Wamsteker K, Lammes FB. A prospective comparison of transvaginal ultrasonography and diagnostic hysteroscopy in the evaluation of patients with abnormal uterine bleeding; the clinical implications. Am J Obstet Gynecol 1995;172:547–52.

[4] van Roessel J, Wamsteker K, Exalto N. Sonographic investigation of the uterus during artificial uterine cavity distention. J Clin Ultrasound 1987;15:439–50.

[5] Syrop CH, Sahakian V. Transvaginal sonographic detection of endometrial polyps with fluid contrast augmentation. Obstet Gynecol 1992;79:1041–3.

[6] Breitkopf D, Goldstein SR, Seeds JW; ACOG Committee on Gynecologic Practice. ACOG technology assessment in obstetrics and gynecology. Number 3, September 2003. Saline infusion sonohysterography. Obstet Gynecol 2003;102:659–62.

[7] de Kroon CD, de Bock GH, Dieben SW, Jansen FW. Saline contrast hysterosonography in abnormal uterine bleeding: a systematic review and meta-analysis. Obstet Gynaecol Surv 2004;59:265–6.

[8] Exalto N, Stappers C, van Raamsdonk LA, Emanuel MH. Gel instillation sonohysterography: first experience with a new technique. Fertil Steril 2007;87(1):152–5.

[9] Bij de Vaate AJ, Brölmann HA, van der Slikke JW, Emanuel MH, Huirne JA. Gel instillation sonohysterography (GIS) and saline contrast sonohysterography (SCSH): comparison of two diagnostic techniques. Ultrasound Obstet Gynecol 2010 Apr;35(4):486–9.

[10] Werbrouck E, Veldman J, Luts J, et al. Detection of endometrial pathology using saline infusion sonography versus gel instillation sonography: a prospective cohort study. Fertil Steril 2011 Jan;95(1):285–8.

[11] Lee C, Salim R, Ofili-Yebovi D, Yazbek J, Davies A, Jurkovic D. Reproducibility of the measurement of submucous fibroid protrusion into the uterine cavity using three-dimensional saline contrast sonohysterography. Ultrasound Obstet Gynecol 2006 Nov;28(6):837–41.

[12] Lethaby A, Puscasiu L, Vollenhoven B. Preoperative medical therapy before surgery for uterine fibroids. Cochrane Database Syst Rev 2017 Nov 15;11:CD000547.

[13] Donnez J, Tomaszewski J, Vázquez F, et al.; PEARL II Study Group. Ulipristal acetate versus leuprolide acetate for uterine fibroids. N Engl J Med 2012 Feb 2;366(5):421–32.

[14] Shen Q, Hua Y, Jiang W, Zhang W, Chen M, Zhu X. Effects of mifepristone on uterine leiomyoma in premenopausal women: a meta-analysis. Fertil Steril 2013 Dec;100(6):1722–6.

[15] Emanuel MH, Wamsteker K. Uterine leiomyomas. In: I Brosens en K Wamsteker, eds. Diagnostic Imaging and Endoscopy in Gynecology. London: WB Saunders; 1997:185–98.

[16] Mazzon I, Favilli A, Cocco P, et al. Does cold loop hysteroscopic myomectomy reduce intrauterine adhesions? A retrospective study. Fertil Steril 2014 Jan;101(1):294–8.

[17] Neuwirth R. A new technique for and additional experience with hysteroscopic resection of submucous fibroids. Am J Obstet Gynecol 1978;131:91–4.

[18] Emanuel MH, Wamsteker K. The intra uterine morcellator: a new hysteroscopic operating technique to remove intrauterine polyps and myomas. J Minim Invasive Gynecol 2005 Jan–Feb;12(1):62–6.

[19] Emanuel MH, Hart A, Wamsteker K, Lammes F. An analysis of fluid loss during transcervical resection of submucous myomas. Fertil Steril 1997 Nov;68(5):881–6.

[20] Duffy SRG. A study of the safety and application of electrosurgery in the treatment of refractory dysfunctional bleeding (academic thesis). University College Cork: National University of Ireland; 1993.

[21] Betjes HE, Hanstede MM, Emanuel MH, Stewart EA. Hysteroscopic myomectomy and case volume hysteroscopic myomectomy performed by high- and low-volume surgeons. J Reprod Med 2009 Jul;54(7):425–8.

[22] Dueholm M, Foreman A, Ingerslev J. Regression of residual tissue after incomplete resection of submucous myomas. Gynaecol Endosc 1998;7:309–14.

[23] Van Dongen H, Emanuel MH, Smeets MJ, Trimbos B, Jansen FW. Follow-up after incomplete hysteroscopic removal of uterine fibroids. Acta Obstet Gynecol Scand 2006;85(12):1463–7.

[24] Shokeir T, El-Shafei M, Yousef H, Allam AF, Sadek E. Submucous myomas and their implications in the pregnancy rates of patients with otherwise unexplained primary infertility undergoing hysteroscopic myomectomy: a randomized matched control study. Fertil Steril 2010 Jul;94(2):724–9. Retraction in: Fertil Steril 2011 Sep;96(3):800.

[25] Pérez-Medina T, Bajo-Arenas J, Salazar F, et al. Endometrial polyps and their implication in the pregnancy rates of patients undergoing intrauterine insemination: a prospective, randomized study. Hum Reprod 2005;20:1632–5.

[26] Bosteels J, Kasius J, Weyers S, Broekmans FJ, Mol BW, D'Hooghe TM. Hysteroscopy for treating subfertility associated with suspected major uterine cavity abnormalities. Cochrane Database Syst Rev 2015 Feb 21;(2):CD009461.

[27] Emanuel MH, Wamsteker K, Hart AA, Metz G, Lammes FB. Long-term results of hysteroscopic myomectomy for abnormal uterine bleeding. Obstet Gynecol 1999 May;93(5 Pt 1):743–8.

[28] Hart R, Molnár BG, Magos A. Long term follow up of hysteroscopic myomectomy assessed by survival analysis. Br J Obstet Gynaecol 1999 Jul;106(7):700–5.

[29] Polena V, Mergui JL, Perrot N, Poncelet C, Barranger E, Uzan S. Long-term results of hysteroscopic myomectomy in 235 patients. Eur J Obstet Gynecol Reprod Biol 2007 Feb;130(2):232–237.

Attilio Di Spiezio Sardo, Fabrizia Santangelo, Claudio Santangelo, Gaetano Riemma, Gloria Calagna and Brunella Zizolfi

26 Hysteroscopic surgery for Mullerian anomalies

26.1 Introduction

Mullerian anomalies result from abnormal formation, fusion, or resorption of the Mullerian duct during embryogenesis (between the 9th and 13th gestational weeks). These anomalies are present in approximately 3–10% of the unselected population and are reported with a wide range of prevalence among subfertile women and in women with a history of recurrent miscarriages [1].

The European Society of Human Reproduction and Embryology (ESHRE) and the European Society for Gynecological Endoscopy (ESGE) have proposed a comprehensive description and categorization of almost all of the currently known anomalies. This classification overcomes the problems of those malformations that could not be classified properly with the previous American Fertility Society system. The ESHRE/ESGE system is designed mainly for clinical orientation and is based on the anatomy of the female genital tract. It defines six classes of uterine malformations [2] (Fig. 26.1).

Nowadays, due to the huge variability of clinical presentation, the identification of a Mullerian anomaly is often accidental. For a long time, bidimensional ultrasound scan and hysterosalpingography were the first-choice imaging diagnostic techniques in this field, but with the introduction of three-dimensional ultrasound (3D-US), the study of Mullerian anomalies has been revolutionized. The 3D-US is a highly reliable, sensitive, and specific technique in the study of these pathologies, especially for the opportunity to study the coronal plane of the uterus [3–8]. Overall, hysteroscopy is an indispensable tool used to explore and analyze the morphology of all the potential involved structures (vaginal canal, uterine cervix, and cavity). The endoscopic evaluation provides quantitative and qualitative information about the malformations, and when integrated with an accurate ultrasound evaluation, it can be considered the best way to define an individual treatment strategy of each case [8].

Indeed, it is not possible to discuss the treatment of Mullerian anomalies through a unique surgical method because the treatment depends on type, complexity, and clinical relevance of the anomaly and sometimes it requires the need of multiple approaches. Due to several advantages, when a Mullerian anomaly is amenable to surgical correction, operative hysteroscopy is the treatment of choice. Hysteroscopy is associated with numerous intraoperative and postoperative benefits: reduced morbidity, absence of a scar on the abdominal wall and uterus, shorter hospital stay, and a faster resumption of daily activities, as well as significant cost reductions. Moreover, this technique results in better reproductive outcomes, thanks to the fact that the hysteroscopic approach is associated with a lower preconception interval after surgery,

https://doi.org/10.1515/9783110535204-026

Class U0 / Normal Uterus

Class U1 / Dysmorphic Uterus

Class U1 / Dysmorphic Uterus

a. T-shaped

b. infantilis

Class U2 / Septate Uterus

Class U2 / Septate Uterus

Class U3 / Bicorporeal Uterus

a. partial

b. complete

a. partial

Class U3 / Bicorporeal Uterus

Class U3 / Bicorporeal Uterus

Class U4 / Hemi - Uterus

b. complete

c. bicorporeal septate

a. with rudimentary cavity

Class U4 / Hemi - Uterus

Class U5 / Aplastic Uterus

Class U5 / Aplastic Uterus

b. without rudimentary cavity

a. with rudimentary cavity

b. without rudimentary cavity

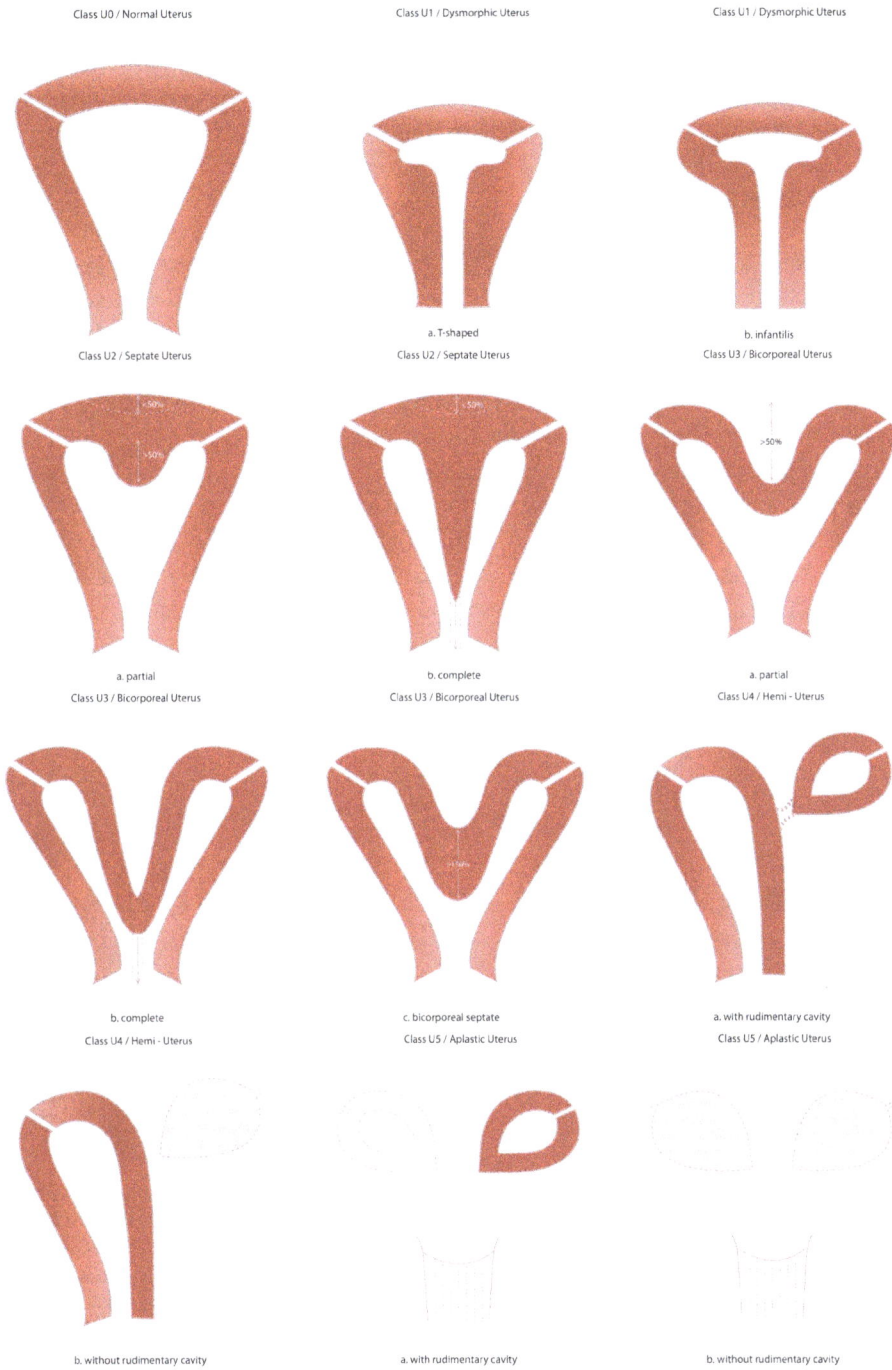

Fig. 26.1: The European Society for Gynecological Endoscopy/European Society of Human Reproduction and Embryology classification of the congenital uterine anomalies.

does not produce a reduction in the volume of the uterine cavity, and does not impli-
cate the need to resort to an elective caesarean section [9–11].

26.2 Dysmorphic uterus (Class U1 sec. ESHRE/ESGE classification)

This definition incorporates all cases of uterus with normal outline but abnormal
lateral wall shape of the uterine cavity (i.e., T-shaped uterus and tubular-shaped
U1a–b). The treatment goals in these cases are designed to improve the volume and
the morphology of the uterine cavity [12, 13] (Fig. 26.2); different methods and instruments have been used, including scissors and a resectoscope with a monopolar hook
or bipolar energy. Using a hooked loop, the surgeon places meticulously parallel longitudinal incisions along the main axis of the uterine cavity, in order to decrease the
centripetal muscular and fibromuscular forces that contribute to stenosis [13, 14].

Recently, a new outpatient technique (Hysteroscopic Outpatient Metroplasty
to Expand Dysmorphic Uteri: the HOME-DU technique) has been proposed by our
group. This technique combines the surgical principles of traditional resectoscopic

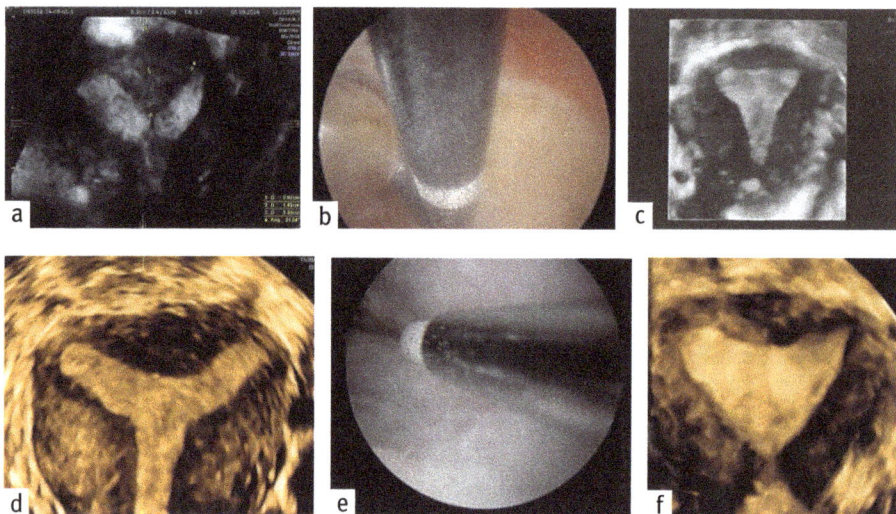

Fig. 26.2: (a) Preoperative evaluation with three-dimensional (3D) ultrasonography of a U2a uterus
with broad base prior to hysteroscopic treatment: septum length: 1.42 cm and myometrial fundal
thickness: 1.34 cm. Based on these measurements, 1.7 cm of the septum need to be resected in order
to produce a fundal notch measuring 1 cm. (b) The novel graduated intrauterine palpator shows that
1.7 cm of the septum has been sectioned. (c) Postoperative 3D ultrasonography evaluation shows
a complete resection of the septum. (d) Preoperative evaluation with 3D ultrasonography of a U1a
"T-Shaped" uterus. (e) Hysteroscopic correction of a T-Shaped uterus with the HOME-DU technique
using miniaturized electrodes. (f) Postoperative 3D ultrasonography evaluation shows an expanded
uterus and restored physiological morphology of the uterine cavity.

surgery and the use of latest innovations of minimally invasive operative hysteroscopy and bipolar technology. HOME-DU is performed under conscious sedation and involves making two incisions of 3–4 mm in depth with a 5-Fr bipolar electrode along the lateral walls of the uterine cavity in the isthmic region, followed by additional incisions placed on the anterior and posterior walls of the fundal region up to the isthmus. At the end of the procedure, a polyethylene oxide-sodium carboxymethylcellulose gel is applied into the uterine cavity, through the inflow channel of the hysteroscope, to prevent intrauterine adhesions [15].

26.3 Septate uterus (Class U2 sec. ESHRE/ESGE classification)

Septate uterus is defined as a uterus with normal outline and an internal indentation at the fundal midline exceeding 50% of the uterine wall thickness.

This indentation is characterized as septum and it could divide partly (U2a) or completely (U2b) the uterine cavity, including in some cases cervix and/or vagina [16].

Hysteroscopic metroplasty has replaced transabdominal metroplasty by enabling a transvaginal approach for the correction of septate uterus and by providing several advantages such as simple and short surgery with a shorter hospitalization time, a decreased need for analgesia, a shorter interval before conception (3–6 months), a lower risk of uterine rupture during pregnancy, and the possibility of planning a vaginal delivery. A combination of these factors makes hysteroscopic metroplasty the gold standard [17].

The traditional 26-Fr resectoscopic treatment of the uterine septum involves the use of straight cutting loops or a Collins electrode, starting to remove the septum from the medial portion and continuing with well-directed smooth movements of the cutting loop, oriented in an antegrade direction [18].

In case of a complete uterine septum with cervical septum, the traditional approach calls for excluding the cervical canal from any resection, in order to reduce the risk of secondary cervical incompetence, thus initiating resection from the isthmic portion of the septum [19]. According to this approach, the cervix of the larger uterine hemicavity is gradually dilated in order to introduce a resectoscope with a classical straight loop, while in the contralateral hemicavity, a curved (Hegar) dilator is inserted, serving as a guide to properly align the first blind incision, which is placed above the internal uterine ostium using an angular cutting loop. In the next step, the septum is incised and fenestrated until revealing the Hegar in the opposite hemicavity, followed by gradual resection toward the fundus using the classical technique. Occasionally, it may be useful to alternate approaching the septum from one wall, followed by the other wall in the contralateral hemicavity.

Some authors suggest resecting both the intrauterine and the cervical septum in a single procedure. This approach starts with resectoscopic removal of the cervical septum, which is then followed by removal of the uterine septum using the classic technique. Currently, there are no data in the literature demonstrating any increase in cervical incompetence in women treated by metroplasty of the uterine and cervical septum [18].

A more recent technique involves using the hysteroscopic approach with miniature instruments (which can be performed both under general anesthesia and in an ambulatory setting), based on the same rules applied in the resectoscopic approach, starting the resection of the septum from its apex (usually with a bipolar electrode) proceeding from one side of the septum to the other, in an alternating fashion; in final stages of office metroplasty, it is possible to use the miniature scissors, allowing a neat finish of resection [20]. An accurate presurgical evaluation with 3D-Transvaginal sonography, together with the use of a graduate intrauterine palpator, facilitates the complete removal of uterine septum, in one surgical step. The graduated intrauterine palpator can improve the accuracy of hysteroscopic metroplasty introducing objective intraoperative criteria: the metroplasty will be stopped when the intrauterine palpator shows that the resected septum corresponds to the presurgical ultrasonographic measurement in order to obtain a fundal notch of 1.0 cm, instead of stopping the metroplasty when the tubal ostia are clearly visible on the same line and/or hemorrhage from small myometrial vessels of the fundus is observed (Figure 26.2) [21, 22]. At the end of the procedure, to prevent intrauterine adhesions, an intrauterine antiadhesive gel is applied into the uterine cavity.

26.4 Robert's uterus (U2bC3V0 sec. ESHRE/ESGE classification)

Robert's uterus is a unique malformation that can be described as a septate uterus with a noncommunicating hemicavity, consisting of a blind uterine horn usually with unilateral hematometra, a contralateral unicornuate uterine cavity, and a normally shaped external uterine fundus. According to the novel classification system of female genital tract anomalies developed by ESHRE/ESGE, Robert's uterus is classified as complete septate uterus with unilateral cervical aplasia (U2bC3V0 anomaly). Traditionally, surgical management of this malformation was performed via an abdominal approach because it seemed the best option to preserve the integrity of the normal hemicavity and to perform a complete endometrectomy to prevent the recurrence of hematometra. The effect of this surgical treatment was very precise, but it caused certain trauma to the uterine wall. Recent studies have shown that hysteroscopy combined with laparoscopy might be a better minimally invasive method for the treatment of Robert's uterus. Therefore, Shi *et al.* noted that ultrasound can be used not only to accurately measure the width and length of the uterine septum but also to properly guide the direction of hysteroscopic electrotomy and indicate the size of septum resection. Traditionally, hysteroscopic metroplasty was performed with 4-mm 30-degree optics, a monopolar resectoscope, and a Collins needle electrode under general anesthesia [23–26].

Recently, a new minimally invasive hysteroscopic technique, guided by ultrasound, has been proposed by our group. During surgery, starting with 5-Fr bipolar electrodes and then continuing with cold scissors, parallel incisions are performed in order to create a communication between the blind uterine hemicavity and the other one to achieve the best anatomical shape of the uterine cavity [23]. As soon as the opening is created, if present, hematometra is evacuated. Subsequently, with 5-Fr bipolar electrodes, the upper portion of the septum is cut, and then, with a 16-Fr mini-resectoscope, the fibrotic tissue of the uterine septum on the anterior and posterior walls is resected. When a normal uterine cavity is obtained, the procedure is stopped. This method significantly reduces the surgical trauma and facilitates a shorter operation time, less bleeding, and rapid postoperative recovery and preservation of the integrity of the uterus, compared with the traditional surgical method [27].

26.5 Hemiuterus (Class U4 sec. ESHRE/ESGE classification)

Hemiuterus is defined as the unilateral uterine development; the contralateral part could be either incompletely formed or absent [16].

Laparotomy is the traditional surgical approach, with a complete removal of the rudimentary horn, if present. However, according to some authors, the hysteroscopic treatment has shown better reproductive prognosis. Using a hysteroscopic approach, the medial wall of the main hemicavity can be incised with a 5-Fr bipolar hook electrode under ultrasound or laparoscopic guidance, thus bringing the main cavity into communication with the accessory horn. Drainage from the accessory hemicavity can be facilitated by leaving *in situ* a Foley for a few days after the operation [28–30].

Generally, the presence of a rudimentary uterine horn that does not communicate with cervical canal causes symptoms characterized by obstruction such as hematometra, menstrual irregularities, and dysmenorrhea, which represent the main indications for surgical correction of this uterine anomaly. However, regardless of whether or not we decide to operate the rudimentary horn for the presence of symptoms, we have also to take in account that if pregnancy occurs in the unicornuate uterus, this event is associated with an increased risk of obstetric complications (miscarriage, cervical incompetence, and preterm delivery). For this reason, the transcervical uterine incision, a novel surgical technique, has been proposed. This procedure consists of a series of incision on the opposite uterine wall of unicornuate horn side designed to widen the narrow uterine cavity [31].

26.6 Vaginal anomalies (Class V1–V2 sec. ESHRE/ESGE classification)

For the treatment of most vaginal abnormalities, hysteroscopy represents the best surgical approach in terms of efficacy and safety [32–35]. The hysteroscopic surgical treatment of the longitudinal vaginal partial or complete septum involves two options of approach: resectoscopic surgery and hysteroscopy with miniature instruments. The resectoscopic treatment involves resection of the septum in an antegrade direction using a straight loop or Collins electrode, similarly to that described for the treatment of the uterine septum. This method appears advantageous compared to the traditional technique (with scissors, after application of Kelly or Kocher forceps) because the magnified video image and the distended vagina allows an enhanced level of safety, avoiding iatrogenic injury to the rectum and bladder [18, 32]. In addition, the electrical energy applied by use of a resectoscope induces a complete occlusion of small vessels of the septum, providing adequate hemostasis. The main limitation of the resectoscopic approach is the need to perform in the operating room and use of general anesthesia [32–34].

With the most recent miniature instruments, this limitation is overcome because the procedure can be performed in an ambulatory setting without the use of anesthesia, including virgin patients [35].

References

[1] Hiersch L, Yeoshoua E, Miremberg H, et al. The association between Mullerian anomalies and short-term pregnancy outcome. J Matern Fetal Neonatal Med. 2016;29(16):2573–8.

[2] Di Spiezio Sardo A, Campo R, Gordts S, et al. The comprehensiveness of the ESHRE/ESGE classification of female genital tract congenital anomalies: a systematic review of cases not classified by the AFS system. Hum Reprod 2015 May;30(5):1046–58.

[3] Vallerie A, Breech L. Update in Mullerian anomalies: diagnosis, management, and outcomes. Curr Opin Obstet Gynecol 2010;22:381–7.

[4] Kupesic S. Clinical implications of sonographic detection of uterine anomalies for reproductive outcome. Ultrasound in Obstet Gynecol 2001;18:387–400.

[5] Byrne J, Nussbaum-Blask A, Taylor WS, et al. Prevalence of Mullerian duct anomalies detected at ultrasound. Am J Med Genet 2000;94:9–12.

[6] Bettocchi S, Ceci O, Nappi L, Pontrelli G, Pinto L, Vicino M. Office hysteroscopic metroplasty: three "diagnostic criteria" to differentiate between septate and bicornuate uteri. J Minim Invasive Gynecol 2007;14(3):324–28.

[7] Pellerito JS, McCarthy SM, Doyle MB, Glickman MG, De Cherney AH. Diagnosis of uterine anomalies: relative accuracy of MR imaging, endovaginal sonography, and hysterosalpingography. Radiology 1992;183(3):795–800.

[8] Woelfer B, Salim R, Banerjee S, Elson J, Regan L, Jurkovic D. Reproductive outcomes in women with congenital uterine anomalies detected by three-dimensional ultrasound screening. Obstet Gynecol 2001;98:1099–103.

[9] Strassman E. Fertility and unification of double uteri. Fertil Steril 1966;17:165–76.

[10] Fayez JA. Comparison between abdominal and hysteroscopic metroplasty. Obstet Gynecol 1986;68:399–403.

[11] Ayhan A, Yucel I, Tuncer Z, Kisnisçi HA. Reproductive performance after conventional metroplasty: an evaluation of 102 cases. Fertil Steril 1992;5:1194–96.

[12] Katz Z, Ben-Arie A, Lurie S, Manor M, Insler V. Beneficial effect of hysteroscopic metroplasty on the reproductive outcome in a 'T-shaped' uterus. Gynecol Obstet Invest 1996;41:41–3.

[13] Garbin O, Ohl J, Bettahar-Lebugle K, Dellenbach P. Hysteroscopic metroplasty in diethylstilboestrol-exposed and hypoplastic uterus: a report on 24 cases. Hum Reprod 1998;13:2751–5.

[14] Fernandez H, Garbin O, Castaigne V, Gervaise A, Levaillant JM. Surgical approach to and reproductive outcome after surgical correction of a T-shaped uterus. Hum Reprod 2011; 26(7):1730–4.

[15] Di Spiezio Sardo A, Florio P, Nazzaro G, et al. Hysteroscopic outpatient metroplasty to expand dysmorphic uteri (HOME-DU technique): a pilot study. Reprod Biomed Online. 2015 Feb;30(2):166–74.

[16] Grimbizis G, Gordts S, Di Spiezio Sardo A, et al. The ESHRE/ESGE consensus on the classification of female genital tract congenital anomalies. Hum Reprod 2013;28(8):2032–44.

[17] Nappi L, Pontis A, Sorrentino F, Greco P, Angioni S. Hysteroscopic metroplasty for the septate uterus with diode laser: a pilot study. Eur J Obstet Gynecol Reprod Biol 2016 Nov;206:32–35.

[18] Nappi C, Di Spiezio Sardo A. State-of-the-art. Hysteroscopic approach to the pathologies of the genital tract. Endopress 2014;10:126–9.

[19] Parsanezhad ME, Alborzi S, Zarei A, et al. Hysteroscopic metroplasty of the complete uterine septum, duplicate cervix, and vaginal septum. Fertil Steril 2006;85(5):1473–7.

[20] Vilos GA. Intrauterine surgery using a new coaxial bipolar electrode in normal saline solution (versapoint): a pilot study. Fertil Steril 1999;72:740–3.

[21] Di Spiezio Sardo A, Zizolfi B, Bettocchi S, et al. Accuracy of hysteroscopic metroplasty with the combination of pre surgical three-dimensional ultrasonography and a novel graduated intrauterine palpator: a randomized controlled trial. J Minim Invasive Gynecol 2015 Nov–Dec;22(6S):S5–6.

[22] Practice Committee of the American Society for Reproductive Medicine. Uterine septum: a guideline. Fertil Steril 2016 Sep 1;106(3):530–40.

[23] Ludwin A, Ludwin I, Martins WP. Robert's uterus: modern imaging techniques and ultrasound-guided hysteroscopic treatment without laparoscopy or laparotomy. Ultrasound Obstet Gynecol 2016;48:526–9.

[24] Ramesh B, Chaithra TM, Desai H, Ghanti R, Daksh S. Management of Robert's uterus by combined hysteroscopic and laparoscopic management: a clinical pearl. Gynecol Surg 2016;13:521–4.

[25] Li J, Yu W, Wang M, Feng LM. Hysteroscopic treatment of Robert's uterus with laparoscopy. J Obstet Gynecol 2015;41:1491–4.

[26] Rosner-Tenerowiez. Hysteroscopic treatment of Robert's uterus. J Minim Invasive Gynecol 2017;24:S1–201.

[27] Di Spiezio Sardo. Hysteroscopic treatment with miniaturized instruments of complete septate uterus with unilateral cervical aplasia (Class U2bC3V0/ESHRE/ESGE Classification) formally named Robert's uterus. Video Abstract, 26th ESGE Annual Congress.

[28] Nogueira U, Candido dos Reis FJ, Campolungo A. Hysteroscopic treatment of unicornuate uterus associated with a cavitary rudimentary horn. Int J Gynecol Obstet 1999;64:77–8.

[29] Dalkalitsis N, Korkontzelos I, Tsanadis G, Stefos T, Lolis D. Unicornuate uterus and uterus didelphys indications and techniques for surgical reconstruction: a review. Clin Exp Obstet Gynecol 2003;30:137–43.

[30] Romano S, Bustan M, Ben-Shlomo I, Shalev E. Case report: a novel surgical approach to obstructed hemiuterus: sonographically guided hysteroscopic correction. Hum Reprod 2000;15(7):1578–9.

[31] Xia EL, Li TC, Sylvia Choi SN, Zhou QY. Reproductive outcome of transcervical uterine incision in unicornuate uterus. Chin Med J (Engl) 2017 Feb 5;130(3):256–61.

[32] Montevecchi L, Valle RF. Resectoscopic treatment of complete longitudinal vaginal septum. Int J Gynaecol Obstet 2004;84(1):65–70.

[33] Patton PE, Novy MJ, Lee OM, Hickok LR. The diagnosis and reproductive outcome after surgical treatment of the complete septate uterus, duplicated cervix and vaginal septum. Am J Obstet Gynecol 2004;190(6):1669–75.

[34] Cetinkaya SE, Kahraman K, Sonmezer M, Atabekoglu C. Hysteroscopic management of vaginal septum in a virginal patient with uterus didelphys and obstructed hemivagina. Fertil Steril 2011;96(1):16–8.

[35] Di Spiezio Sardo A, Bettocchi S, Bramante S, Guida M, Bifulco G, Nappi C. Office vaginoscopic treatment of an isolated longitudinal vaginal septum: a case report. J Minim Invasive Gynecol 2007 Jul–Aug;14(4):512–5.

Martin Hirsch, Ertan Sarıdoğan and Peter O'Donovan

27 Avoiding complications in hysteroscopic surgery

27.1 Introduction

The use of hysteroscopy has increased from a diagnostic tool to an operative proce-dure over the last few decades due to advances in technology, surgical skill, and ultra-sound diagnostic capabilities. Hysteroscopy is a time and cost-efficient outpatient or ambulatory procedure sparing patients from major abdominal surgery in the areas of benign and reproductive gynecology. Despite its commonality, hysteroscopic surgery has recognized complications, which can be serious and life-threatening.

Risk is related to many aspects of surgical decision making, including patient selection, procedure selection, practitioner skill, and instrument usage. This chapter will focus on the procedure-related risks. These risks are broadly divided into early and delayed complications. Early complications covered include embolization (rare), fluid overload (up to 5%) [1–4], hemorrhage (0.6%), infection (0.01–1.62%), and perfo-ration (0.12–3.00%) [3]. Delayed complications include intrauterine adhesions (IUAs) and infertility [4].

27.2 Complications

27.2.1 Air/gas embolization

Operative hysteroscopy can expose large venous vessels to pressurized fluid or gas distension media. Embolization occurs when air or gas enters the venous circula-tion during operative hysteroscopy. Air can enter during the insertion of the hys-teroscope, if the inflow tubing is not primed with fluid or due to the presence of air bubbles in the distension medium [5]. Gas embolism occurs due to gases such as carbon dioxide, carbon monoxide, and evaporative gases, which are produced secondary to hysteroscopic electrosurgery [6]. This rare complication can be life-threatening [7]. In the conscious patient, this presents with dyspnea or chest pain, and in the anaesthetized patient, a reduction in oxygen saturations followed by cir-culatory collapse [8]. Management of this acute life-threatening condition requires prompt recognition and moving the patient into the left lateral position with five degrees downward head tilt. This favors movement of air within the right ventricle toward the apex of the ventricle. Aspiration of the emboli has been described with insertion of a central venous catheter from the jugular vein into the right ventricle or performing cardiocentesis [9].

https://doi.org/10.1515/9783110535204-027

27.2.2 Fluid overload

Fluid distension media are required to adequately visualize the uterine cavity to facilitate operative hysteroscopy. Fluid absorption can occur via direct intravasation of fluid when vessels are exposed during resection of myoma or endometrium or via peritoneal absorption from retrograde spillage of distension media during hysteroscopy. Excessive fluid absorption results in intravascular hypervolemia. In addition, if hypotonic distension media such as glycine 1.5% or sorbitol 3% are used, dilutional hyponatremia could develop. Symptoms such as headaches, nausea, vomiting, and fatigue are experienced when plasma sodium levels fall below 125 nmol/l. More severe hemodilution and hyponatremia with sodium levels below 120 mmol/l cause a change in the osmotic pressure and water being drawn into the brain cells, resulting in cerebral edema and neurological problems, coma, seizures, and even death. When isotonic distention media such as normal saline or lactated ringer are used, electrolyte disturbances are less likely to occur. However, hypervolemia can still lead to pulmonary edema and congestive cardiac failure. Due to a reduced risk of hyponatremia, isotonic distension media are considered safer compared to hypotonic media.

The incidence of this complication varies, and intra-operative risk factors include high distension media pressure, low mean arterial pressure, deep myometrial surgical penetration, prolonged surgery, large sized myoma, vascular myomas, and large uterine cavity. These risks are compounded with the following pre-operative factors: hypotonic electrolyte free distension media, premenopausal status, and preexisting cardiovascular or renal disease.

The management of suspected fluid overload includes insertion of a urinary catheter, strict fluid balance monitoring, assessment or serum electrolytes, fluid restriction, and consideration of diuretic usage. The management of symptomatic hypervolemic hyponatremia requires high-dependency care and 3% hypertonic sodium chloride to restore sodium levels in conjunction with the previously described conservative measures.

Preventing fluid overload can be achieved by pre- and intraoperative steps. Pre-operative usage of gonadotrophin-releasing hormone agonists (GnRHa) can reduce the size of the myoma and the time required to resect it. Intraoperatively it is recommended to adhere closely to cutoff levels of fluid deficit during surgery. These are set at 1000 ml deficit with hypotonic solution and 2500 ml deficit with isotonic solution [2]. Additional intraoperative measures include intracervical injection of diluted vasopressin to temporarily induce vasoconstriction, maintaining the intrauterine pressure as low as possible to allow adequate visualization while below mean arterial pressure.

27.2.3 Hemorrhage

Intraoperative bleeding is common and can result from iatrogenic trauma to vessels within the endometrium, myometrium, myoma, and pelvis. The risk of hemorrhage during operative hysteroscopy is between 0.16% and 0.61%. Troublesome bleeding is usually associated with resection of endometrium and fibroids compared to resection of polyp or simple adhesiolysis. Uterine perforation with injury to uterine or pelvic vessels can cause severe bleeding, potentially accounting for the highest rates of hemorrhage associated with adhesiolysis rather than myoma resection in some published series [10].

The swift recognition and management of hemorrhage are essential. Hemorrhage associated with an intrauterine cause without perforation can be managed with administration of antifibrinolytic agents (tranexamic acid), intracervical vasoconstrictors (synthetic vasopressin), uterotonic agents (misoprostol), intrauterine balloon tamponade (30 ml Foley catheter balloon), and bimanual uterine compression. In rare situations where bleeding does not resolve with conservative or medical measures, further interventions such uterine artery embolization or hysterectomy may be necessary. Hemorrhage associated with uterine perforation requires laparoscopic or laparotomic investigation and treatment. A Uterine perforation can usually be sutured at laparoscopy to control bleeding.

The prevention of hemorrhage can be achieved by minimizing the risk of perforation (see perforation) and the preoperative use of GnRHa and intraoperative use of intracervical synthetic vasopressin. The 3-month preoperative usage of GnRHa agents reduces the myoma volume and the time required for resection [11, 12].

27.2.4 Infection

Infection is an uncommon complication following operative hysteroscopy. The risk of infection is between 0.01% and 1.42% [13, 14]. The most frequent sources of infection include endometritis (0.9%) and urinary tract infection (0.6%) [14]. Women with hydrosalpinges are at increased risk of tubo-ovarian abscess following hysteroscopy and should be given prophylactic antibiotics.

The routine use of prophylactic antibiotics is not recommended in the absence of hydrosalpinges to reduce the risk of infection following operative hysteroscopy [15].

27.2.5 Perforation

Uterine perforation is a serious and common risk of hysteroscopy affecting up to 1.6% of procedures [16]. This leads to a loss in uterine cavity distension pressure and suboptimal views.

Uterine perforation and intraabdominal passage of the perforating instrument can lead to immediate and delayed complications. Immediate complications include injury of the bladder, bowel, ureter, and major blood vessels. The risk of visceral injury varies depending on the nature of the perforating instrument, with increased risk associated with sharp or electrosurgical devices.

A large German survey of over 21,000 operative hysteroscopies observed 25 (0.12%) perforations, of which 5 (20%) had coexisting injury to the bladder or bowel. The majority (68%) of these perforations occurred during the procedure and were not related to entry [13].

Risk factors for uterine perforation include increasing parity, recent pregnancy, small postmenopausal uterus, tight postmenopausal cervix, IUA, pyometra, endometritis, position/attitude of the uterus (retroversion, acute anteversion, or retroflexion), and uterine anomalies [17].

Management of uterine perforation with a blunt instrument or cold device of 5 mm or less, without ensuing hemorrhage, can be conservative with overnight admission and observation. Uterine perforation with an instrument greater than 5 mm, that is sharp, or electrosurgical requires immediate investigation with laparoscopy to exclude or manage injury. Delayed risks of uterine perforation include a greater risk of uterine rupture during pregnancy [18].

The prevention of uterine perforation has limited evidence that directly supports the usage of one technique. The use of misoprostol 400 mcg preoperatively has been shown to reduce the need for dilatation, cervical trauma, and operative time, which are proxy measures for risk of perforation [19].

27.2.6 Intrauterine adhesions

IUAs are a serious complication of hysteroscopic surgery. They are associated with amenorrhea, infertility, and recurrent pregnancy loss. There are limited data assessing the risk of IUA due to difficulties diagnosing and classifying adhesions. The risk of IUA formation following operative hysteroscopy appears lowest with procedures confined to the endometrium, such as polyp removal, and greatest following procedures extending to the myometrium and resection of multiple submucosal myoma [20]. The risk of iatrogenic IUA-associated infertility needs to be balanced against the reduced success of spontaneous or assisted conception in women with infertility-associated submucosal myoma prior to surgery. The risk and benefits of myoma surgery need careful consideration and counseling among a population of women with infertility and submucosal myoma.

The usage of intrauterine devices or estrogen therapy following hysteroscopic metroplasty or myomectomy in the prevention of IUA has inconsistent and conflicting results. There has not been reported harm or deterioration in adhesions associated with these postoperative strategies compared to control groups, and therefore, they are frequently used in clinical practice [21–24]. Data from randomized trials suggest that the use of gel antiadhesion agents reduces risk of adhesion formation after intrauterine surgery, although the long-term benefit on fertility still remains unknown [4].

27.3 Conclusion

Hysteroscopy is moving away from being a diagnostic tool toward a common operative procedure. This has been facilitated by increasingly accessible and accurate non-invasive diagnostic tests such as ultrasound and magnetic resonance imaging. This increase in operative hysteroscopy will lead to a proportional rise in the number of complications seen, but concomitant advances in technology and equipment may reduce complications. It is essential that clinicians performing hysteroscopy are aware of how to recognize, manage, and prevent complications where possible.

References

[1] A Scottish audit of hysteroscopic surgery for menorrhagia: complications and follow up. BJOG An Int J Obstet Gynaecol 1995;102:249–254.

[2] Umranikar S, Clark TJ, Saridogan E, et al. BSGE/ESGE guideline on management of fluid distension media in operative hysteroscopy. Gynecol Surg 2016;13(4):289–303.

[3] Aas-Eng MK, Langebrekke A, Hudelist G. Complications in operative hysteroscopy—is prevention possible? Acta Obstet Gynecol Scand 2017;96(12):1399–1403.

[4] Abbott JA, Munro MG, Singh SS, et al. AAGL practice report: practice guidelines on intrauterine adhesions developed in collaboration with the European Society of Gynaecological Endoscopy (ESGE). Gynecol Surg 2017;14(1):6.

[5] Brooks PG. Venous air embolism during operative hysteroscopy. J Am Assoc Gynecol Laparosc 1997;4(3):399–402.

[6] Imasogie N, Crago R, Leyland NA, Chung F. Probable gas embolism during operative hysteroscopy caused by products of combustion. Can J Anesth 2002;49(10):1044–7.

[7] Shveiky D, Rojansky N, Revel A, Benshushan A, Laufer N, Shushan A. Complications of hysteroscopic surgery: "beyond the learning curve." J Minim Invasive Gynecol 2007;14(2):218–22.

[8] Stoloff DR, Isenberg RA, Brill AI. Venous air and gas emboli in operative hysteroscopy. J Am Assoc Gynecol Laparoscop 2001;8(2):181–92.

[9] American College of Obstetricians and Gynecologists. ACOG technology assessment in obstetrics and gynecology, number 4, August 2005: hysteroscopy. Obstet Gynecol 2005;106(2):439–42.

[10] Agostini A, Cravello L, Desbrière R, Maisonneuve AS, Roger V, Blanc B. Hemorrhage risk during operative hysteroscopy. Acta Obstet Gynecol Scand 2002;81(9):878–81.

[11] Bizzarri N, Ghirardi V, Remorgida V, Venturini PL, Ferrero S. Three-month treatment with triptorelin, letrozole and ulipristal acetate before hysteroscopic resection of uterine myomas: prospective comparative pilot study. Eur J Obstet Gynecol Reprod Biol 2015;192:22–6.

[12] Muzii L, Boni T, Bellati F, et al. GnRH analogue treatment before hysteroscopic resection of submucous myomas: a prospective, randomized, multicenter study. Fertil Steril 2010;94(4):1496–9.

[13] Aydeniz B, Gruber IV, Schauf B, Kurek R, Meyer A, Wallwiener D. A multicenter survey of complications associated with 21 676 operative hysteroscopies. Eur J Obstet Gynecol Reprod Biol 2002;104(2):160–4.

[14] Agostini A, Cravello L, Shojai R, Ronda I, Roger V, Blanc B. Postoperative infection and surgical hysteroscopy. Fertil Steril 2002;77(4):766–8.

[15] ACOG Practice Bulletin No. 195: prevention of infection after gynecologic procedures. Obstet Gynecol 2018;131(6):e172–e189.

[16] Agostini A, Cravello L, Bretelle F, Shojai R, Roger V, Blanc B. Risk of uterine perforation during hysteroscopic surgery. J Am Assoc Gynecol Laparosc 2002;9(3):264–7.

[17] Shakir F, Diab Y. The perforated uterus. The Obstetrician & Gynaecologist 2013;15:256–61.

[18] Sentilhes L, Sergent F, Roman H, Verspyck E, Marpeau L. Late complications of operative hysteroscopy: predicting patients at risk of uterine rupture during subsequent pregnancy. Eur J Obstet Gynecol Reprod Biol 2005;120(2):134–8.

[19] Oppegaard KS, Lieng M, Berg A, Istre O, Qvigstad E, Nesheim BI. A combination of misoprostol and estradiol for preoperative cervical ripening in postmenopausal women: a randomised controlled trial. BJOG An Int J Obstet Gynaecol 2010;117(1):53–61.

[20] Taskin O, Sadik S, Onoglu A, et al. Role of endometrial suppression on the frequency of intrauterine adhesions after resectoscopic surgery. J Am Assoc Gynecol Laparosc 2000;7(3):351–4.

[21] Yu X, Yuhan L, Dongmei S, Enlan X, Tinchiu L. The incidence of post-operative adhesion following transection of uterine septum: a cohort study comparing three different adjuvant therapies. Eur J Obstet Gynecol Reprod Biol 2016;201:61–4.

[22] Lin X, Wei M, Li TC, et al. A comparison of intrauterine balloon, intrauterine contraceptive device and hyaluronic acid gel in the prevention of adhesion reformation following hysteroscopic surgery for Asherman syndrome: a cohort study. Eur J Obstet Gynecol Reprod Biol 2013;170(2):512–6.

[23] Lin XN, Zhou F, Wei ML, et al. Randomized, controlled trial comparing the efficacy of intrauterine balloon and intrauterine contraceptive device in the prevention of adhesion reformation after hysteroscopic adhesiolysis. Fertil Steril 2015;104(1):235–40.

[24] Tonguc EA, Var T, Yilmaz N, Batioglu S. Intrauterine device or estrogen treatment after hysteroscopic uterine septum resection. Int J Gynecol Obstet 2010;109(3):226–9.

Mary Connor

28 Endometrial ablation techniques for heavy menstrual bleeding

28.1 Introduction

Endometrial ablation (EA) is an established treatment for heavy menstrual bleeding (HMB). The number of hysterectomies for this indication has significantly fallen since EA and the levonorgestrel-releasing intrauterine device (LNG-IUS) became readily available. However, despite undergoing apparently successful treatment, some women still require additional intervention for their HMB, including hysterectomy. Indications for the procedure given our current knowledge are presented. Also discussed are the short- and long-term complications associated with EA. Many current ablation devices offer treatment of such short duration that therapy in an outpatient setting is a realistic option; the implications of this are considered.

28.2 Historical perspective

Hysteroscopic transcervical EA and transcervical resection of the endometrium for the management of HMB were introduced into clinical gynecological practice in 1985. The principle of the techniques is the destruction of the endometrium and its basal layer by electrical or laser energy delivered under direct vision, with a consequent reduction or even cessation of menstrual blood loss. Simplification of EA arose with the development of second-generation devices providing simultaneous treatment of all of the endometrium. Since 2003, more EA procedures than hysterectomies have been performed in England for the surgical treatment of HMB, and from 2005, more than half of these were with second-generation devices [1].

A meta-analysis showed that second-generation devices are at least as effective when compared with first-generation techniques, as similar rates of patient dissatisfaction were seen following either treatment (12% vs. 11%; odds ratio [OR], 1.2; 95% confidence interval [CI], 0.9–1.6, $p = 0.2$) [2].

28.3 Indications for second-generation EA

Treatment of HMB with second-generation devices is firmly established [3] and is recommended as first-line surgical treatment when medical therapy, including the use of the LNG-IUS, has been unsuccessful, the woman's family is complete, and the uterine cavity is of normal size and shape [4]. The procedures are quick to perform,

https://doi.org/10.1515/9783110535204-028

associated with fewer complications than either hysterectomy or first-generation ablation, and have a short recovery time [2]. A role for first-generation resection and ablation continues but is generally confined to the treatment of abnormal shaped cavities or as an adjunct to HMB therapy following resection of an intrauterine fibroid.

With a normal uterine cavity and absence of fibroids of a significant size and rejection or failure of the LNG-IUS, the choice is often between EA and hysterectomy. When discussing the options with a patient, it is important to consider the probable specific advantages and disadvantages for them, in particular the likelihood of requiring further treatment for HMB. The increased risks associated with hysterectomy should also be explained, including an increased chance of additional surgery for other conditions, such as pelvic floor repair [5].

The age of the woman at the time of presentation will have an impact upon the long-term effectiveness of EA and is discussed below [6, 7]. Consequently, patients younger than 35 years should be made aware that for they have an increased risk of additional treatment for HMB at some stage following EA.

Patients for whom amenorrhea is an important goal must be advised that a reduction in menstrual loss is expected following EA rather than a total absence of vaginal bleeding. If this is not acceptable, then hysterectomy may be preferable.

It is expected that cramp-like pelvic pain associated with the passage of menstrual blood and clots will improve with reduction in bleeding. However, pain due to endometriosis or pre-existing adenomyosis, as indicated by a history of dyspareunia or postcoital ache, is unlikely to improve and may even become worse. Adenomyosis was recognized as an important cause of first-generation ablation failure [8]. Severe dyspareunia, whatever the cause, is therefore a reason for advising against EA; hysterectomy or persisting with the LNG-IUS are likely to be more effective treatments.

28.4 Risk factors for treatment failure

The likelihood of satisfactory treatment with EA must be discussed with patients. One definition of successful treatment of HMB is the lack of need for further therapy, whether medical or surgical. The most significant risk factor for further treatment is age at the time of the initial therapy [6, 7]. In a review of over 3600 women who had undergone EA in North Carolina, 21% subsequently underwent hysterectomy, with a further 3.9% having another uterine conserving procedure [6]. Women who were aged 45 years or younger were 2.1 times more likely to have a hysterectomy than women over 45 years of age (95% CI, 1.8–2.4); those who were 40 years or younger were over 40% at risk of subsequently having a hysterectomy and the risk of hysterectomy continued throughout the 8 years of follow-up. In this study, the type of EA and the presence or absence of fibroids were not significant risk factors.

A study of both first- and second-generation EA procedures performed between 2000 and 2011 in England looked at the time until further treatment and whether repeat EA or hysterectomy [7]. Using a national administrative database, it was established that among the cohort of nearly 115,000 women, at least 16.7% of women had further treatment within 5 years, with 13.5% undergoing a hysterectomy. The risk of further treatment was again greater for women who were younger at the time of initial treatment; when comparing women under 35 years of age, this was 26.9%, but for women 45 years or more, only 10.4%, with a hazard ratio (HR) of 2.83 (95% CI, 2.67–2.99). It was noted that reintervention rates were higher than reported in many single-device studies or RCTs between devices.

A cause of treatment failure, besides persistence or reemergence of HMB, is persistent pelvic pain. The latter may be due to adenomyosis, endometriosis, hematometra, or posttubal sterilization syndrome [8]. Endometrium may not be fully treated, with the area around the cornua particularly vulnerable (Fig. 28.1). Blood released

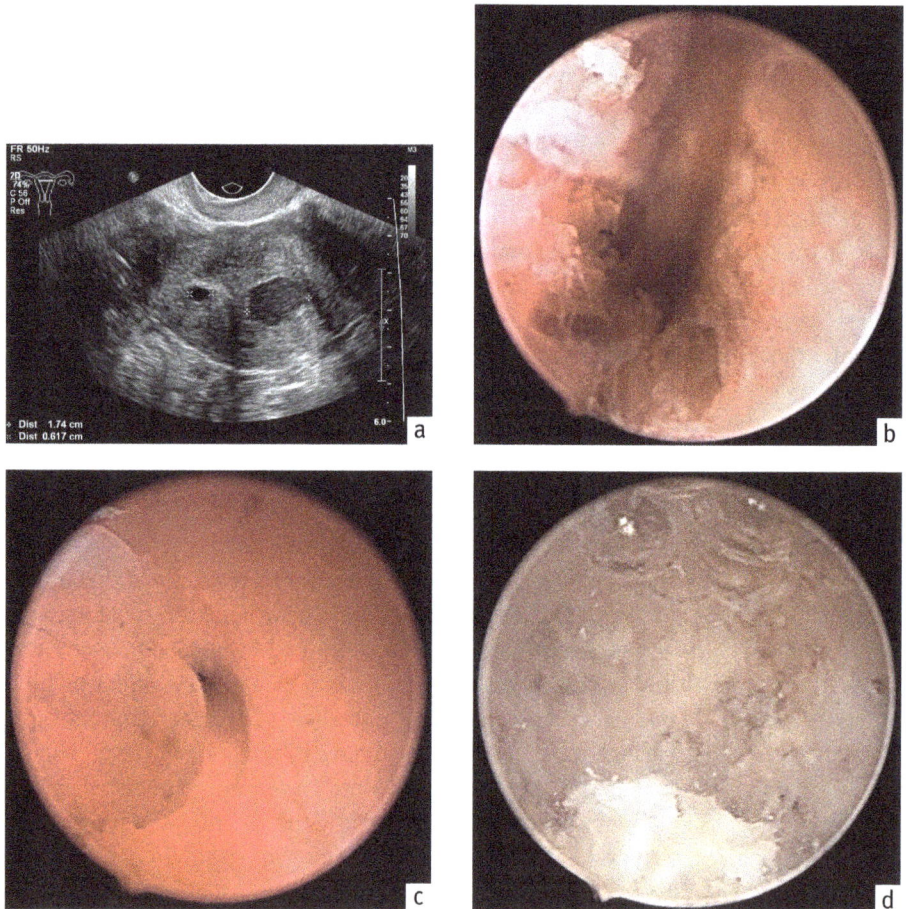

Fig. 28.1: (a) Ultrasound scan image showing transverse section of two areas of hematometra at uterine fundus. (b) Blood from hematometra released under Ultrasound scan control. (c) Viable endometrium around exposed left cornua. (d) Endometrium following repeat ablation.

during subsequent menstruation is trapped due to uterine adhesions and retrograde flow down the fallopian tubes is blocked.

An investigation of dissatisfaction rates of women following hysterectomy, EA with either first- and second-generation techniques, and LNG-IUS when used for treatment of HMB concluded that hysterectomy was associated with least dissatisfaction [2]. However, the dissatisfaction rates for all treatments were low and absolute differences were small. Predictors of reduced dissatisfaction for second-generation devices were identified as shorter uterine cavity length (≤8 cm vs >8 cm; OR, 0.6; CI, 0.4–0.9; p = 0.02), with a trend for absence of fibroids and endometrial polyps.

28.5 Comparison of second-generation devices

There are a number of different techniques for producing global endometrial destruction. A study compared second-generation devices for which sufficient high-quality information was available using the technique of network meta-analysis and combined direct and indirect estimates for treatment effect [9]. The main outcome measures were amenorrhea, heavy bleeding, and patient dissatisfaction. Results from direct evidence and network meta-analysis showed increased rates of amenorrhea at 12 months following bipolar radio frequency and microwave (Microsulis) ablation compared with thermal balloon therapies (OR, 2.51; 95% CI, 1.53–4.12, p < 0.001, and 1.66, 1.01–2.71, p = 0.05, respectively). However, there were no other significant differences between these devices, and these were the ones most commonly used at the time.

Of note, in their conclusion, the authors comment that rates of dissatisfaction and heavy bleeding are consistently low for the second-generation devices and are therefore an "excellent conservative alternative" to hysterectomy for women with HMB.

28.6 Complications of EA

Adverse events due to EA include those associated with the actual procedure and ones that arise at a later date. The need for additional treatment, whether within 12 months or several years, may be considered a complication and has been explored above. It is very important that the manufacturer's instructions are followed when undertaking the device and that the person performing the procedure has received appropriate training [10].

There are some absolute contraindications applicable to all devices and include active pelvic infection, the presence of premalignant or malignant endometrial disease, previous midline uterine surgery, or classical Caesarean section. Caution also needs to be exercised with a smaller- or larger-than-average uterus (<4 cm cavity length or >12 cm); previous abdominal surgery or severe infection, as bowel may be adherent to the uterine fundus and at risk of thermal damage; and previous caesarean section where the myometrial thickness is less than 8 mm. Most second-generation devices are not suitable for use following a previous EA; laparoscopic control is advisable when this circumstance occurs.

The United States Food and Drug Administration Manufacturer and User Facility Device Experience (MAUDE) database provides information about complications that have arisen with use of determined as the denominators are unknown or unconfirmed. However, the database highlights the types of incidents that can happen, the circumstances in which they occurred, and if there are trends.

Gurtcheff and Sharp (2003) analyzed reports following use of global EA devices and found complications occurred with all the devices in common use at the time (see Tab. 28.1) [11].

Serious complications included uterine perforation, the need for laparotomy, thermal bowel injury, sepsis, intensive care admission, adnexal or uterine necrosis, hemorrhage, and the death of a patient. Less serious problems were endometritis, hematometra, and other thermal injury. Some patients suffered several complications; one had hemorrhage with uterine perforation that was managed by laparotomy and emergency hysterectomy. The authors highlighted their concern that they failed to find any reports of uterine perforation or bowel injury associated with a global EA device published in the medical literature between 1990 and 2003, the period of their investigation.

Tab. 28.1: Complications following global endometrial ablation reported to the MAUDE database [11].

Type of complication	NovaSure (n = 4 patients)	HydroThermablator (n = 3 patient)	ThermaChoice (n = 50 patients)	Her option (n = 5 patients)	Total
Major	7	4	24	3	40
Death	0	0	1	0	1
Bowel burn	2	1	5	0	8
Other burns	0	2	7	0	9
Sepsis	1	0	1	1	3
Leading to laparotomy	3	1	8	0	12
ICU admission	1	0	1	1	3
Adnexal/uterine necrosis	0	0	1	1	2
Hemorrhage	0	0	2	0	2
Minor	4	1	38	2	45
Endometritis	2	0	4	0	6
Uterine perforation	2	1	25	2	30
Hematometra	0	0	9	0	9

MAUDE = Manufacturer and User Facility Device Experience.

A subsequent paper that reviewed the MAUDE database between 2003 and 2006 observed similar types of incidents but a fall in the number reported even though the number of procedures had risen [12]. They considered that this may reflect greater operator experience with the devices, better training of operators, and increased safety measures by the manufacturers. However, serious perioperative complications still occurred and a significant proportion were due to operator error and not following operating instructions.

28.7 Pregnancy following EA

A criterion for undertaking EA is completed family, as the aim is to destroy the endometrium. However, endometrial destruction may be incomplete or not permanent, and if contraception is inadequate, pregnancies may occur [13–15]. The risk of pregnancy appears to be higher in women who have cyclical bleeding following ablation [13]. Termination of the pregnancy can be complicated, and some authors recommend surgical procedures are conducted under ultrasound control [14] or preferably a medical procedure is offered [15].

The pregnancies have a high risk of problems, with ectopic pregnancies in 3–13% [14, 15], and those that continue are at increased risk of intrauterine growth retardation and fetal anomalies such as limb defects and prematurity. For the mother, the risks of serious complications are higher with possible placenta increta and caesarean hysterectomy; uterine rupture and maternal death have also been reported [15].

The requirement for adequate contraception until menopause following EA must be stressed.

28.8 Endometrial cancer following EA

Concern has been expressed about the development of endometrial cancer in women who have undergone EA, particularly that the diagnosis may be delayed or even missed. One study offers some reassurance. The time to diagnosis in women who developed endometrial cancer following EA ($n = 3$) was compared with that of those who presented with the disease after medical management of HMB ($n = 601$); there was no evidence of delay [16]. Also, the incidence of cancer following EA was not significantly different (HR, 0.45; 95% CI, 0.05–1.40; $p = 0.17$).

28.9 Analgesia for second-generation EA

There are several possible venues for the provision of EA services. General anesthesia in a day case setting is common, and sometimes, conscious sedation is made available in an outpatient clinic, but both require the presence of an anesthetist. The narrow insertion size and the short duration of active treatment of many of the second-generation EA devices support local anesthetic outpatient services, and the acceptability of this to patients has been demonstrated [17–19].

Preprocedural oral analgesia, including nonsteroidal anti-inflammatory drugs, when tolerated, local anesthetic infiltration of the cervix or a paracervical block, and sometimes the addition of patient-controlled nitrous oxide (Entonox) are routinely provided [17–20]. However, it is recognized that fundal pain may still be experienced because the upper half of the uterine cavity is not reached by anesthetic delivered to the cervix [20, 21]. As a consequence, the use of fundal analgesia was explored for use during outpatient EA [22]. In a randomized, double-blind, placebo-controlled trial, cornual analgesia was shown to significantly reduce procedural pain scores for both a balloon and radiofrequency ablation (1.44; 95% CI, −2.65 to −0.21) [21]. They acknowledge that including bupivacaine may be unnecessary.

More evidence is required to optimize the outpatient experience; some studies show improvement in posttreatment pain rather than during the procedure [18]. Munro and Brooks comment that there is evidence for the effectiveness of paracervical anesthesia during treatment, but not for other techniques [20]. They conclude that it remains necessary to determine the ideal techniques for intracervical and paracervical anesthesia, including depth of insertion, the optimal agents, and time to attain the maximal anesthetic effect.

References

[1] Reid P. Endometrial ablation in England—coming of age? An examination of hospital episode statistics 1989/1990 to 2004/2005. Eur J Obstet Gynecol Reprod Biol 2007;135:191–4.

[2] Bhattacharya S, Middleton LJ, Tsourapas A, et al. Hysterectomy, endometrial ablation and Mirena® for heavy menstrual bleeding: a systematic review of clinical effectiveness and cost-effectiveness analysis. Health Technol Assess 2011;15:1–252.

[3] Lethaby A, Sheppard S, Cooke I, Farquhar C. Endometrial resection and ablation versus hysterectomy for heavy menstrual bleeding. Cochrane Database Syst Rev 1999;2:CD000329.

[4] National Collaborating Centre for Women's and Children's Health, National Institute for Health and Clinical Excellence. Heavy Menstrual Bleeding. Clinical Guideline No. 44. London: NICE; 2007. Available at: http://www.nice.org.uk/CG44.

[5] Cooper K, Lee A, Chien P, Raja E, Timmaraju V, Bhattacharya S. Outcomes following hysterectomy or endometrial ablation for heavy menstrual bleeding: retrospective analysis of hospital episode statistics in Scotland. BJOG 2011;118:1171–9.

[6] Longinotti MK, Jacobson GF, Hung YY, Learman LA. Probability of hysterectomy after endometrial ablation. Obstet Gynecol 2008;112:1214–20.

[7] Bansi-Matharu L, Gurol-Urganci I, Mahmood TA, et al. Rates of subsequent surgery following endometrial ablation among English women with menorrhagias: population-based cohort study. BJOG 2013;120:1500–7.

[8] McCausland AM, McCausland VM. Long-term complications of endometrial ablation: cause, diagnosis, treatment and prevention. J Minim Invasive Gynecol 2007;14(4):399–406.

[9] Daniels JP, Middleton LJ, Champaneria R, et al; International Heavy Menstrual Bleeding IPD Meta-analysis Collaborative Group. Second generation endometrial ablation techniques for heavy menstrual bleeding: network meta-analysis. BMJ 2012;344:e2564.

[10] Medicines and Healthcare products Regulatory Agency, Royal College of Obstetricians and Gynaecologists, and British Society for Gynaecological Endoscopy. Guidance on the responsibilities of manufacturers, the regulator and clinicians with respect to endometrial ablation. 2011. http://webarchive.nationalarchives.gov.uk/20141206133509/http://www.mhra.gov.uk/home/groups/clin/documents/publication/con108727.pdf (Accessed 21 November 2017).

[11] Gurtcheff SE, Sharp HT. Complications associated with global endometrial ablation: the utility of the MAUDE database. Obstet Gynecol 2003;102(6):1278–82.

[12] Della Badia C, Nyirjesy P, Atogho A. Endometrial ablation devices: review of a manufacturer and user facility device experience database. J Minim Invasive Gynecol 2007;14(4):436–44.

[13] Hare AA, Olah KS. Pregnancy following endometrial ablation: a review article. J Obstet Gynaecol 2005;25:108–114.

[14] Xia E, Li TC, Dan Y, et al. The occurrence and outcome of 39 pregnancies after 1621 cases of transcervical resection of endometrium. Hum Reprod 2006;21(12):3282–6.

[15] Laberge PY. Serious and deadly complications from pregnancy after endometrial ablation: two case reports and review of the literature. J Gynecol Obstet Biol Reprod 2008;37:609–13.

[16] Dood RL, Gracia CR, Sammel MD, et al. Endometrial cancer after endometrial ablation versus medical management of abnormal uterine bleeding. J Minim Invasive Gynecol 2014;21(5):744–52.

[17] Marsh F, Thewlis J, Duffy S. Thermachoice endometrial ablation in the outpatient setting, without local anesthesia or intravenous sedation: a prospective cohort study. Fertil Steril 2005;83(3):715–20.

[18] Chapa HO, Antonetti AG, Bakker K. Ketorolac-mepivacaine lower uterine block for in-office endometrial ablation: a randomized, controlled trial. J Reprod Med 2010;55(11–12):464–8.

[19] Clark TJ, Samuels N, Malick S, Middleton L, Daniels J, Gupta J. Bipolar radiofrequency compared with thermal balloon endometrial ablation in the office: a randomized controlled trial. Obstet Gynecol 2011;117(5):109–18.

[20] Munro MG, Brooks PG. Use of local anesthesia for office diagnostic and operative hysteroscopy. J Minim Invasive Gynecol 2010;17:709–18.

[21] Kumar V, Tryposkiadis K, Gupta JK. Hysteroscopic local anesthetic intrauterine cornual block in office endometrial ablation: a randomized controlled trial. Fertil Steril 2016;105(2):474–80.

[22] Skensved H. Global-local anaesthesia: combining paracervical block with intramyometrial prilocaine in the fundus significantly reduces patients' perception of pain during radio-frequency endometrial ablation (Nova-Sure1) in an office setting. Gynecol Surg 2012;9:207–12.

Index

https://doi.org/10.1515/9783110535204-029